WORKBOOK TO ACCOMPANY

GETTING STARTED
IN THE
COMPUTERIZED
MEDICAL OFFICE

Fundamentals and Practice

Second Edition

Cindy Correa

Former Educational Coordinator and Curricula Developer for
City University of New York at Queens College—Allied Health Program/CEP

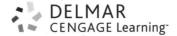

DELMAR
CENGAGE Learning™

Australia • Brazil • Japan • Korea • Mexico • Singapore • Spain • United Kingdom • United States

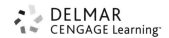

Workbook to Accompany Getting Started in the Computerized Medical Office: Fundamentals and Practice, Second Edition
Cindy Correa

Vice President, Career and Professional Editorial: Dave Garza

Director of Learning Solutions: Matthew Kane

Senior Acquisitions Editor: Rhonda Dearborn

Managing Editor: Marah Bellegarde

Senior Product Manager: Sarah Prime

Editorial Assistant: Lauren Whalen

Vice President, Career and Professional Marketing: Jennifer Baker

Marketing Director: Wendy E. Mapstone

Senior Marketing Manager: Nancy Bradshaw

Marketing Coordinator: Erica Ropitzky

Production Director: Carolyn Miller

Senior Content Project Manager: Stacey Lamodi

Senior Art Director: Jack Pendleton

Senior Technology Product Manager: Mary Colleen Liburdi

For product information and technology assistance, contact us at
Cengage Learning Customer & Sales Support, 1-800-354-9706

For permission to use material from this text or product, submit all requests online at **www.cengage.com/permissions.**
Further permissions questions can be e-mailed to
permissionrequest@cengage.com

Library of Congress Control Number: 2010920752

ISBN-13:978-1-4354-3851-4

ISBN-10:1-4354-3851-5

Delmar
5 Maxwell Drive
Clifton Park, NY 12065-2919
USA

Cengage Learning is a leading provider of customized learning solutions with office locations around the globe, including Singapore, the United Kingdom, Australia, Mexico, Brazil, and Japan. Locate your local office at: **international.cengage.com/region**

Cengage Learning products are represented in Canada by Nelson Education, Ltd.

To learn more about Delmar, visit **www.cengage.com/delmar**
Purchase any of our products at your local college store or at our preferred online store **www.cengagebrain.com**

Notice to the Reader

Publisher does not warrant or guarantee any of the products described herein or perform any independent analysis in connection with any of the product information contained herein. Publisher does not assume, and expressly disclaims, any obligation to obtain and include information other than that provided to it by the manufacturer. The reader is expressly warned to consider and adopt all safety precautions that might be indicated by the activities described herein and to avoid all potential hazards. By following the instructions contained herein, the reader willingly assumes all risks in connection with such instructions. The publisher makes no representations or warranties of any kind, including but not limited to, the warranties of fitness for particular purpose or merchantability, nor are any such representations implied with respect to the material set forth herein, and the publisher takes no responsibility with respect to such material. The publisher shall not be liable for any special, consequential, or exemplary damages resulting, in whole or part, from the readers' use of, or reliance upon, this material.

Printed in the United States of America
1 2 3 4 5 6 7 12 11 10

CONTENTS

ABOUT THE WORKBOOK

This workbook is designed to accompany the book *Getting Started in the Computerized Medical Office: Fundamentals and Practice, Second Edition.* The purpose of this workbook is to provide additional practice through supplemental exercises and review of concepts and terms discussed in the book. The workbook may be used to gain more experience using Medical Office Simulation Software (MOSS) 2.0, as a review tool to reinforce skills learned in the book, or as an evaluation tool to monitor student progress and understanding, or even as minitests or quizzes by the instructor.

HOW TO USE THE WORKBOOK

This workbook follows the units and course work in the same order as they are presented in the book. Students may work on each unit as the material from the book is completed; it is not necessary to finish the entire book before beginning to use the workbook. This is left to the discretion of the instructor and/or student and the lesson plan that is followed. Additionally, the workbook can be reserved for use only as a tool for testing students at any point of the coursework, and includes a comprehensive final examination. The patients used in the workbook are different from those used in the book so that they are easily identified on reports, and instructors have the flexibility of adding their own exercises with patients they create to suit the goals of the course.

FEATURES

Exercises in the workbook are called *Building Skills* and appear in the approximate order as presented in the book so that instructors and students may follow the material easily, either concurrently, or in logical sequence if done at a later time or as a test. All exercises are clearly numbered and identified as to the task to be completed. Instructions are included where applicable for further clarification.

Review Exercises

Concepts and terminology from the book are reviewed with exercises presented as multiple choice, true/false, matching, labeling, and short answer questions.

Building Skills: Practical Exercises

Supplemental exercises in the workbook that utilize MOSS are presented with instructions and a numbered sequence designed to guide students through steps already learned in the book. *Critical Thinking* exercises are found at the end of select Building Skills sections and contain less guidance, allowing students to think through steps and concepts more independently.

Figures and Answer Keys

The workbook offers screen shots and figures that allow students to check their work when using MOSS. All review exercises consisting of multiple choice, true/false, matching, labeling, and short answer questions have answer keys available in the Instructor's Manual.

Comprehensive Testing

The workbook provides one final examination focusing on the student's proficiency using MOSS to complete tasks common in the administrative medical office. The final examination is independent of the workbook exercises, and is intended as a stand-alone resource for evaluating the student's hands-on use of practice management software.

ABOUT THE AUTHOR

Cindy Correa has an extensive background in curricula development for medical career programs at technical colleges and continuing education departments of university programs. During her time in medical office and administrative hospital positions, she worked as a medical biller, transcriptionist, clinical medical assistant, and office manager. She has developed, written, and taught courses in medical terminology, medical billing, administrative and clinical medical assisting certificate programs, medical transcription, and numerous medical and business computer lab courses.

Chapter Assignment Sheets

U N I T **1**

Introduction to Computers

BUILDING SKILLS 1-1: COMPONENTS OF THE WINDOWS DESKTOP

Instructions: Label the parts of the Windows Desktop in Figure WB1-1. Provide a brief description of the purpose of each component in the spaces below corresponding to each label number.

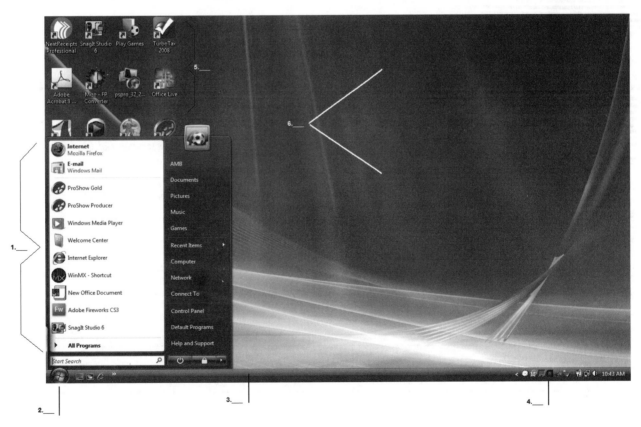

Figure WB1-1 *(Screen shot reprinted by permission from Microsoft Corporation.)*

3

1. _____

_____

_____

2. _____

_____

_____

3. _____

_____

_____

4. _____

_____

_____

5. _____

_____

_____

6. _____

_____

_____

BUILDING SKILLS 1-2: COMPONENTS OF AN APPLICATIONS WINDOW

Instructions: Label the parts of an applications window, using the Internet Explorer browser shown in Figure WB1-2. Provide a brief description of the purpose of each component in the spaces below corresponding to each label number.

1. _____

_____

_____

2. _____

_____

_____

3. _____

_____

_____

4. _____

_____

_____

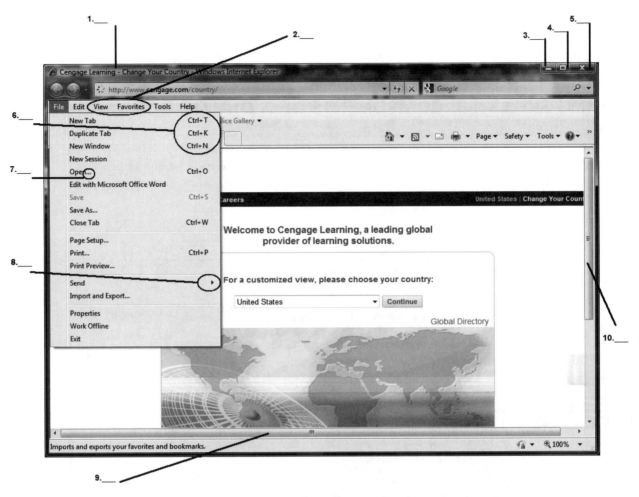

Figure WB1-2 *(Screen shot reprinted by permission from Microsoft Corporation.)*

5. _____

6. _____

7. _____

8. _____

9. _____

10. _____

_____

_____

BUILDING SKILLS 1-3: COMPONENTS OF A DIALOG BOX

Instructions: Label the parts of the dialog boxes shown in Figures WB1-3 and WB1-4. Provide a brief description of the purpose of each component in the spaces below corresponding to each label number.

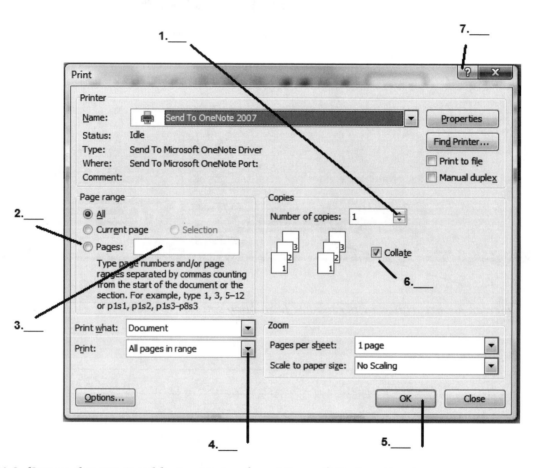

Figure WB1-3 *(Screen shot reprinted by permission from Microsoft Corporation.)*

1. _____

_____

2. _____

_____

3. _____

_____

4. _____

_____

5. _____

_____

6. _____

_____

7. _____

_____

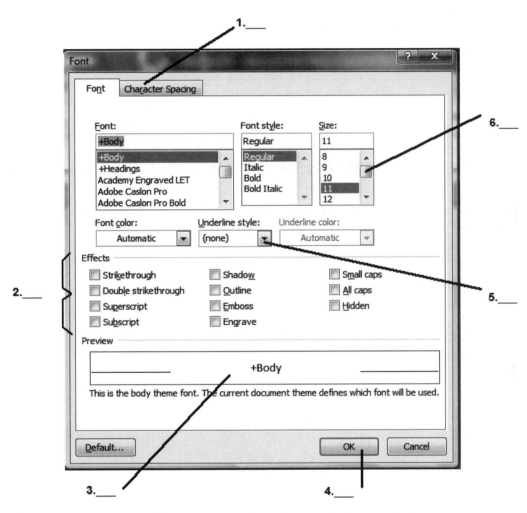

Figure WB1-4 *(Screen shot reprinted by permission from Microsoft Corporation.)*

1. _____

_____

_____

2. _____

_____

_____

3. _____
   _____
   _____

4. _____
   _____
   _____

5. _____
   _____
   _____

6. _____
   _____
   _____

BUILDING SKILLS 1-4: COMPONENTS OF A DIALOG BOX REVIEW

Instructions: Referring back to Figure WB1-4, label as many different components of the dialog box as you can. Describe the function of any component not shown previously.

_____
_____
_____
_____
_____

U N I T **2**

Medical Practice Management Software

BUILDING SKILLS 2-1: COMPONENTS OF A PRACTICE MANAGEMENT SOFTWARE REVIEW

Instructions: For each of the components of practice management software listed below, provide a brief description of the main purpose or function for each.

1. Appointment Scheduling System

_____
_____
_____
_____
_____

2. Patient Registration System

_____
_____
_____
_____
_____

3. File Maintenance System

_____
_____
_____
_____
_____

4. Procedure Posting System

_____

_____

_____

_____

_____

5. Insurance Billing System

_____

_____

_____

_____

_____

6. Posting Payments System

_____

_____

_____

_____

_____

7. Patient Billing System

_____

_____

_____

_____

_____

8. Report Generation System

_____

_____

_____

_____

_____

BUILDING SKILLS 2-2: USING A PRACTICE MANAGEMENT SOFTWARE APPLICATION IN THE MEDICAL OFFICE

Instructions: For each of the following office tasks, match the practice management software system from the list that would be utilized to complete the task with software.

Appointment Scheduling System   Patient Registration System   File Maintenance System

Procedure Posting System   Insurance Billing System   Posting Payments System

Patient Billing System   Report Generation System

1. _____ A patient mails a $55.00 personal check to the office for a balance due on their account.

2. _____ An established patient has provided you with their new home address and phone number.

3. _____ Information on all patients with 60 days past-due accounts is needed to send collection letters.

4. _____ One insurance company check with payments for 10 patients arrives in the office mail.

5. _____ A patient who was seen by Dr. Heath in the hospital calls the office one week later to visit the doctor in follow-up.

6. _____ An insurance payment is posted, leaving a $45.00 remainder balance due from the patient.

7. _____ A batch of Medicare claims has been prepared and is ready to be submitted.

8. _____ A new patient has submitted their registration form and an insurance card to the front desk 15 minutes before their appointment time.

9. _____ A medical biller is ready to input procedures completed at Community Hospital over the past week by Dr. Schwartz.

10. _____ A patient calls the office and does not remember the date and time they were to see Dr. Heath in the month of May.

11. _____ At the beginning of the year, five CPT codes and three ICD codes need to be updated.

12. _____ A new patient has to change the time of his visit with Dr. Schwartz on October 3.

13. _____ The office manager would like to review all balances receivable from claims sent to a certain insurance company.

14. _____ The address for a new office location that is frequently used for patient referrals needs to be added to the database.

15. _____ A patient is ready to check out after an office visit and gives the front-desk staff a superbill containing services provided today by Dr. Schwartz.

BUILDING SKILLS 2-3: HEALTH INSURANCE PORTABILITY AND ACCOUNTABILITY ACT (HIPAA) REVIEW

Instructions: Select the correct answer for each of the following.

1. The main purpose of HIPAA is

    a. the protection of a patient's rights.

    b. the security and privacy of health information.

    c. to increase the documentation requirements for medical offices.

    d. to protect the physician from lawsuits.

2. For the purpose of HIPAA, hospitals, physicians, health care plans, clearinghouses, and other medical providers and services are referred to as

    a. covered entities.

    b. acceptable health care providers.

    c. authorized professional entities for providing care.

    d. None of the above.

3. HIPAA requires that all patients

    a. must be provided with a written privacy notice by providers.

    b. must have a written explanation of privacy rights and practices.

    c. must sign a written privacy form.

    d. A and C.

    e. All of the above.

4. The Business Associate Agreement assures that

    a. PHI will be safeguarded.

    b. PHI will be used for a particular stated purpose.

    c. PHI can be disclosed in a certain manner.

    d. A and B.

    e. All of the above.

5. If a patient reviews PHI, finds inaccuracies, and is denied changes to the record, the denial must be

    a. provided in an affidavit.

    b. documented in the patient's file.

    c. provided in a written statement to the patient.

    d. No action is required.

6. When health care providers are using PHI related to treatment, there are

    a. limits to the amount of PHI that can be disclosed.

    b. no limits to the PHI disclosed if related to treatment.

    c. limits that only the minimal amount of information is permitted to be disclosed for any reason.

    d. None of the above.

7. Every covered entity must designate a person who is responsible for developing and implementing privacy policies and procedures. This person is known as the

    a. office manager.

    b. main provider of the facility or service.

    c. privacy officer.

    d. None of the above.

8. If a patient wants copies of their protected health information, the covered entity can be charged a reasonable fee to provide those copies.

    a. True

    b. False

9. As long as there is a designated person to handle privacy policies, covered entities are not required to train staff members about the privacy rules, policies, and procedures of the covered entity.

    a. True

    b. False

10. Claim submissions, insurance claim payments, and remittance advice information are not subject to HIPAA guidelines and privacy regulations.

    a. True

    b. False

U N I T **3**

Basic Management Concepts for Medical Administrative Staff

BUILDING SKILLS 3-1: EXPLORING CAREERS IN THE FRONT AND BACK OFFICE

The following list contains positions and titles that may exist in the medical and administrative hospital offices where you will be working. You may now be training for one of these careers; others may be positions to aspire to with further training or experience. Depending on the medical office and specialty you will be working in, you may be part of a facility with a diversified health care team. It is often surprising how what one may think of as a traditional role, such as nurses working only in hospitals, is actually not accurate. Nurses have a wide range of facilities and environments where they can work. As an example, it is not unusual for registered nurses to have specialized roles working alongside surgeons in private practice, such as in cardiovascular and thoracic surgery. Nurse practitioners and physician assistants may work with obstetric patients and their prenatal needs, freeing the physician for high-risk cases and time in the delivery room. Often, orthopedic surgeons have orthopedic technicians on staff, providing joint injections, cast removals, and other specialized tasks. Many medical offices have phlebotomists, X-ray, and laboratory technicians on staff.

Instructions: Using the Internet, visit the Web site for the Occupational Outlook Handbook, current edition, at: http://www.bls.gov/OCO/ to research the various medical-office careers listed below, and the information indicated for each. Use the Search box at the top right of the Web site to find the titles listed in A–M below. If required, a hard copy of the Occupational Outlook Handbook, or other similar publications, may be used from the library.

For each title, provide a brief description for each of the following areas with your findings:

1. *The nature of the work and typical work environment*

2. *Job outlook*

3. *Average earnings*

4. *Required training*

5. *Professional organizations and/or associations*

    A. Medical Assistants (Administrative)

    B. Receptionists and Information Clerks (Medical)

    C. Secretaries and Administrative Assistants (Medical)

    D. Medical Transcriptionists

    E. Medical Records and Health Information Technicians

    F. Physician Assistants

    G. Licensed Practical and Licensed Vocational Nurses

    H. Registered Nurses (and Nurse Practitioners)

    I. Medical and Health Services Managers

    J. Clinical Laboratory Technologists and Technicians

    K. Radiologic Technologists and Technicians

    L. Physical and Occupational Therapist Assistants and Aides

    M. Physical and Occupational Therapists

BUILDING SKILLS 3-2: SCHEDULING APPOINTMENTS FOR ESTABLISHED PATIENTS USING MOSS

Instructions: Start MOSS and then click on the Appointment Scheduling button located at the Main Menu. Schedule appointments as indicated for each of the established patients below. Screen shots are provided to check your work.

A. Naomi Yamagata

> 30 minutes for an office visit with Dr. Schwartz
> Reason note: Shortness of breath and chest pain
> Date: 10/22/2009
> Time: 11:00 a.m.

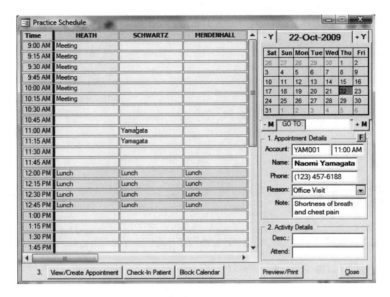

(Delmar/Cengage Learning.)

B. Caitlin Barryroe

> 30 minutes for an office visit with Dr. Heath
> Reason note: Pain when urinating
> Date: 10/22/2009
> Time: 10:30 a.m.

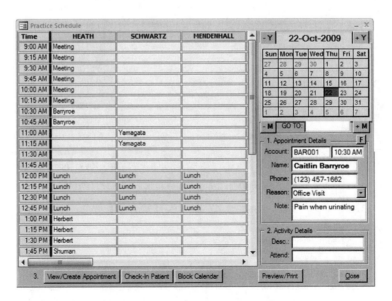

(Delmar/Cengage Learning.)

C. Gabrielle Camille calls in for her child, Emery Camille

15 minutes for an office visit with Dr. Schwartz
Reason note: Ear pain and sore throat
Date: 10/22/2009
Time: 3:00 p.m.

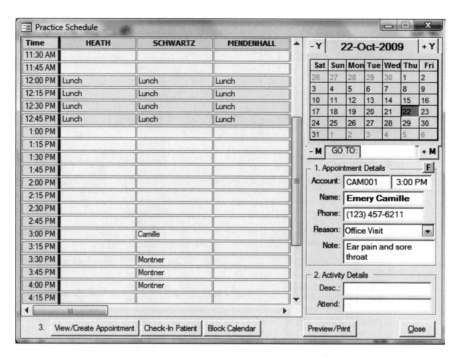

(Delmar/Cengage Learning.)

D. Aimee Bradley

30 minutes for an office visit with Dr. Schwartz
Reason note: Sore throat and fever
Date: 10/22/2009
Time: 4:30 p.m.

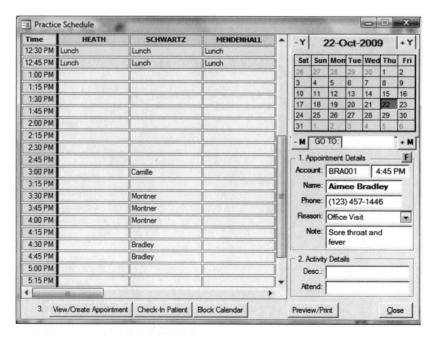

(Delmar/Cengage Learning.)

E. Nancy Herbert

45 minutes for an office visit with Dr. Heath
Reason note: Follow-up COPD, needs medication refills
Date: 10/22/2009
Time: 1:00 p.m.

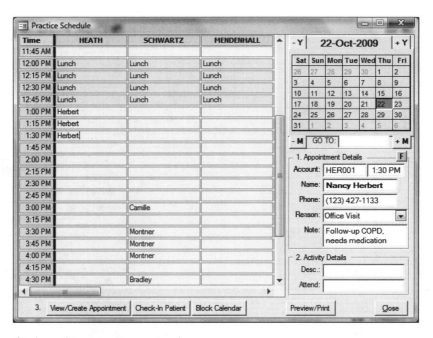

(Delmar/Cengage Learning.)

F. Deanna Hartsfeld

30 minutes for an office visit with Dr. Heath
Reason note: Recheck high cholesterol and blood pressure
Date: 10/22/2009
Time: 3:30 p.m.

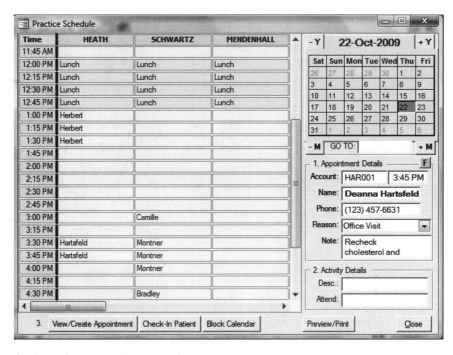

(Delmar/Cengage Learning.)

G. Anthony Rizzo calls in for his teenage child, Tina Rizzo

30 minutes for an office visit with Dr. Heath
Reason note: Allergies, sneezing, and persistent cough
Date: 10/22/2009
Time: 5:00 p.m.

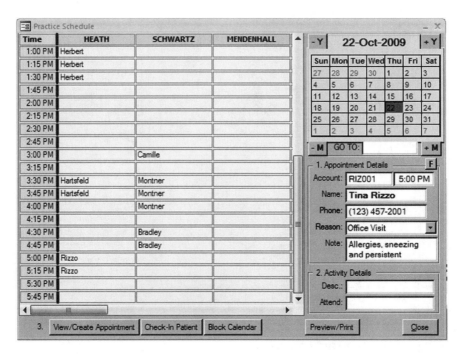

(Delmar/Cengage Learning.)

H. Joel Royzin

45 minutes with Dr. Heath
Reason note: PVD and DM
Date: 10/22/2009
Time: 2:15 p.m.

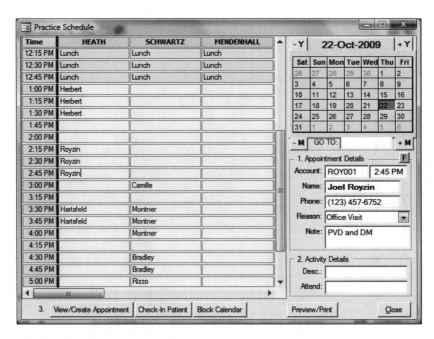

(Delmar/Cengage Learning.)

I. Derek Wallace

> 15 minutes with Dr. Heath
> Reason note: Follow-up UTI
> Date: 10/22/2009
> Time: 11:00 a.m.

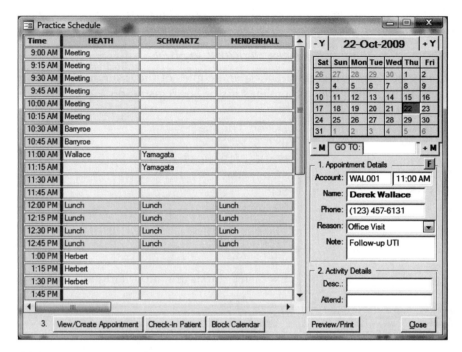

(Delmar/Cengage Learning.)

J. Alan Shuman

> 30 minutes with Dr. Heath
> Reason note: COPD
> Date: 10/22/2009
> Time: 1:45 p.m.

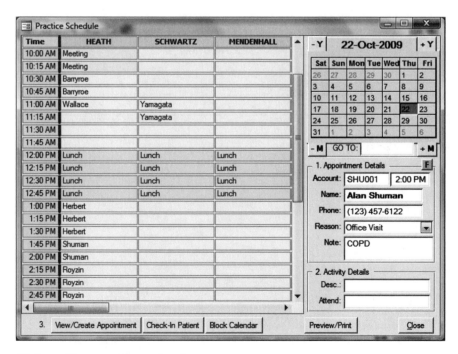

(Delmar/Cengage Learning.)

BUILDING SKILLS 3-3: SCHEDULING APPOINTMENTS FOR NEW PATIENTS USING MOSS

Instructions: Each patient below has been screened via telephone for name, daytime telephone number, insurance coverage, and reason for visit. Screen shots are provided to check your work.

1. *Be certain Feedback Mode is turned off in MOSS. Search the database to be sure the patient is not already in the system, and then create an account with the basic information given.*

2. *Schedule appointments for the date and times indicated in MOSS.*

   NOTE: The remainder of the required information and copies of the insurance cards will be obtained at the time of the office visit when the patient completes his or her registration form.

   A. Name: Devon Trimble
       Date of Birth: 08/25/1972
       Daytime telephone: Work – (123) 537-2210
       Insurance: Signal HMO
       Guarantor and policyholder: Self
       Duration of visit: 60 minutes
       Doctor: Heath
       Date: 10/27/2009
       Time: 3:00 p.m.

       Reason for visit: Excessive thirst, urination, fatigue

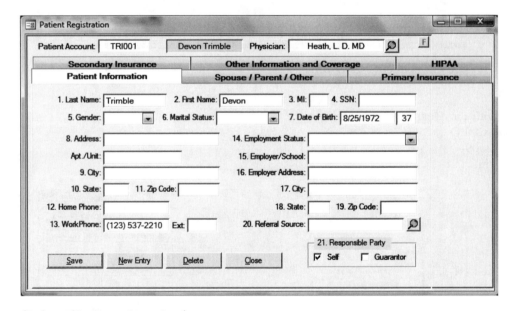

   (Delmar/Cengage Learning.)

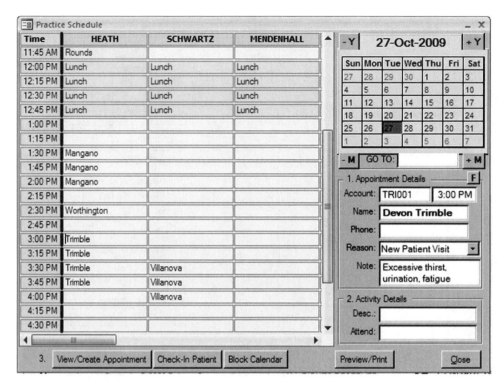

(Delmar/Cengage Learning.)

B. Name: Wynona Sheridan
   Date of Birth: 06/05/1984
   Daytime telephone: Work – (123) 537-0211 ext. 6
   Insurance: ConsumerONE HRA
   Guarantor and policyholder: Self
   Duration of visit: 45 minutes
   Doctor: Heath
   Date: 10/27/2009
   Time: 4:00 p.m.
   Reason for visit: Possible flu, diarrhea, and vomiting

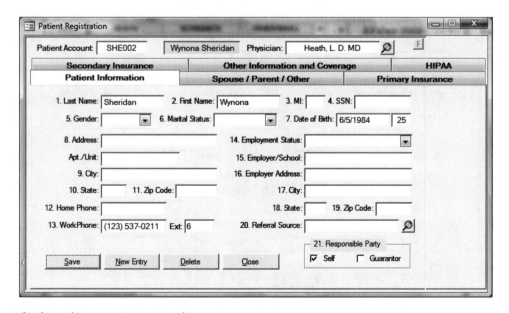

(Delmar/Cengage Learning.)

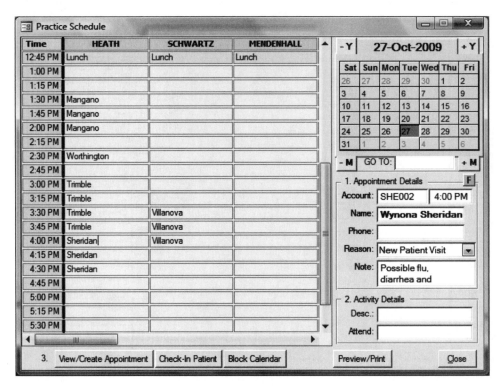

(Delmar/Cengage Learning.)

C. Name: Harold Engleman
   Date of Birth: 10/28/1948
   Daytime telephone: Work – (123) 970-5000
   Primary Insurance: FlexiHealth PPO – Out-of-Network
   Secondary Insurance: None
   Guarantor and policyholder: Self
   Duration of visit: 60 minutes
   Doctor: Schwartz
   Date: 10/22/2009
   Time: 10:00 a.m.
   Reason for visit: Heartburn, hypertension

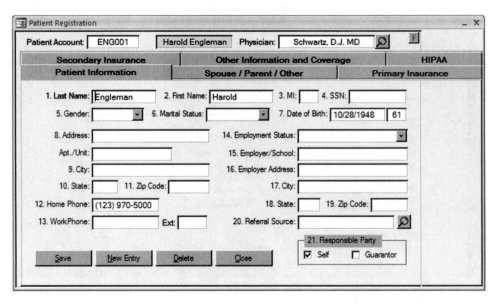

(Delmar/Cengage Learning.)

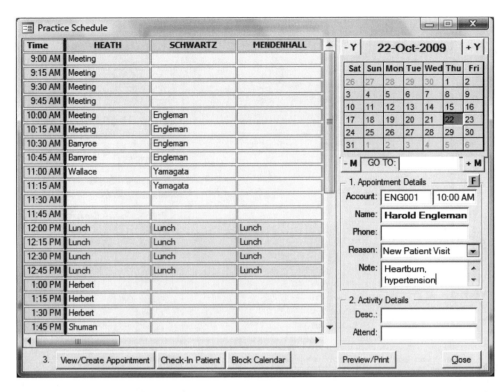

(Delmar/Cengage Learning.)

BUILDING SKILLS 3-4: MODIFYING SCHEDULED APPOINTMENT DETAILS USING MOSS

Instructions: Complete the appointment modifications as required by each patient situation below. Screen shots are provided to check your work.

A. Caitlin Barryroe calls the office to say she was called into work on 10/22/2009. She needs to change her appointment. She can take an early lunch on Friday, 10/23/2009, and see the doctor around 11:30 a.m. Reschedule the appointment with Dr. Heath.

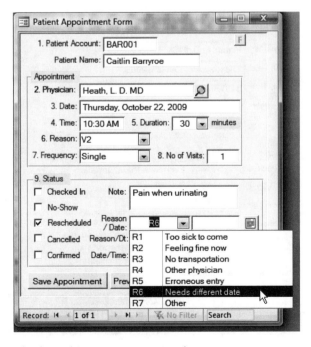

(Delmar/Cengage Learning.)

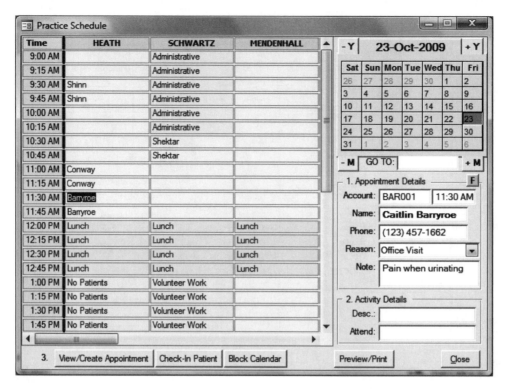

(Delmar/Cengage Learning.)

B. Dr. Heath receives preliminary blood test results from Patient Trimble's doctor, taken just before the patient moved to Douglasville a couple of weeks back. The patient's glucose is over 600, and he requests that you call the patient and have him come in sooner for his appointment, if possible. After contacting the patient, he confirms that he is available in the afternoon on 10/20/2009. Reschedule his appointment from 10/27/2009 at 1:00 p.m. to 10/20/2009 at 3:00 p.m., and then inform the physician. All other appointment details remain the same.

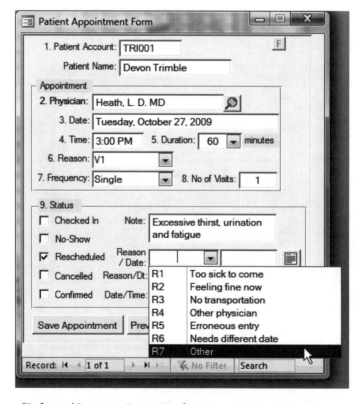

(Delmar/Cengage Learning.)

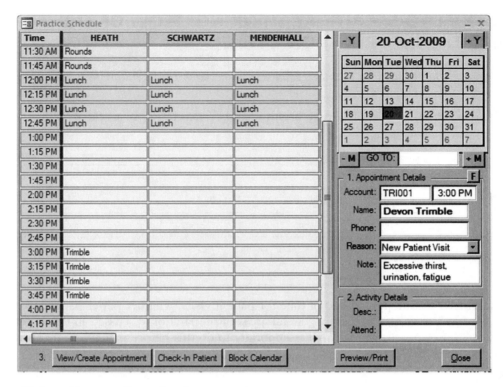

(Delmar/Cengage Learning.)

C. A call is received on 10/19/2009 from the Admissions Coordinator at Retirement Inn Nursing Home to advise Dr. Heath that Patient Joel Royzin has been accepted as a resident to the home. His move-in date will be 10/23/2009. The patient has been experiencing complications after his foot amputation for PVD, and requires assistance with self-care. She is requesting that Dr. Heath please visit the patient at the nursing home in follow-up, call in current medications and treatment orders, and cancel the office appointment scheduled for 10/22/2009 at 2:15 p.m. Check your work with the screen shot below and assure that the appointment has been removed from the schedule.

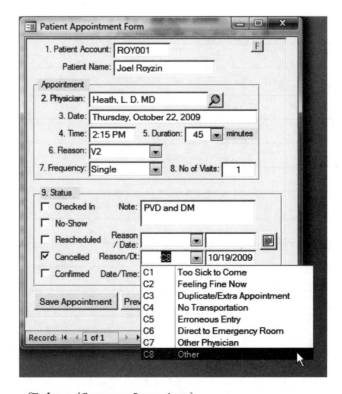

(Delmar/Cengage Learning.)

BUILDING SKILLS 3-5: CRITICAL THINKING: FLOW OF THE OFFICE AND THE INFORMATION CYCLE

Instructions: Working individually or in small groups, discuss each of the following topics or questions and provide answers as indicated for each.

1. Provide specific examples of how electronic health records software improves the overall efficiency in a medical-office environment.

_____

_____

_____

_____

_____

_____

2. Every medical office must prepare ahead of time for patient visits, whether paper patient records or electronic health records are used. List the six general areas of preparation discussed in this book, and provide at least one detail for each area as to why it is important to do this before patients come to the office.

A. _____

_____

_____

_____

_____

B. _____

_____

_____

_____

_____

C. _____

_____

_____

_____

_____

D. _____

_____

_____

_____

_____

E. _____

_____

_____

_____

_____

F. _____

_____

_____

_____

_____

3. Describe three important items or tasks that should be obtained from every new patient who visits the office. (Hint: These may be obtained or done ahead of time, or at the time of visit.)

A. _____

_____

_____

_____

B. _____

_____

_____

_____

C. _____

_____

_____

_____

4. Think about new or established patients checking out after completing visits with the physician in the medical office. As a front-office staff member, describe specific details you may be responsible for when checking the patient out as he or she is leaving.

_____

_____

_____

_____

_____

_____

_____

5. Describe the importance of the work completed by the front-desk staff as it relates to the later work done by the medical-billing staff. How can the front-desk staff improve cash flow in the medical office?

_____

_____

_____

_____

_____

_____

_____

_____

_____

_____

_____

_____

UNIT **4**

Fundamentals of Medical Insurance

BUILDING SKILLS 4-1: UNDERSTANDING TYPES OF HEALTH INSURANCE PLANS

Instructions: Indicate what type of insurance plan is described in each of the following examples.

1. _____ A patient can visit any in-network physician, but must pay an annual $500.00 deductible and a $40.00 copayment at each physician visit.

2. _____ A patient can visit any physician he or she wishes to, subject to an annual deductible of $2,000.00 and a 10% co-insurance on the approved amount for physician services.

3. _____ A patient can visit any physician in a network and pay a $40.00 copayment at each visit. The patient can also choose to visit any physician outside the network, subject to an annual deductible and 50% co-insurance of the approved amount for physician services.

4. _____ Providing supplemental coverage, these private plans are offered by insurance companies and cover portions of medical bills that are not covered by Medicare Parts A, B, and D, such as deductibles, co-insurance, and other select services.

5. _____ These are plans offered by private insurance companies and health service organizations that provide benefits for everything covered under Original Medicare, and that may offer additional benefits.

6. _____ A federally administered health insurance available to qualifying persons aged 65 and over, or any qualifying person with end-stage renal disease or amyotrophic lateral sclerosis (Lou Gehrig's disease), or an eligible person on long-term disability.

7. _____ A type of plan that focuses on reducing costs by limiting access to health care, usually through a gatekeeper and in-network providers, and is intended to encourage patients to seek care early to prevent the need for more intensive care later.

8. _____ A federally and state-funded health program for eligible individuals and families with low incomes and resources.

Instructions: Respond to the questions presented in the space that follow.

9. Explain reasons why some patients may prefer to use Original Medicare and a supplemental insurance over a Medicare Advantage plan.

10. Explain how HRA-type plans differ from the more traditional structure of current day HMOs and PPOs. Note some of the advantages and disadvantages when comparing these plans.

BUILDING SKILLS 4-2: PRACTICING WITH INDEMNITY INSURANCE PAYMENTS AND ADJUSTMENTS

Instructions: For each situation below, provide the answers as indicated for each.

A. A patient has an indemnity health insurance plan with a $250.00 deductible and a 20% co-insurance on the allowed amount for covered services. If the deductible has already been met for the year, calculate the amount the patient must pay out-of-pocket to a physician who does not participate with his plan for the service below:

Standard fee:	$348.00
Allowed:	$286.00
Insurance Paid:	$228.80
Co-insurance:	$57.40
Answer:	_____

B. A patient has an indemnity health insurance plan with a $500.00 deductible and a 20% co-insurance on the allowed amount for covered services. If the deductible has already been met for the year, calculate the amount the patient must pay out-of-pocket to a physician who does not participate with his plan for the service below:

Standard fee:	$268.40
Allowed:	$188.70
Answer:	_____

C. A patient has an indemnity health insurance plan with a $250.00 deductible and a 20% co-insurance on the allowed amount for covered services. There is still $75.00 left of the deductible that must be met. Calculate the amount the patient must pay out-of-pocket to a physician who participates with his plan for the service below, and the total amount that is to be adjusted:

Standard fee: $348.00

Participation discount: $62.00

Insurance paid: $168.80

Applied to deductible: $75.00

Co-insurance: $42.20

Answer: _____

D. A patient has an indemnity health insurance plan with a $250.00 deductible and a 10% co-insurance on the allowed amount for covered services. There is still $250.00 left of the deductible that must be met. Calculate the amount the patient must pay out-of-pocket to a physician who participates with his plan for the service below, and the total amount that is to be adjusted:

Standard fee: $150.00

Participation discount: $32.00

Insurance paid: 0.00

Answer: _____

E. A patient has an indemnity health insurance plan with a deductible that has been met and a 10% co-insurance on the allowed amount for covered services. Calculate the amount the patient must pay out-of-pocket to a nonparticipating physician for the service below:

Standard fee: $196.40

Allowed: $142.60

Insurance paid: $128.34

Answer: _____

BUILDING SKILLS 4-3: PRACTICING WITH MANAGED CARE PAYMENTS AND ADJUSTMENTS

Instructions: For each situation below, provide the answers as indicated for each.

A. A patient has a PPO health insurance plan with a $40.00 copayment due at each physician visit. Calculate the amount the patient must pay out-of-pocket to an in-network physician for the following service:

Submitted fee:	$422.00
PPO discount:	$103.60
Patient copay:	$40.00
Insurance paid:	$278.40
Answer:	_____

B. A patient has a PPO health insurance plan with a $40.00 copayment at each visit. Calculate the amount the insurance will pay, assuming that the PPO plan pays at 100% after the discount and copayment is applied, for the following service:

Submitted fee:	$150.00
PPO Discount:	$32.53
Answer:	_____

C. A patient has a POS health plan with a $50.00 copayment at each visit. The plan pays 100% after the discount and copayment are applied. Calculate the insurance payment for the following service:

Submitted fee:	$232.00
POS/PPO discount:	$25.44
Answer:	_____

D. A patient has an HMO health insurance plan with a $20.00 copayment at each visit. The HMO pays 100 percent of the allowed amount, less the patient copayment. Calculate the insurance payment for the following service:

Submitted fee:	$245.00
Allowed amount:	$156.76
Answer:	_____

BUILDING SKILLS 4-4: PRACTICING WITH MEDICARE PAYMENTS AND ADJUSTMENTS

Instructions: For each service below, provide the answers as indicated. Hint: Review the Medicare PAR and NON-PAR situations discussed in Unit 4.

A. Patient A has Medicare and receives a service with a standard fee of $198.00. The deductible has been met. Her physician is PAR with Medicare and is required to accept assignment. How much will the adjustment be for the following service?:

Standard fee:	$198.00
Medicare Approved:	$156.00
Medicare pays (80%):	$124.80
Patient co-insurance (20%):	$31.20
Adjustment:	_____

B. Patient B has Medicare and receives a service with a standard fee of $467.00. The deductible has been met. Her physician is PAR with Medicare and is required to accept assignment. For the following service, calculate the adjustment, the patient co-insurance, and the amount Medicare will pay at 80%

Standard fee:	$467.00
Medicare Approved:	$351.60
Medicare Adjustment:	_____
Medicare Payment:	_____
Patient Co-Insurance:	_____

C. Patient C has Medicare and receives a service with a standard fee of $467.00. His physician is PAR with Medicare and is required to accept assignment. For the following service, calculate the total amount the patient will pay out-of-pocket.

Standard fee:	$467.00
Medicare Approved:	$351.60
Deductible applied:	$85.00
Medicare paid:	$213.28
Patient out-of-pocket:	_____

D. Patient D, a Medicare patient, receives a service with a standard fee of $125.00. His physician is NON-PAR with Medicare and accepts assignment. For the service below, what is the total out-of-pocket that the patient must pay?

Standard fee:	$125.00
Medicare Approved:	$103.25 (Reduced 5%)

Medicare pays (80%): $82.60

Patient co-insurance $20.65
(20%):

Patient out-of-pocket: _____

E. Patient E, a Medicare patient, receives a service with a standard fee of $268.00. His physician is NON-PAR with Medicare and accepts assignment on this service. What is the total out-of-pocket amount that the patient must pay? The service below shows the standard fee, and the reduced Medicare-approved amount. Medicare pays 80 percent of the approved fee for the service.

Standard fee: $268.00

Medicare Approved: $204.80

Patient out-of-pocket: _____

F. Patient F, a Medicare patient, receives a service with a standard fee of $268.00. His physician is NON-PAR with Medicare and does not accept assignment. What is the total out-of-pocket amount the patient must pay for the following service?

Standard fee: $268.00

Limiting charge (cap): $235.75

Medicare Approved: $205.00
                       (Reduced 5%)

Medicare pays (80%): $164.00

Patient co-insurance $41.00
(20%):

Patient out-of-pocket: _____

G. Patient G, a Medicare patient, receives a service with a standard fee of $183.00. Her physician is NON-PAR with Medicare and does not accept assignment. Her deductible has been met. What is the total out-of-pocket amount the patient must pay for the following service?

Standard fee: $183.00

Charge limit (cap): $165.95

Medicare Approved: $144.30

Patient out-of-pocket: _____

U N I T **5**

Patient Registration and Data Entry

BUILDING SKILLS 5-1: THE PATIENT REGISTRATION PROCESS

Instructions: Using the blank lines below, list seven important tasks discussed in this book that the front-desk staff must complete for new patient registration before the back-office staff can take the patient back for a doctor's visit.

1. _____

    _____

2. _____

    _____

3. _____

    _____

4. _____

    _____

5. _____

    _____

6. _____

    _____

7. _____

    _____

Instructions: Answer the questions as indicated.

8. Discuss some ways that a patient's marital status, employment status, or financial situation may impact his or her ability to pay for medical expenses.

Marital status: _____

_____

_____

_____

_____

Employment status: _____

_____

_____

_____

_____

Financial status: _____

_____

_____

_____

_____

9. Discuss some of the differences when obtaining patient information from new patients versus established patients who visit the office to see the physician.

_____

_____

_____

_____

_____

_____

_____

_____

_____

_____

10. How does using practice management software assist medical staff with the patient registration process?

_____

_____

_____

_____

_____

_____

_____

BUILDING SKILLS 5-2: PRACTICE REGISTERING NEW OFFICE PATIENTS

Instructions: Be sure the Feedback Mode is turned off in MOSS. For each of the new patients who follow, complete the following tasks:

1. *Greet and then check in each patient on the appointment schedule in MOSS to indicate they have arrived. Obtain signature and document HIPAA privacy policy from patient or guarantor.*

2. *Check the copy of the insurance card against the insurance information on the registration form for accuracy.*

3. *Refer to the registration form and enter all data as it pertains to each patient in MOSS. (Hint: Do not forget to include copayment information on the insurance screen where applicable.)*

4. *Verify eligibility of insurance benefits using MOSS.*

New Patient Devon Trimble

Today's Date:	October 20, 2009
Appointment time:	3:00 p.m.
Physician:	Dr. Heath

Refer to Source Documents WB5-1 and WB5-2 in the back of the workbook

Check your work with Figures WB5-1, WB5-2, WB5-3 and WB5-4.

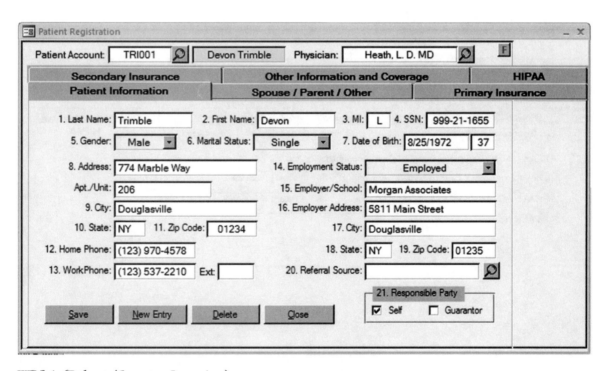

Figure WB5-1 *(Delmar/Cengage Learning)*

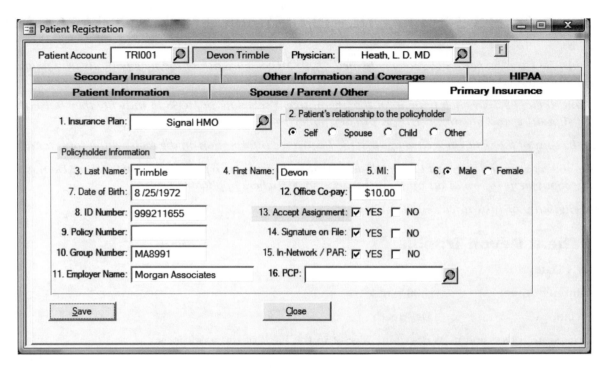

Figure WB5-2 *(Delmar/Cengage Learning)*

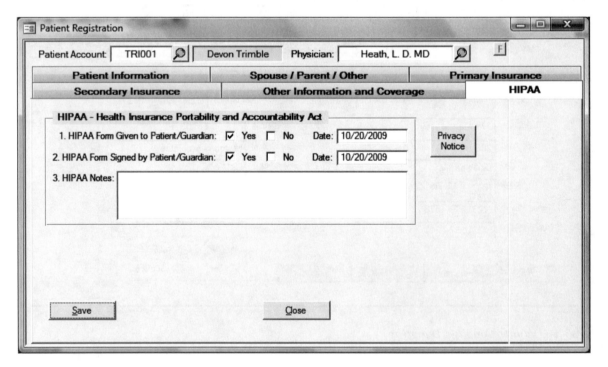

Figure WB5-3 *(Delmar/Cengage Learning)*

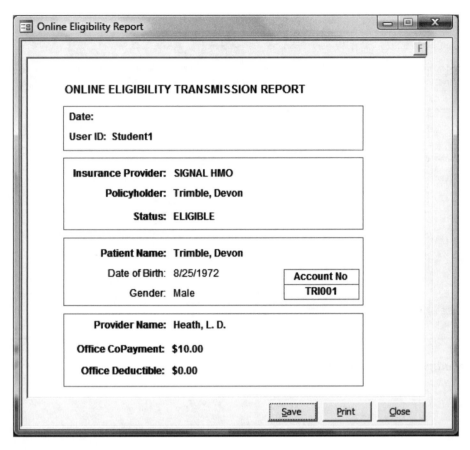

Figure WB5-4 *(Delmar/Cengage Learning)*

New Patient Wynona Sheridan

Today's Date: October 27, 2009

Appointment time: 4:00 p.m.

Physician: Dr. Heath

Refer to Source Documents WB5-3 and WB5-4 in the back of the workbook.

Check your work with Figures WB5-5, WB5-6, WB5-7, and WB5-8.

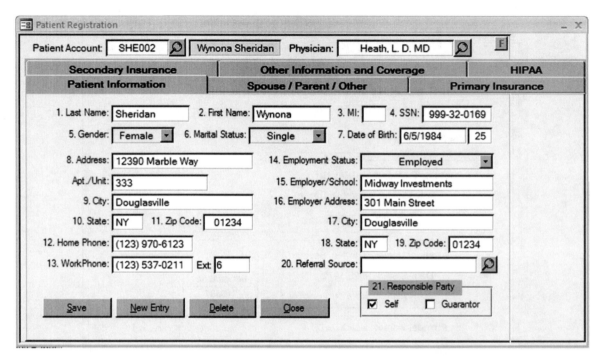

Figure WB5-5 *(Delmar/Cengage Learning)*

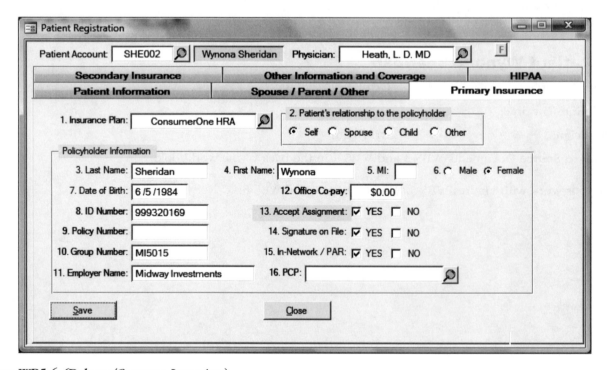

Figure WB5-6 *(Delmar/Cengage Learning)*

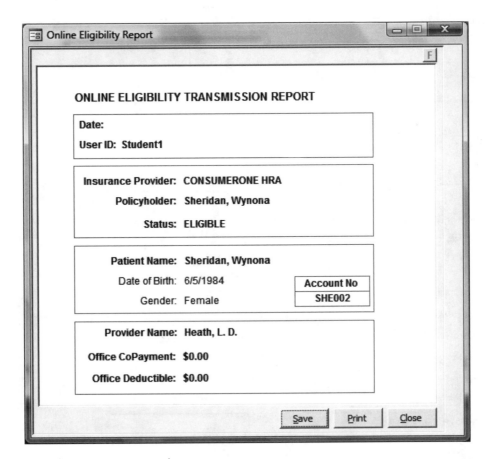

Figure WB5-7 *(Delmar/Cengage Learning)*

Figure WB5-8 *(Delmar/Cengage Learning)*

New Patient Harold Engleman

Today's Date: October 22, 2009

Appointment time: 10:00 a.m.

Physician: Dr. Schwartz

Refer to Source Documents WB5-5 and WB5-6 in the back of the workbook.

Check your work with Figures WB5-9, WB5-10, WB5-11, and WB5-12.

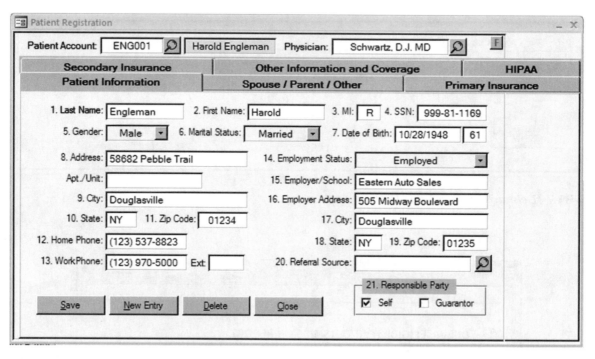

Figure WB5-9 *(Delmar/Cengage Learning)*

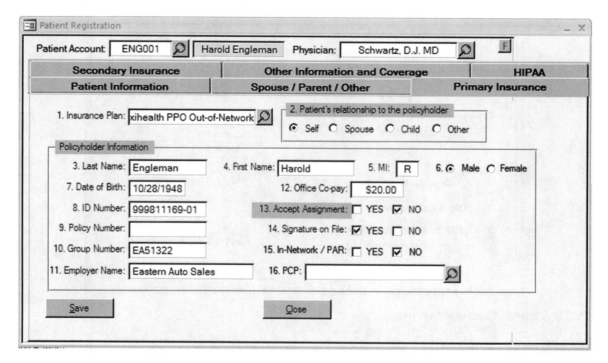

Figure WB5-10 *(Delmar/Cengage Learning)*

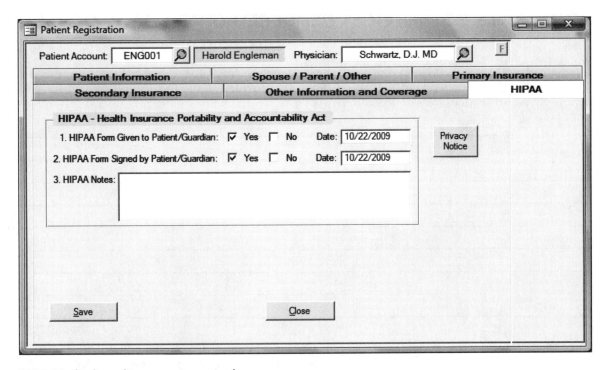

Figure WB5-11 *(Delmar/Cengage Learning)*

Figure WB5-12 *(Delmar/Cengage Learning)*

BUILDING SKILLS 5-3: SERVICES RENDERED OUTSIDE THE OFFICE

Instructions: Answer the following questions as indicated.

1. Describe examples of how patient information might be provided to the medical-office staff for patients receiving physician services outside the office.

    _____

    _____

    _____

    _____

    _____

    _____

    _____

    _____

    _____

2. Describe the four main types of facilities outside the office where physicians commonly provide patient services, as discussed in this book. For each, give a brief summary on the type of patient care provided by each facility.

    A. _____

    _____

    _____

    _____

    B. _____

    _____

    _____

    _____

    C. _____

    _____

    _____

    _____

    D. _____

    _____

    _____

    _____

3. Sometimes, medical-office staff will need to do a little extra to obtain complete information on patients who received physician services outside the office. Explain the various resources which the staff may check or use in order to complete patient information where needed.

_____
_____
_____
_____
_____
_____
_____
_____
_____
_____
_____
_____
_____
_____
_____
_____
_____
_____
_____
_____

BUILDING SKILLS 5-4: PRACTICE REGISTERING NEW PATIENTS WHO RECEIVED EMERGENCY ROOM SERVICES BY THE PHYSICIAN

Instructions: Be sure the Feedback Mode is turned off in MOSS. Dr. Heath was one of three physicians on duty in the emergency room at Community General Hospital on 11/11/2009 from 6:00 p.m. until 6:00 a.m. Do the steps below for each of the following patients who received physician services CPT 99282. Follow any additional instructions included with each patient case study.

1. *Search the MOSS database, and then enter each new patient in the system using the Emergency Care and Treatment form.*

2. *Enter the procedure and diagnostic codes on the Outside Service Log, Source Document WB5-7 in the back of the workbook, in preparation for medical insurance billing. (Hint: Continue the Reference Number in sequence for each entry.)*

Emergency Room Patient Dennis Johnsen

Today's Date: November 12, 2009

Physician: Dr. Heath

Refer to Source Documents WB5-8 and WB5-9 in the back of the workbook.

Additional Instructions:

1. *Read the Emergency Care and Treatment form turned in to you by Dr. Heath on the morning of 11/12/2009 (Source Document WB5-8). Check the information against the insurance card copy that accompanies this form (Source Document WB5-9).*

2. *Enter patient registration information in MOSS as needed and check insurance eligibility using MOSS.*

3. *Enter the date of service, physician name, facility name, procedure, and diagnosis(es) for this patient onto the log in preparation for billing (Source Document WB5-7).*

Check your work with Figures WB5-13, WB5-14, WB5-15, and WB5-16.

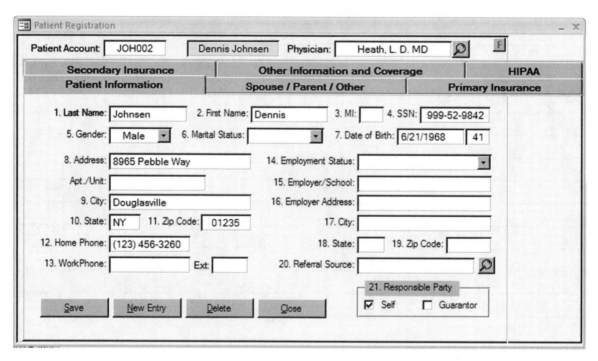

Figure WB5-13 *(Delmar/Cengage Learning)*

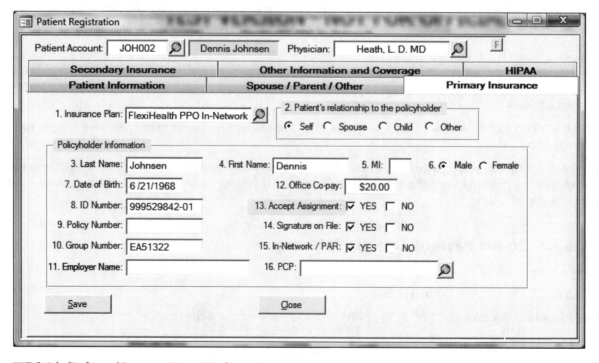

Figure WB5-14 *(Delmar/Cengage Learning)*

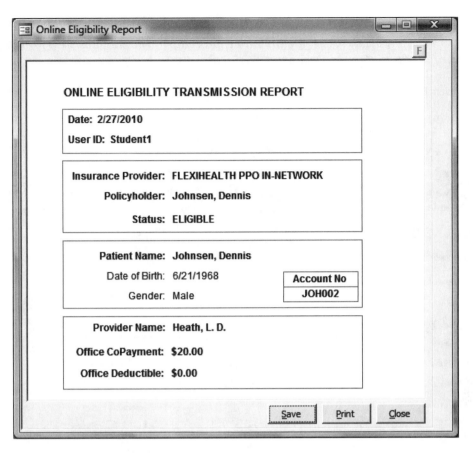

Figure WB5-15 *(Delmar/Cengage Learning)*

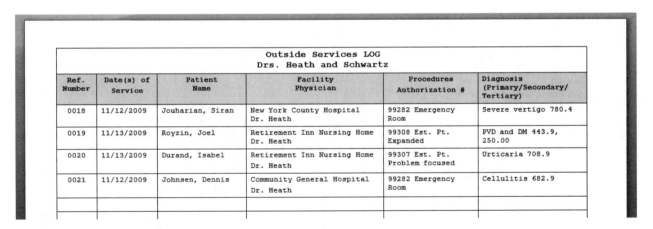

Figure WB5-16 *(Delmar/Cengage Learning)*

Emergency Room Patient William Bernardo

Today's Date: November 12, 2009

Physician: Dr. Heath

Refer to Source Documents WB5-10, WB5-11, and WB5-12 in the back of the workbook.

Additional Instructions:

1. *Read the Emergency Care and Treatment form turned in to you by Dr. Heath on the morning of 11/12/2009 (Source Document WB5-10). Check the information against the insurance card copies that accompany this form (Source Documents WB5-11 and WB5-12).*

2. Enter patient registration information in MOSS as needed and check insurance eligibility using MOSS.

3. Enter the date of service, physician name, facility name, procedure, and diagnosis(es) for this patient onto the log in preparation for billing (Source Document WB5-7).

Check your work with Figures WB5-17, WB5-18, WB5-19, WB5-20, and WB5-21.

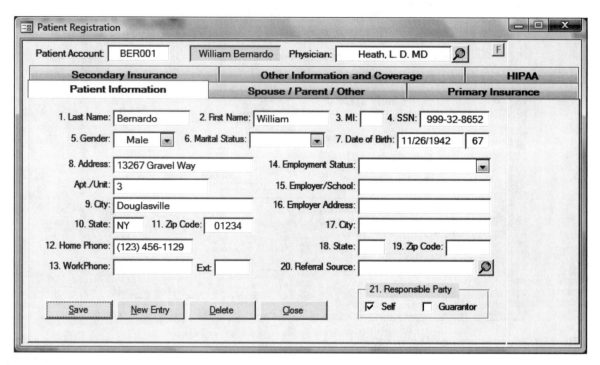

Figure WB5-17 *(Delmar/Cengage Learning)*

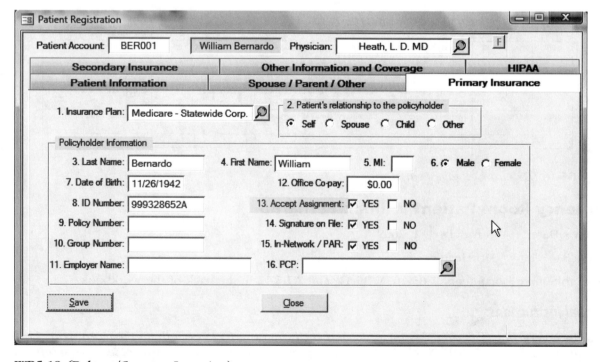

Figure WB5-18 *(Delmar/Cengage Learning)*

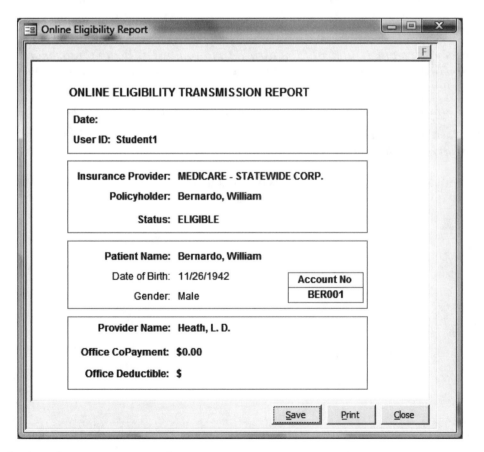

Figure WB5-19 *(Delmar/Cengage Learning)*

Figure WB5-20 *(Delmar/Cengage Learning)*

Ref. Number	Date(s) of Service	Patient Name	Facility Physician	Procedures Authorization #	Diagnosis (Primary/Secondary/Tertiary)
			Outside Services LOG		
			Drs. Heath and Schwartz		
0018	11/12/2009	Jouharian, Siran	New York County Hospital Dr. Heath	99282 Emergency Room	Severe vertigo 780.4
0019	11/13/2009	Royzin, Joel	Retirement Inn Nursing Home Dr. Heath	99308 Est. Pt. Expanded	PVD and DM 443.9, 250.00
0020	11/13/2009	Durand, Isabel	Retirement Inn Nursing Home Dr. Heath	99307 Est. Pt. Problem focused	Urticaria 708.9
0021	11/09/2009	Johnsen, Dennis	Community General Hospital Dr. Heath	99282 Emergency Room	Cellulitis 682.9
0022	11/09/2009	Bernardo, William	Community General Hospital Dr. Heath	99282 Emergency Room	COPD and CHF 496, 428.0

Figure WB5-21 *(Delmar/Cengage Learning)*

Emergency Room Patient Janet Souza

Today's Date: November 12, 2009

Physician: Dr. Heath

Refer to Source Documents WB5-13 and WB5-14 in the back of the workbook.

Additional Instructions:

1. *Read the Emergency Care and Treatment form turned in to you by Dr. Heath on the morning of 11/12/2009 (Source Document WB5-13). Check the information against the insurance card copy that accompanies this form (Source Document WB5-14).*

2. *Enter patient registration information in MOSS as needed and check insurance eligibility using MOSS.*

3. *Enter the date of service, physician name, facility name, procedure, and diagnosis(es) for this patient onto the log in preparation for billing (Source Document WB5-7).*

Check your work with Figures WB5-22, WB5-23, WB5-24, and WB5-25.

Figure WB5-22 *(Delmar/Cengage Learning)*

Figure WB5-23 *(Delmar/Cengage Learning)*

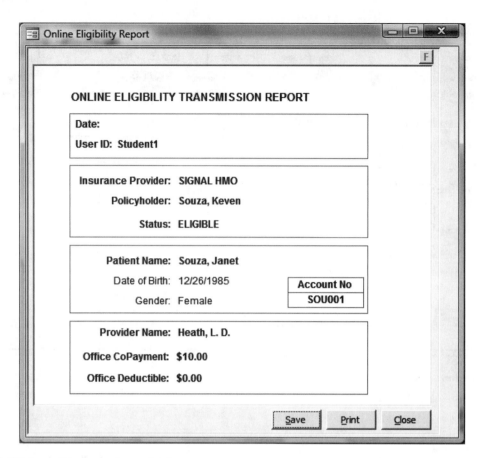

Figure WB5-24 *(Delmar/Cengage Learning)*

Ref. Number	Date(s) of Service	Patient Name	Facility Physician	Procedures Authorization #	Diagnosis (Primary/Secondary/Tertiary)
			Outside Services LOG **Drs. Heath and Schwartz**		
0018	11/12/2009	Jouharian, Siran	New York County Hospital Dr. Heath	99282 Emergency Room	Severe vertigo 780.4
0019	11/13/2009	Royzin, Joel	Retirement Inn Nursing Home Dr. Heath	99308 Est. Pt. Expanded	PVD and DM 443.9, 250.00
0020	11/13/2009	Durand, Isabel	Retirement Inn Nursing Home Dr. Heath	99307 Est. Pt. Problem focused	Urticaria 708.9
0021	11/09/2009	Johnsen, Dennis	Community General Hospital Dr. Heath	99282 Emergency Room	Cellulitis 682.9
0022	11/09/2009	Bernardo, William	Community General Hospital Dr. Heath	99282 Emergency Room	COPD, CHF 496, 428.0
0023	11/10/2009	Souza, Janet	Community General Hospital Dr. Heath	99282 Emergency Room	Gastroenteritis 558.9

Figure WB5-25 *(Delmar/Cengage Learning)*

BUILDING SKILLS 5-5: PRACTICE REGISTERING NEW PATIENTS WHO RECEIVED HOSPITAL SERVICES BY THE PHYSICIAN

Dr. Heath and Dr. Schwartz are the attending on-call physicians for the hospital and will see patients in the emergency room, clinic, or in consultation for another physician. If medically necessary, they will request consultations with specialists for patients who are being admitted, or for situations that arise during a patient's hospitalization that require a specialist.

Instructions: The following patients were admitted to Community General Hospital and will need to be searched in the MOSS database, and then entered in the system. The procedure and diagnostic codes will be entered on the billing log, Source Document WB5-7 in the back of the workbook. Be sure the Feedback Mode is turned off in MOSS before proceeding.

Hospital Admission for Karen Ross

Today's Date: November 17, 2009

Physician: Dr. Heath

Refer to Source Document WB5-15 in the back of the workbook.

Additional Instructions:

1. *Review the Record of Admission form received from Dr. Heath (Source Document WB5-15).*

2. *Enter patient registration information in MOSS, as much as can be obtained from the form.*

3. *Enter the date of service, physician name, facility name, procedure, and diagnosis(es) for this patient onto the log in preparation for billing (Source Document WB5-7).*

Check your work with Figures WB5-26, WB5-27, WB5-28, and WB5-29.

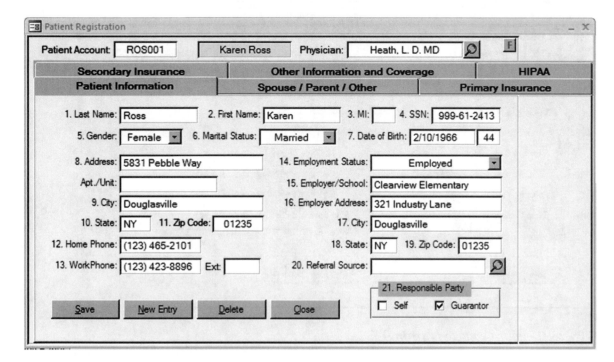

Figure WB5-26 *(Delmar/Cengage Learning)*

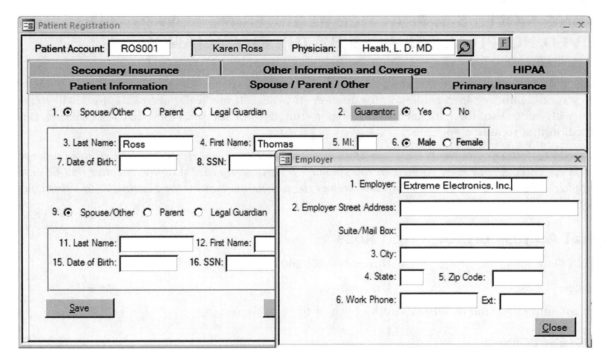

Figure WB5-27 *(Delmar/Cengage Learning)*

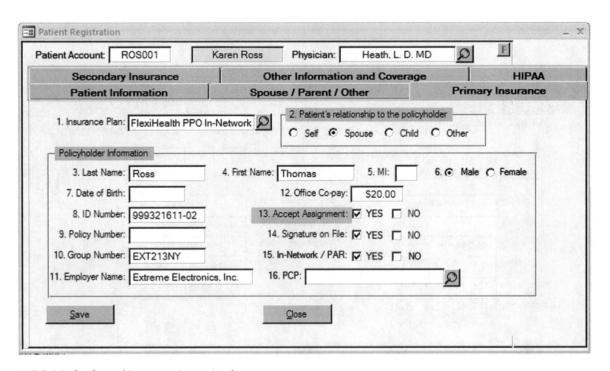

Figure WB5-28 *(Delmar/Cengage Learning)*

			Outside Services LOG Drs. Heath and Schwartz			
Ref. Number	Date(s) of Service	Patient Name	Facility Physician	Procedures Authorization #	Diagnosis (Primary/Secondary/ Tertiary)
0018	11/12/2009	Jouharian, Siran	New York County Hospital Dr. Heath	99282 Emergency Room	Severe vertigo 780.4
0019	11/13/2009	Royzin, Joel	Retirement Inn Nursing Home Dr. Heath	99308 Est. Pt. Expanded	PVD and DM 443.9, 250.00
0020	11/13/2009	Durand, Isabel	Retirement Inn Nursing Home Dr. Heath	99307 Est. Pt. Problem focused	Urticaria 708.9
0021	11/09/2009	Johnsen, Dennis	Community General Hospital Dr. Heath	99282 Emergency Room	Cellulitis 682.9
0022	11/09/2009	Bernardo, William	Community General Hospital Dr. Heath	99282 Emergency Room	COPD, CHF 496, 428.0
0023	11/10/2009	Souza, Janet	Community General Hospital Dr. Heath	99282 Emergency Room	Gastroenteritis 558.9
0024	11/17/2009	Ross, Karen	Community General Hospital Dr. Heath	99221 Initial Hospital Care	DM and HTN 250.00 401.9

Figure WB5-29 *(Delmar/Cengage Learning)*

Hospital Admission for Sean McKay

Today's Date: November 20, 2009

Physician: Dr. Heath

Refer to Source Document WB5-16 in the back of the workbook.

Additional Instructions:

1. *Review the Record of Admission form received from Dr. Heath (Source Document WB5-16).*

2. *Enter patient registration information in MOSS as needed.*

3. *Enter the date of service, physician name, facility name, procedure, and diagnosis(es) for this patient onto the log in preparation for billing (Source Document WB5-7).*

Check your work with Figures WB5-30, WB5-31, and WB5-32.

Figure WB5-30 *(Delmar/Cengage Learning)*

Figure WB5-31 *(Delmar/Cengage Learning)*

Ref. Number	Date(s) of Service	Patient Name	Facility Physician	Procedures Authorization #	Diagnosis (Primary/Secondary/ Tertiary)
			Outside Services LOG Drs. Heath and Schwartz		
0018	11/12/2009	Jouharian, Siran	New York County Hospital Dr. Heath	99282 Emergency Room	Severe vertigo 780.4
0019	11/13/2009	Royzin, Joel	Retirement Inn Nursing Home Dr. Heath	99308 Est. Pt. Expanded	PVD and DM 443.9, 250.00
0020	11/13/2009	Durand, Isabel	Retirement Inn Nursing Home Dr. Heath	99307 Est. Pt. Problem focused	Urticaria 708.9
0021	11/09/2009	Johnsen, Dennis	Community General Hospital Dr. Heath	99282 Emergency Room	Cellulitis 682.9
0022	11/09/2009	Bernardo, William	Community General Hospital Dr. Heath	99282 Emergency Room	COPD, CHF 496, 428.0
0023	11/10/2009	Souza, Janet	Community General Hospital Dr. Heath	99282 Emergency Room	Gastroenteritis 558.9
0024	11/17/2009	Ross, Karen	Community General Hospital Dr. Heath	99221 Initial Hospital Care	DM and HTN 250.00 401.9
0025	11/20/2009	McKay, Sean	Community General Hospital Dr. Heath	99221 Initial Hospital Care	Viral Inf. Dehydration 079.99 276.51

Figure WB5-32 *(Delmar/Cengage Learning)*

Hospital Admission for Mark Hedensten

Today's Date: November 22, 2009

Physician: Dr. Schwartz

Refer to Source Document WB5-17 in the back of the workbook.

Additional Instructions:

1. *Review the Record of Admission form received from Dr. Schwartz (Source Document WB5-17).*

2. *Enter patient registration information in MOSS as needed.*

3. *Enter the date of service, physician name, facility name, procedure, and diagnosis(es) for this patient onto the log in preparation for billing (Source Document WB5-7).*

Check your work with Figures WB5-33, WB3-34, and WB5-35.

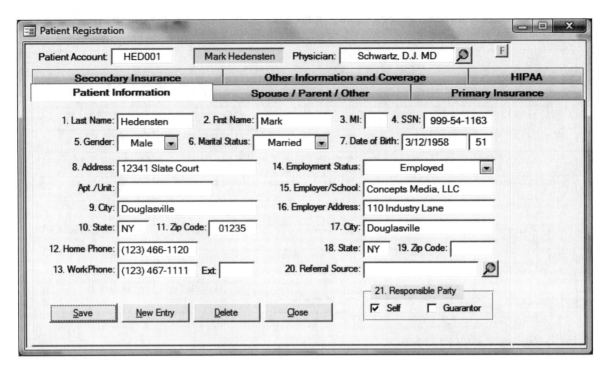

Figure WB5-33 *(Delmar/Cengage Learning)*

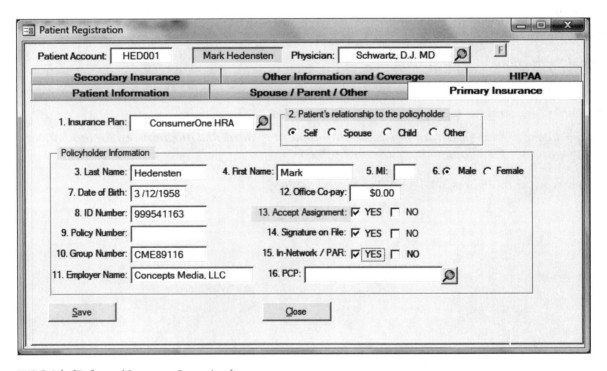

Figure WB5-34 *(Delmar/Cengage Learning)*

			Outside Services LOG Drs. Heath and Schwartz		
Ref. Number	Date(s) of Service	Patient Name	Facility Physician	Procedures Authorization #	Diagnosis (Primary/Secondary/ Tertiary)
0018	11/12/2009	Jouharian, Siran	New York County Hospital Dr. Heath	99282 Emergency Room	Severe vertigo 780.4
0019	11/13/2009	Royzin, Joel	Retirement Inn Nursing Home Dr. Heath	99308 Est. Pt. Expanded	PVD and DM 443.9, 250.00
0020	11/13/2009	Durand, Isabel	Retirement Inn Nursing Home Dr. Heath	99307 Est. Pt. Problem focused	Urticaria 708.9
0021	11/09/2009	Johnsen, Dennis	Community General Hospital Dr. Heath	99282 Emergency Room	Cellulitis 682.9
0022	11/09/2009	Bernardo, William	Community General Hospital Dr. Heath	99282 Emergency Room	COPD, CHF 496, 428.0
0023	11/10/2009	Souza, Janet	Community General Hospital Dr. Heath	99282 Emergency Room	Gastroenteritis 558.9
0024	11/17/2009	Ross, Karen	Community General Hospital Dr. Heath	99221 Initial Hospital Care	DM and HTN 250.00 401.9
0025	11/20/2009	McKay, Sean	Community General Hospital Dr. Heath	99221 Initial Hospital Care	Viral Inf. Dehydration 079.99 276.51
0026	11/22/2009	Hedensten, Mark	Community General Hospital Dr. Schwartz	99221 Initial Hospital Care	Angina and PVC 413.9 427.69

Figure WB5-35 *(Delmar/Cengage Learning)*

U N I T **6**

Procedure Posting Routines

BUILDING SKILLS 6-1: MANAGING PATIENTS AT THE FRONT DESK

Instructions: For each of the case studies that follow, complete the tasks as indicated for each patient.

New Patient Devon Trimble – October 20, 2009

Patient Trimble is at the front desk, ready to check out after his visit with Dr. Heath. Review the superbill returned to you (refer to Source Document WB6-1 in the back of the workbook). Answer the following questions.

Cover the answers using the tear-off bookmark from the cover of your textbook. Check your work before entering data into MOSS to be sure you have correctly interpreted the source documents.

A.	Identify the procedures marked on the Superbill.	99204, 80053, 81002
B.	Identify the diagnoses marked on the Superbill.	250.00
C.	Which procedures go with which diagnosis?	All procedures were done for diagnosis 250.00.
D.	Did the patient make a payment?	Yes, $10.00
E.	When does Dr. Heath want to see the patient back in the office?	In 2 weeks

Complete the following front-desk tasks for Patient Trimble:

1. Post the procedures using MOSS for 10/20/2009.

2. Post the payment of $10.00 using Source Document WB6-2.

3. Schedule an appointment in two weeks with Dr. Heath for a 15-minute follow-up visit. The patient tells you that 11/03/2009 at 1:00 p.m. is convenient.

Check your work with Figures WB6-1, WB6-2, WB6-3, and WB6-4.

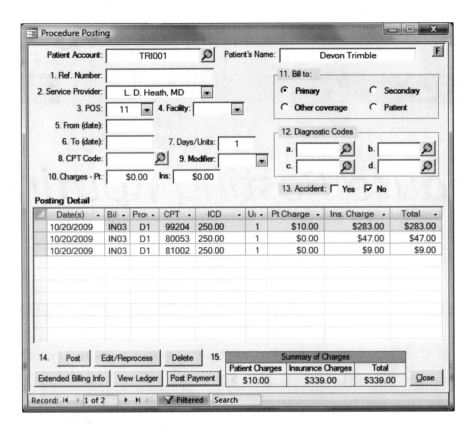

Figure WB6-1 *(Delmar/Cengage Learning)*

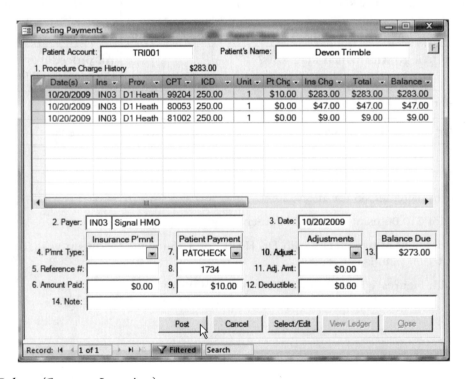

Figure WB6-2 *(Delmar/Cengage Learning)*

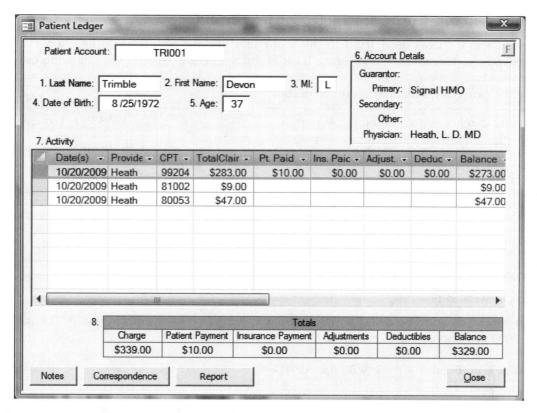

Figure WB6-3 *(Delmar/Cengage Learning)*

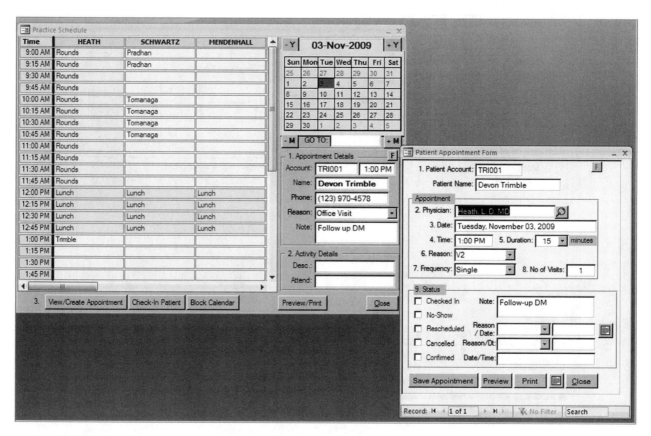

Figure WB6-4 *(Delmar/Cengage Learning)*

New Patient Harold Engleman – October 22, 2009

Patient Engleman is at the front desk, ready to check out after his visit with Dr. Schwartz. Review the superbill returned to you, Source Document WB6-3 in the back of the workbook. Answer the following questions:

A.	Identify the procedures marked on the Superbill.	99205
B.	Identify the diagnoses marked on the Superbill.	Dx 1: 530.81, Dx 2: 401.9
C.	Which procedures go with which diagnosis?	Both diagnoses go with 99205.
D.	Did the patient make a payment?	No payment
E.	When does Dr. Schwartz want to see the patient back in the office?	In 1 month

Complete the following front-desk tasks for Patient Engleman:

1. Post the procedures using MOSS for 10/22/2009.

2. There is no payment to post.

3. Schedule an appointment in one month with Dr. Schwartz for a 15-minute follow-up visit. The patient tells you that 11/24/2009 at 10:30 a.m. is convenient.

Check your work with Figures WB6-5, WB6-6, and WB6-7.

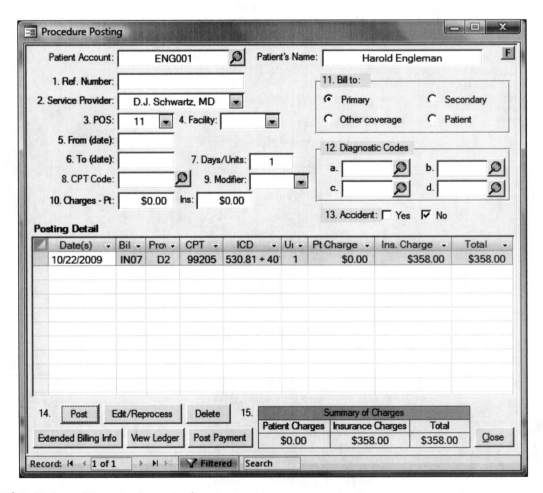

Figure WB6-5 *(Delmar/Cengage Learning)*

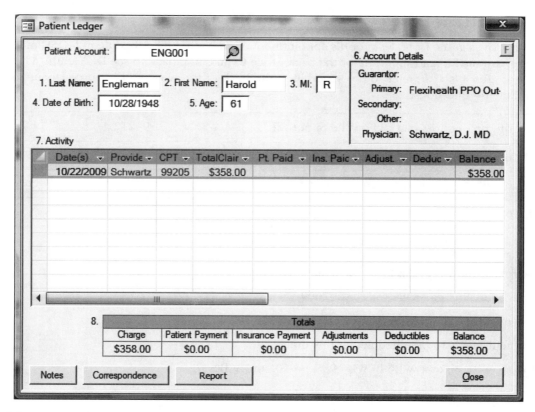

Figure WB6-6 *(Delmar/Cengage Learning)*

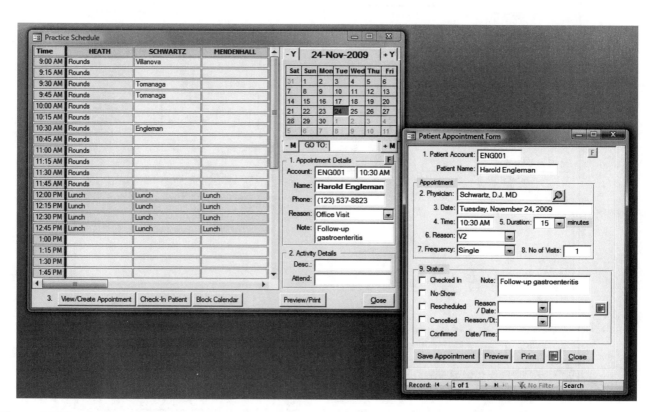

Figure WB6-7 *(Delmar/Cengage Learning)*

Established Patient Derek Wallace – October 22, 2009

Patient Wallace arrives at the front desk for his appointment. Find him on the schedule in MOSS and mark him as checked-in. Prepare his file and superbill for the back office to take him back to see Dr. Heath. When he returns to the front desk after his visit, refer to the superbill in the back of the workbook, Source Document WB6-4. Answer the following questions:

A.	Identify the procedures marked on the Superbill.	99212
B.	Identify the diagnoses marked on the Superbill.	599.0
C.	Which procedures go with which diagnosis?	Office visit for diagnosis 599.0
D.	Did the patient make a payment?	Yes, $20.00
E.	When does Dr. Heath want to see the patient back in the office?	As needed

Complete the following front-desk tasks for Patient Trimble:

1. Post the procedures using MOSS for 10/22/2009.

2. Post the payment of $20.00 using Source Document WB6-5.

3. No appointment needs to be scheduled at this time.

Check your work with Figures WB6-8, WB6-9, WB6-10, and WB6-11.

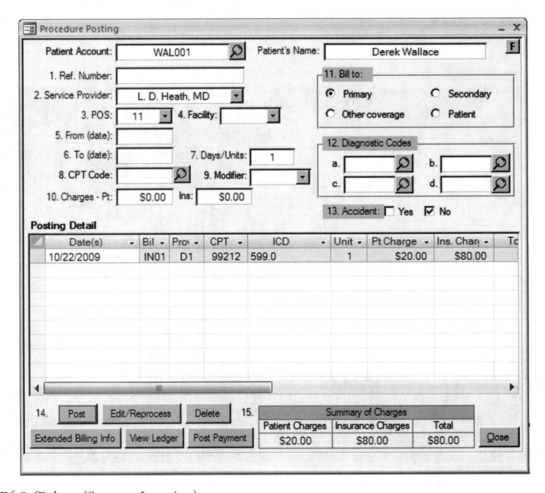

Figure WB6-8 *(Delmar/Cengage Learning)*

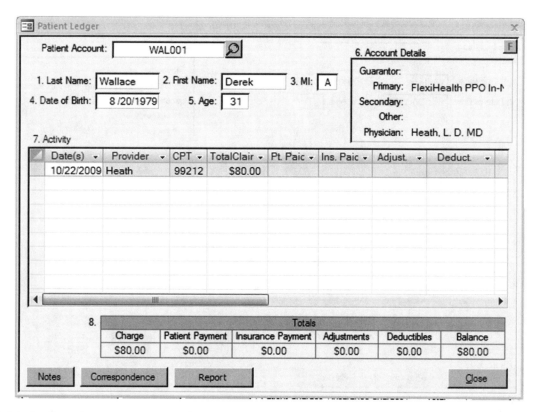

Figure WB6-9 *(Delmar/Cengage Learning)*

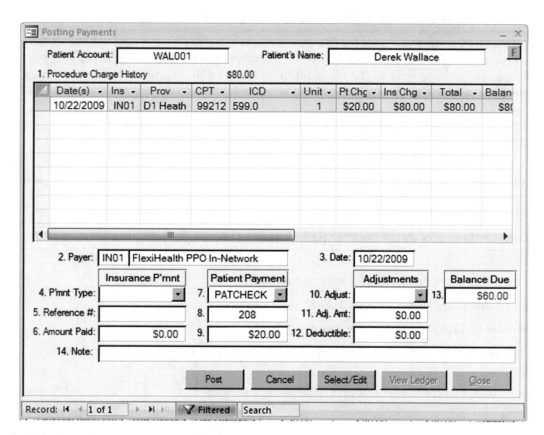

Figure WB6-10 *(Delmar/Cengage Learning)*

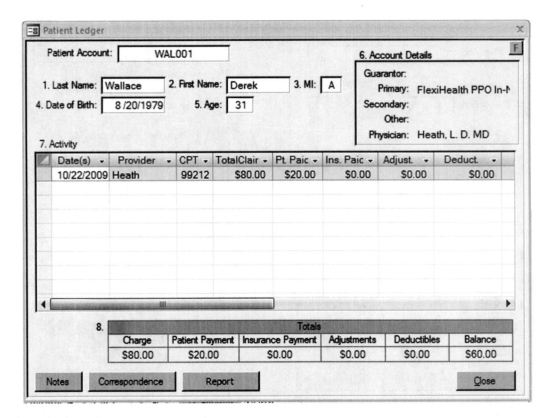

Figure WB6-11 *(Delmar/Cengage Learning)*

Established Patient Naomi Yamagata – October 22, 2009

Patient Yamagata arrives at the front desk for her appointment. Find her on the schedule in MOSS and mark her as checked-in. Prepare her file and superbill for the back office to take her back to the doctor. When she returns to the front desk after her visit, refer to the superbill in the back of the workbook, Source Document WB6-6. Answer the following questions:

A.	Identify the procedures marked on the Superbill.	99214
B.	Identify the diagnoses marked on the Superbill.	493.90
C.	Which procedures go with which diagnosis?	Office visit for diagnosis 493.90
D.	Did the patient make a payment?	Yes, $10.00
E.	When does Dr. Schwartz want to see the patient back in the office?	In 2 weeks

Complete the following front-desk tasks for Patient Yamagata:

1. Post the procedures using MOSS for 10/22/2009.

2. Post the payment of $10.00 cash to the account.

3. Schedule a 15-minute follow-up visit in two months. The patient tells you that 11/5/2009 at 11:15 a.m. is convenient.

Check your work with Figures WB6-12, WB6-13, WB6-14, and WB6-15.

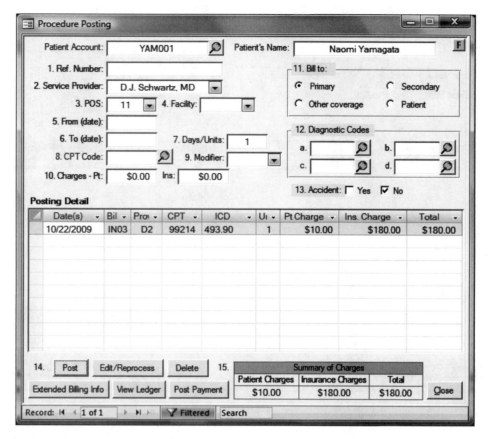

Figure WB6-12 *(Delmar/Cengage Learning)*

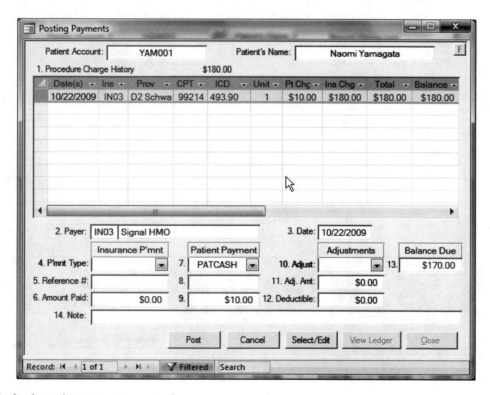

Figure WB6-13 *(Delmar/Cengage Learning)*

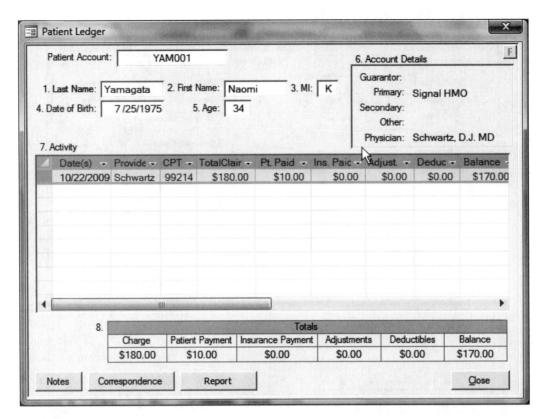

Figure WB6-14 *(Delmar/Cengage Learning)*

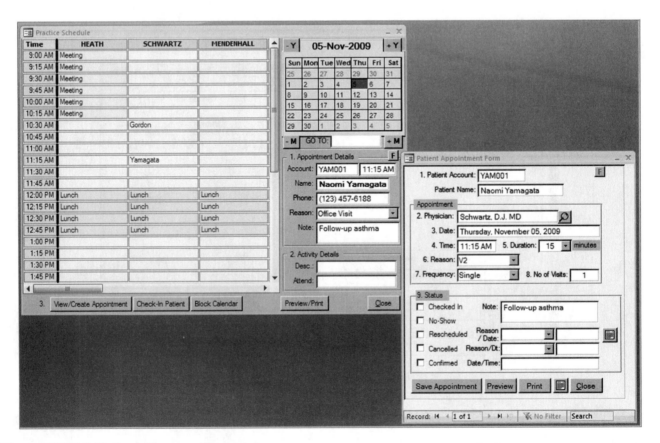

Figure WB6-15 *(Delmar/Cengage Learning)*

Established Patient Nancy Herbert – October 22, 2009

Patient Herbert arrives at the front desk for her appointment. Find her on the schedule in MOSS and mark her as checked-in. Prepare her file and superbill for the back office to take her back to see Dr. Heath. When she returns to the front desk after her visit, refer to the superbill in the back of the workbook, Source Document WB6-7. Answer the following questions:

A.	Identify the procedures marked on the Superbill.	99215, 80053, 85014
B.	Identify the diagnoses marked on the Superbill.	496, 401.9, 285.9
C.	Which procedures go with which diagnosis?	99215 – all 3 diagnoses, 80053 – all 3 diagnoses, 85014 – ICD 285.9
D.	Did the patient make a payment?	No payment was made
E.	When does Dr. Heath want to see the patient back in the office?	In 3 months

Complete the following front-desk tasks for Patient Herbert:

1. Post the procedures using MOSS for 10/22/2009. (Hint: Be certain to use the extended billing when posting laboratory procedures, and provide CLIA number 01D0886230 where indicated. Medicare requires this number be provided when services are provided in an authorized laboratory in a physician's office.)

2. Schedule an appointment in three months with Dr. Heath for a 30-minute visit. The patient tells you that 01/22/2010 at 10:00 a.m. is convenient.

Check your work with Figures WB6-16, WB6-17, WB6-18, WB6-19, WB6-20, and WB6-21.

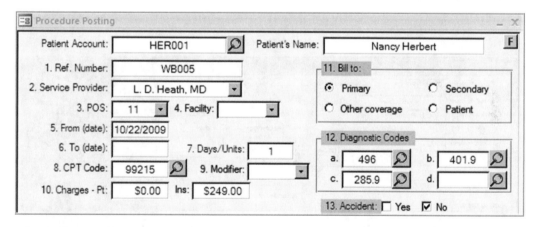

Figure WB6-16 *(Delmar/Cengage Learning)*

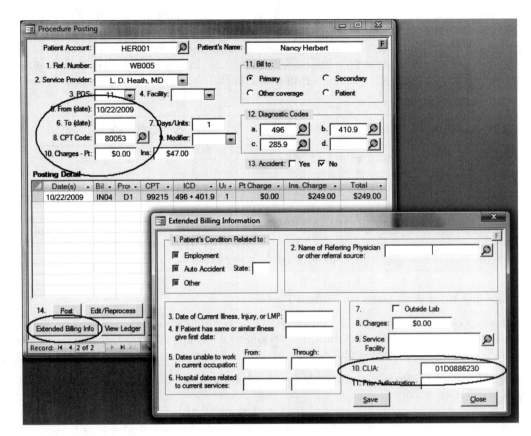

Figure WB6-17 *(Delmar/Cengage Learning)*

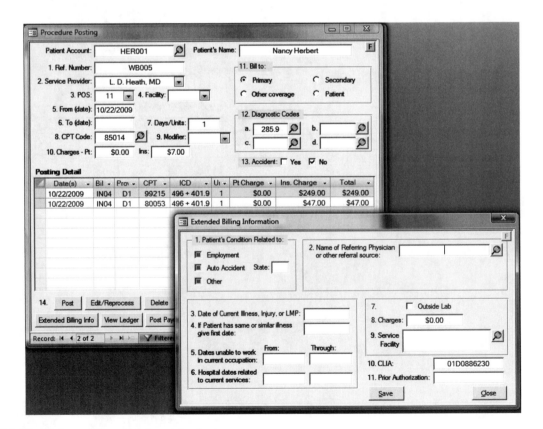

Figure WB6-18 *(Delmar/Cengage Learning)*

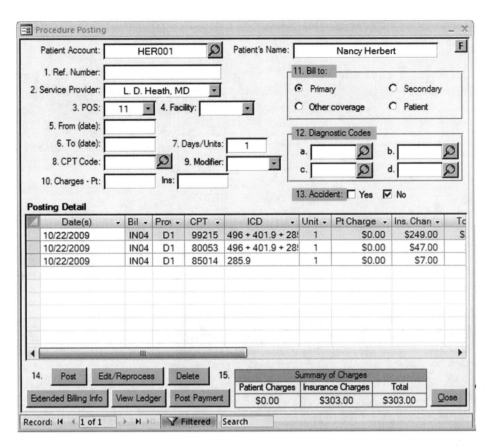

Figure WB6-19 *(Delmar/Cengage Learning)*

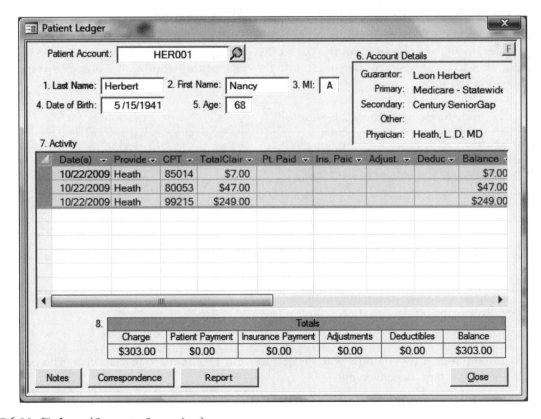

Figure WB6-20 *(Delmar/Cengage Learning)*

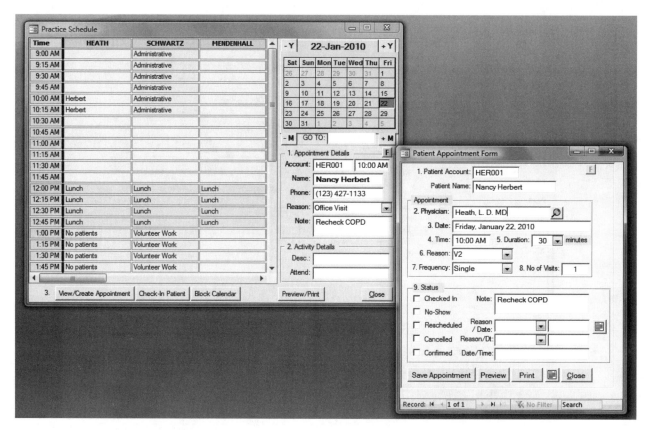

Figure WB6-21 *(Delmar/Cengage Learning)*

Established Patient Alan Shuman – October 22, 2009

Patient Shuman arrives at the front desk for his appointment. Find him on the schedule in MOSS and mark him as checked-in. Prepare his file and superbill for the back office to take him back to see Dr. Heath. When he returns to the front desk after his visit, refer to the superbill in the back of the workbook, Source Document WB6-8. Answer the following questions:

A.	Identify the procedures marked on the Superbill.	99215, 90658, 90772
B.	Identify the diagnoses marked on the Superbill.	496, 438.9
C.	Which procedures go with which diagnosis?	99215 – all diagnoses, 90658 and 90772 for ICD 496
D.	Did the patient make a payment?	Yes, $20.00
E.	When does Dr. Heath want to see the patient back in the office?	In 2 months

Complete the following front-desk tasks for Patient Shuman:

1. Post the procedures using MOSS for 10/22/2009.

2. Post the payment of $20.00 using Source Document WB6-9.

3. Schedule an appointment in two months with Dr. Heath for a 15-minute follow-up visit. The patient tells you that 12/22/2009 at 1:00 p.m. is convenient.

Check your work with Figures WB6-22, WB6-23, WB6-24, and WB6-25.

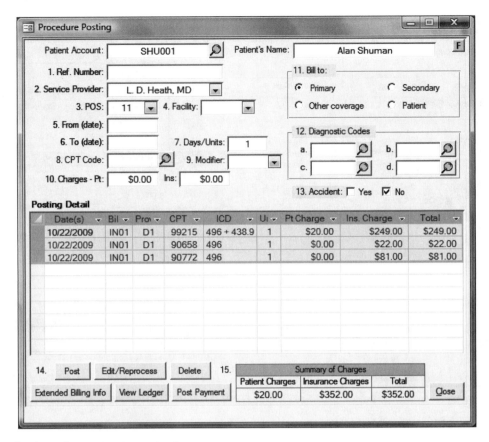

Figure WB6-22 *(Delmar/Cengage Learning)*

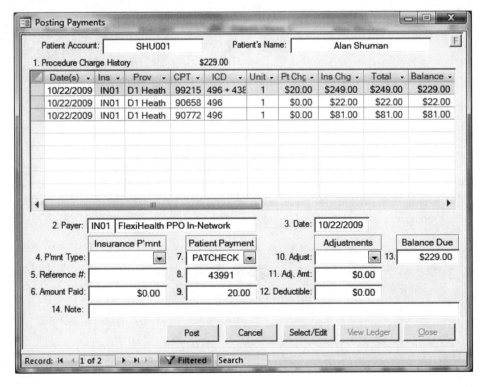

Figure WB6-23 *(Delmar/Cengage Learning)*

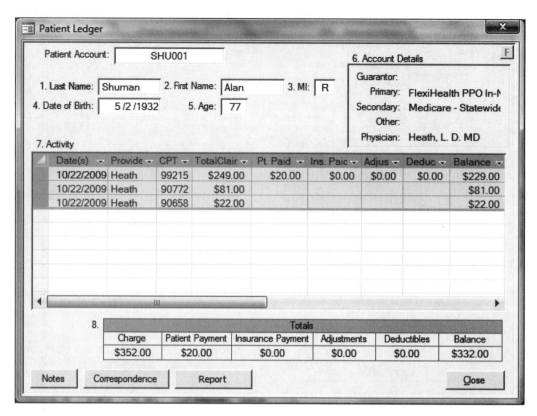

Figure WB6-24 *(Delmar/Cengage Learning)*

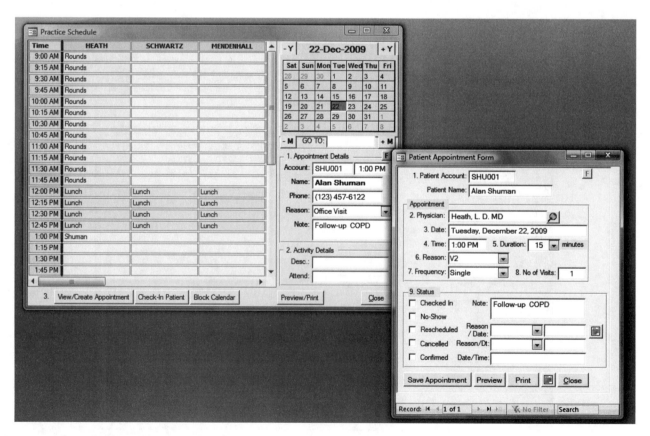

Figure WB6-25 *(Delmar/Cengage Learning)*

Established Patient Emery Camille – October 22, 2009

Gabrielle Camille arrives at the front desk with her son, Emery, for his appointment. Find him on the schedule in MOSS and mark him as checked-in. Prepare his file and superbill for the back office to take him back to see Dr. Schwartz. When she returns to the front desk after Emery's visit, refer to the superbill in the back of the workbook, Source Document WB6-10. Answer the following questions:

A.	Identify the procedures marked on the Superbill.	99213, 85031
B.	Identify the diagnoses marked on the Superbill.	382.9, 079.99
C.	Which procedures go with which diagnosis?	99213 – all diagnoses, 85031 for ICD 382.9
D.	Did the patient make a payment?	Yes, $10.00
E.	When does Dr. Schwartz want to see the patient back in the office?	In 1 week

Complete the following front-desk tasks for Patient Camille:

1. Post the procedures using MOSS for 10/22/2009.

2. Post the payment of $10.00 using Source Document WB6-11.

3. Schedule an appointment in one week with Dr. Schwartz for a 15-minute follow-up visit. The patient's mother, Gabrielle, tells you that 10/29/2009 at 3:30 p.m., after school, is convenient.

Check your work with Figures WB6-26, WB6-27, WB6-28, and WB6-29.

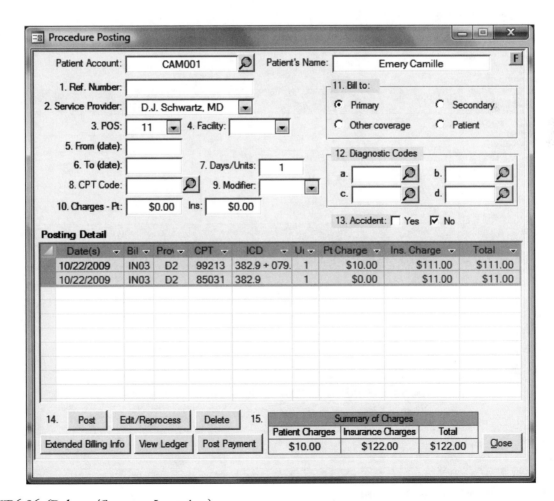

Figure WB6-26 *(Delmar/Cengage Learning)*

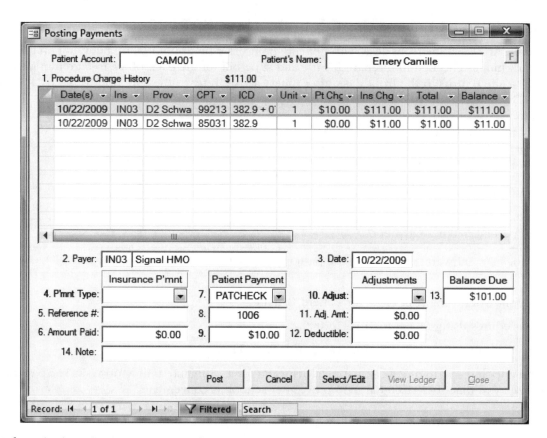

Figure WB6-27 *(Delmar/Cengage Learning)*

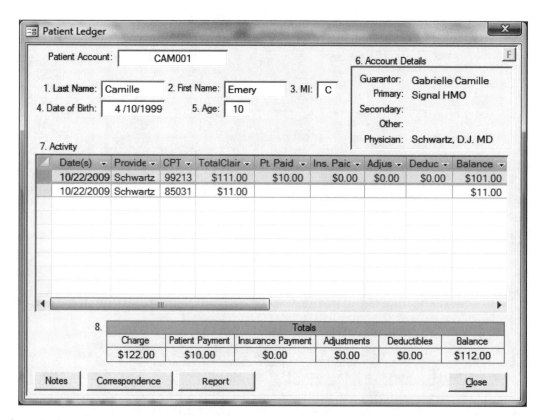

Figure WB6-28 *(Delmar/Cengage Learning)*

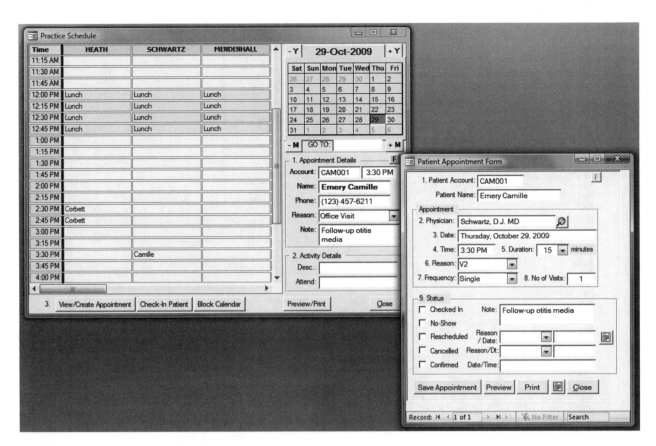

Figure WB6-29 *(Delmar/Cengage Learning)*

Established Patient Deanna Hartsfeld – October 22, 2009

Deanna Hartsfeld arrives at the front desk for her appointment. Find her on the schedule in MOSS and mark her as checked-in. Prepare her file and superbill for the back office to take her back to see Dr. Heath. When she returns to the front desk after her visit, refer to the superbill in the back of the workbook, Source Document WB6-12. Answer the following questions:

A.	Identify the procedures marked on the Superbill.	99214, 80053
B.	Identify the diagnoses marked on the Superbill.	272.0, 401.9
C.	Which procedures go with which diagnosis?	99214 – all diagnoses, 80053 for ICD 272.0
D.	Did the patient make a payment?	There was no payment made at this time.
E.	When does Dr. Heath want to see the patient back in the office?	In 2 months

Complete the following front-desk tasks for Patient Hartsfeld:

1. Post the procedures using MOSS for 10/22/2009. (Hint: Be certain to use the extended billing when posting laboratory procedures, and provide CLIA number 01D0886230 where indicated. Medicare requires this number be provided when services are provided in an authorized laboratory in a physician's office.)

2. Schedule an appointment in two months with Dr. Heath for a 15-minute recheck visit. The patient tells you that 12/22/2009 at 2:45 p.m. is convenient.

Check your work with Figures WB6-30, WB6-31, and WB6-32.

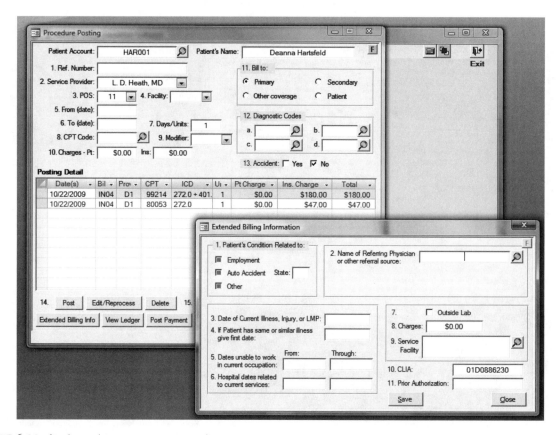

Figure WB6-30 *(Delmar/Cengage Learning)*

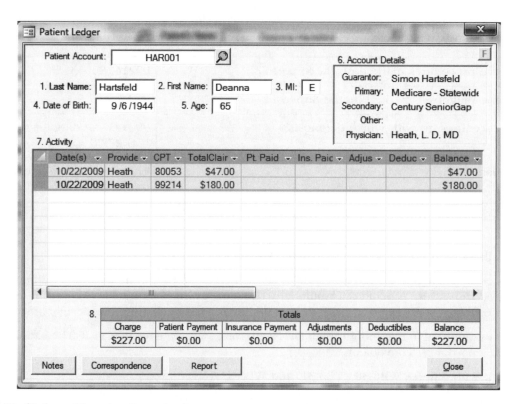

Figure WB6-31 *(Delmar/Cengage Learning)*

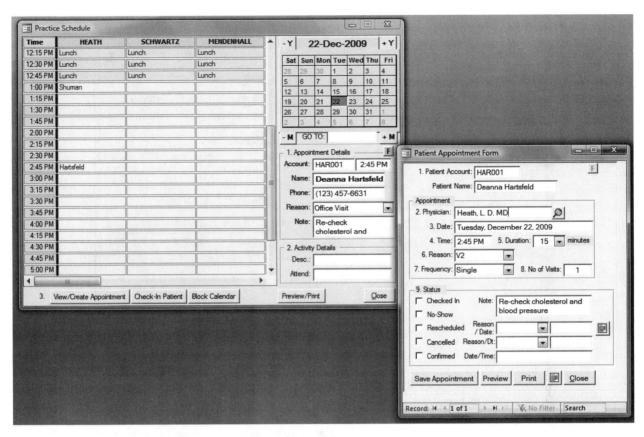

Figure WB6-32 *(Delmar/Cengage Learning)*

Established Patient Aimee Bradley – October 22, 2009

Aimee Bradley arrives at the front desk for her appointment. Find her on the schedule in MOSS and mark her as checked-in. Prepare her file and superbill for the back office to take her back to see Dr. Schwartz. When she returns to the front desk after her visit, refer to the superbill in the back of the workbook, Source Document WB6-13. Answer the following questions:

A.	Identify the procedures marked on the Superbill.	99214, 87081
B.	Identify the diagnoses marked on the Superbill.	463, 462
C.	Which procedures go with which diagnosis?	99214 – all diagnoses, 87081 for ICD 462
D.	Did the patient make a payment?	There was no payment made at this time.
E.	When does Dr. Schwartz want to see the patient back in the office?	In 3 weeks

Complete the following front-desk tasks for Patient Bradley:

1. Post the procedures using MOSS for 10/22/2009.

2. Schedule an appointment in three weeks with Dr. Schwartz for a 15-minute follow-up visit. The patient tells you that 11/12/2009 at 3:00 p.m. is convenient.

Check your work with Figures WB6-33, WB6-34, and WB6-35.

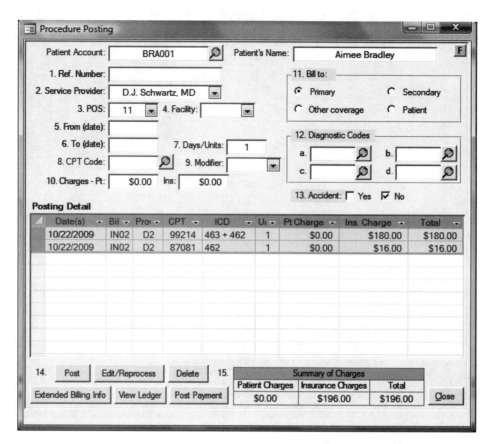

Figure WB6-33 *(Delmar/Cengage Learning)*

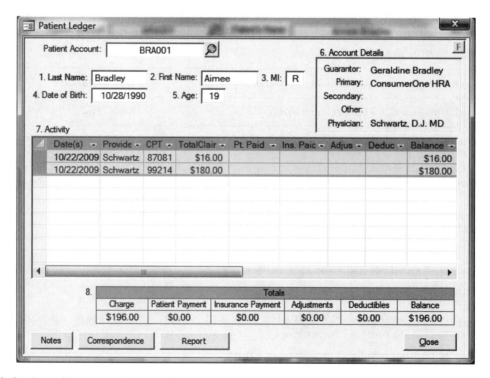

Figure WB6-34 *(Delmar/Cengage Learning)*

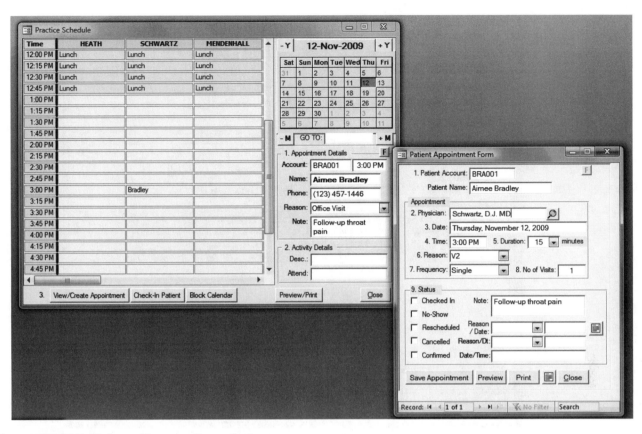

Figure WB6-35 *(Delmar/Cengage Learning)*

Established Patient Tina Rizzo – October 22, 2009

Tina Rizzo arrives with her father, Anthony, for her appointment. Find her on the schedule in MOSS and mark her as checked-in. Prepare her file and superbill for the back office to take her back to see the doctor. When she returns to the front desk after her visit, refer to the superbill in the back of the workbook, Source Document WB6-14. Answer the following questions:

A.	Identify the procedures marked on the Superbill.	99214, 85031, 36415
B.	Identify the diagnoses marked on the Superbill.	477.9, 782.1
C.	Which procedures go with which diagnosis?	99214 – all diagnoses, 85031 for all diagnoses, 36415 for ICD 782.1
D.	Did the patient make a payment?	There was no payment made at this time.
E.	When does Dr. Heath want to see the patient back in the office?	In 2 weeks

Complete the following front-desk tasks for Patient Rizzo:

1. Post the procedures using MOSS for 10/22/2009.

2. Schedule an appointment in two weeks with Dr. Heath, for a 15-minute follow-up visit. The patient's father tells you that 11/5/2009 at 3:45 p.m. is convenient.

Check you work with Figures WB6-36, WB6-37, and WB6-38.

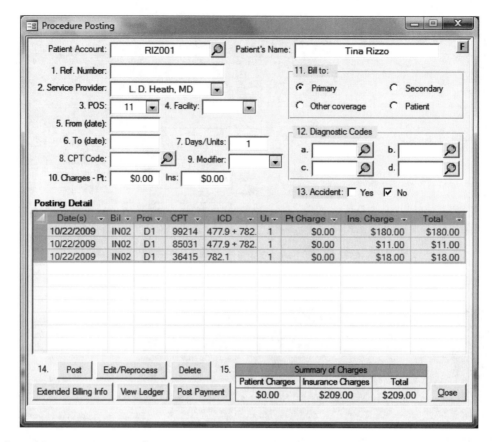

Figure WB6-36 *(Delmar/Cengage Learning)*

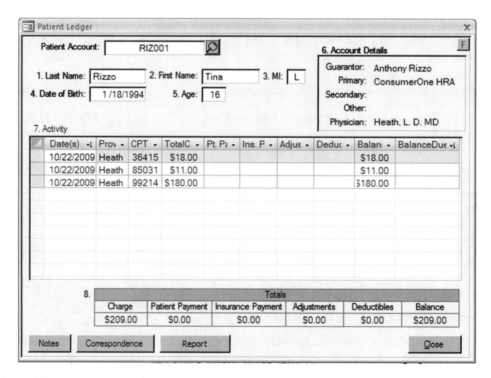

Figure WB6-37 *(Delmar/Cengage Learning)*

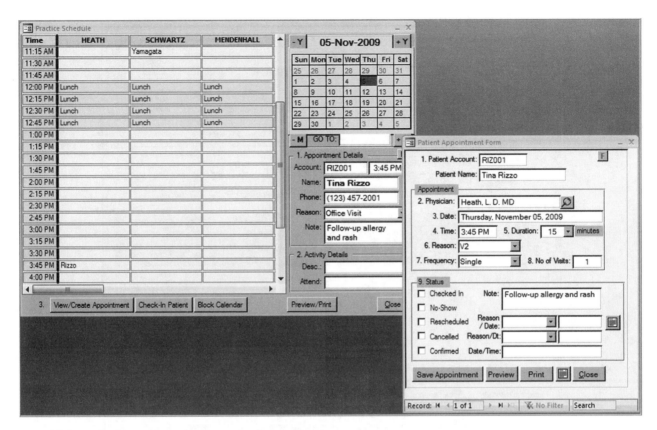

Figure WB6-38 *(Delmar/Cengage Learning)*

Critical Thinking: Established Patient Caitlin Barryroe – 10/23/2009

Instructions: You are the front-desk medical assistant on 10/23/2009 at Douglasville Medicine Associates. Complete the check-in and check-out process for Patient Barryroe, as indicated below:

A. Check in the patient on the appointment schedule in MOSS.

B. Check out the patient, using the information found on the superbill, Source Document WB6-15 in the back of the workbook. Post all procedures as indicated.

C. Post the payment using the check found on Source Document WB6-16 in the back of the workbook.

D. Schedule a 15-minute follow up appointment as indicated on the superbill with the patient's doctor. The patient advises you she is available any Wednesday, Thursday, or Friday in the morning before 10:00 a.m. She must be at work by 11:00 a.m. each morning.

Check your work with Figures WB6-39, WB6-40, WB6-41, and WB6-42.

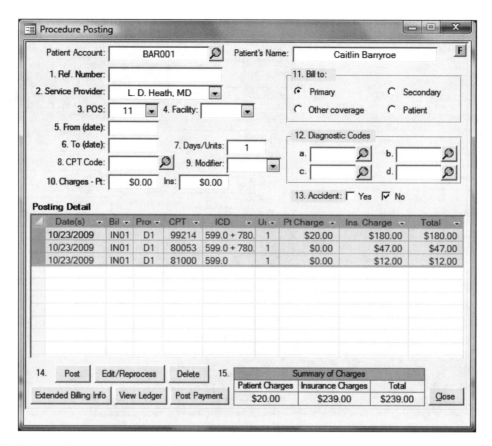

Figure WB6-39 *(Delmar/Cengage Learning)*

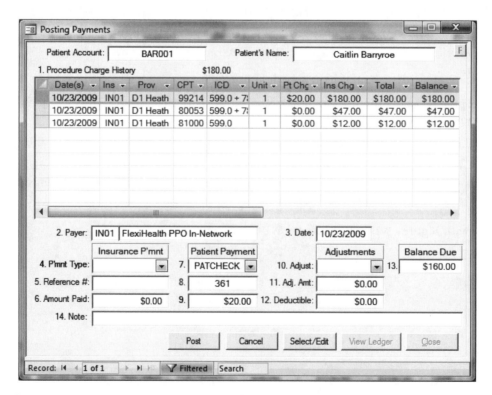

Figure WB6-40 *(Delmar/Cengage Learning)*

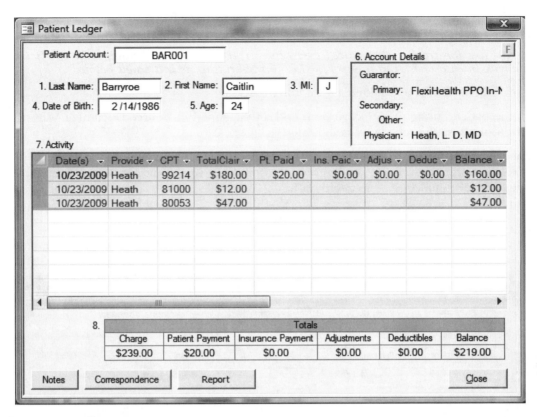

Figure WB6-41 *(Delmar/Cengage Learning)*

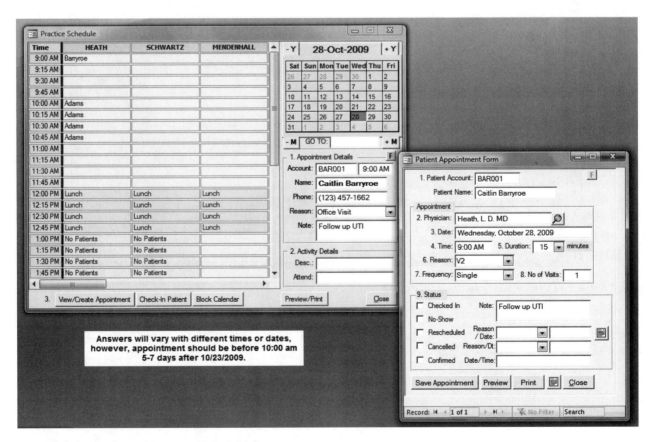

Figure WB6-42 *(Delmar/Cengage Learning)*

Critical Thinking: New Patient Wynona Sheridan – 10/27/2009

Instructions: You are the front-desk medical assistant on 10/27/2009 at Douglasville Medicine Associates. Complete the check-in and check-out process for Patient Sheridan, as indicated below:

A. Check in the patient on the appointment schedule in MOSS.

B. Check out the patient, using the information found on the superbill, Source Document WB6-17 in the back of the workbook. Post all procedures as indicated.

C. Schedule a 15-minute follow-up appointment as indicated on the superbill with the patient's doctor. The patient advises you she is available any morning the following week, but not in the afternoons. She prefers late morning, closer to lunch time, to avoid traffic.

Check your work with Figures WB6-43, WB6-44, and WB6-45.

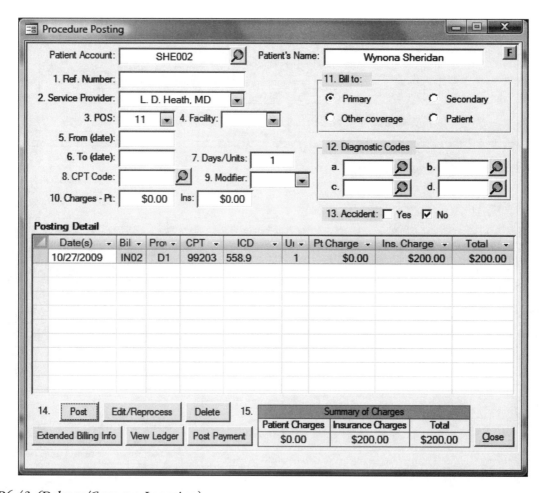

Figure WB6-43 *(Delmar/Cengage Learning)*

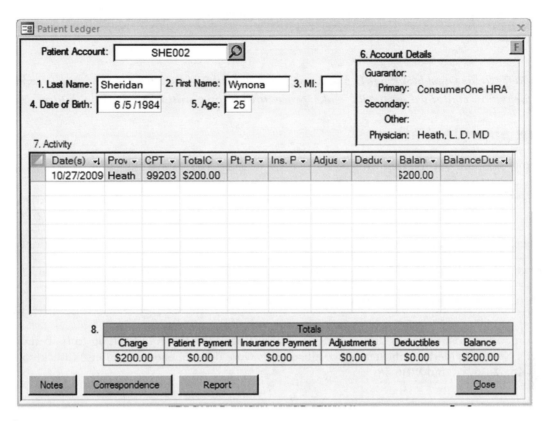

Figure WB6-44 *(Delmar/Cengage Learning)*

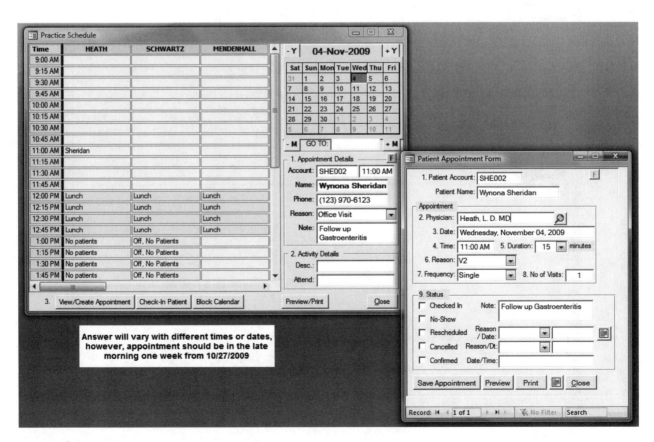

Figure WB6-45 *(Delmar/Cengage Learning)*

BUILDING SKILLS 6-2: POSTING CHARGES FOR SERVICES OUTSIDE THE OFFICE

Instructions: Refer to the Outside Services Log you completed in Unit 5 of the workbook (Source Document WB5-7). Using the information contained on the log, enter procedures in preparation for medical billing.

ER Patient Siran Jouharian

Before entering data, answer the following:

A.	What is the reference number and date of service?	Reference #0018, Date of Service: 11/12/2009
B.	At which facility did the physician provide services?	New York County Hospital
C.	Which diagnostic and procedure codes will be used to enter procedures?	CPT 99282 and ICD 780.4
D.	Which physician provided the service(s)?	Dr. Heath

You are now ready to post the procedures in MOSS. (Hint: Check the Extended Billing to be certain the facility where services were provided is indicated, since all services were done outside the office.) Check your work with Figures WB6-46, WB6-47, and WB6-48.

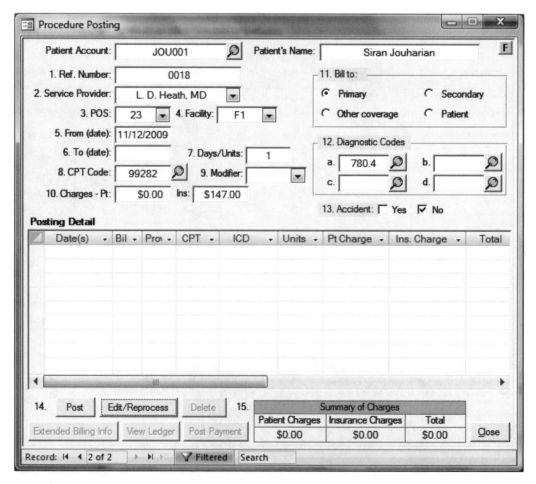

Figure WB6-46 *(Delmar/Cengage Learning)*

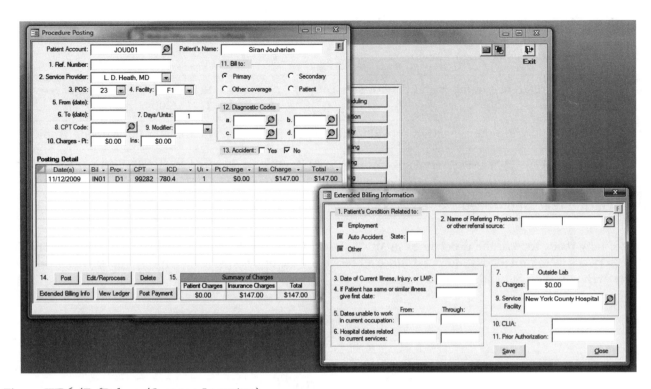

Figure WB6-47 *(Delmar/Cengage Learning)*

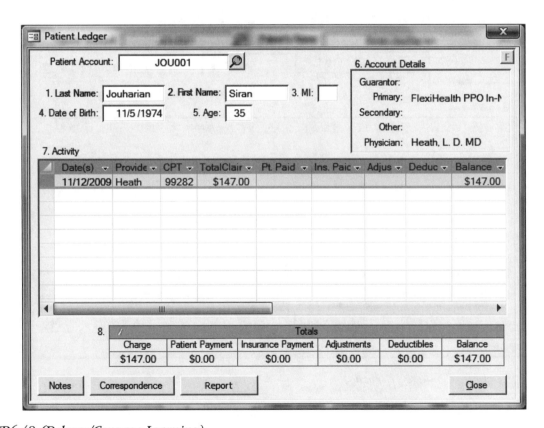

Figure WB6-48 *(Delmar/Cengage Learning)*

Nursing Home Patient Joel Royzin

Before entering data, answer the following:

A.	What is the reference number and date of service?	Reference #0019, Date of Service: 11/13/2009
B.	At which facility did the physician provide services?	Retirement Inn Nursing Home
C.	Which diagnostic and procedure codes will be used to enter procedures?	CPT 99308 and ICD 443.9, 250.00
D.	Which physician provided the service(s)?	Dr. Heath

You are now ready to post the procedures in MOSS. (Hint: Check the Extended Billing to be certain the facility where services were provided is indicated, since all services were done outside the office.) Check your work with Figures WB6-49, WB6-50, and WB6-51.

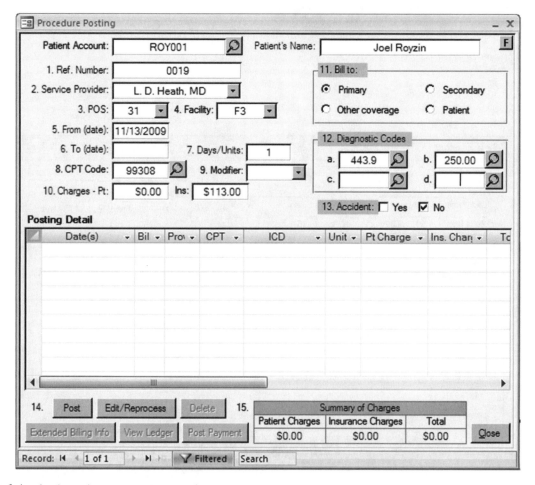

Figure WB6-49 *(Delmar/Cengage Learning)*

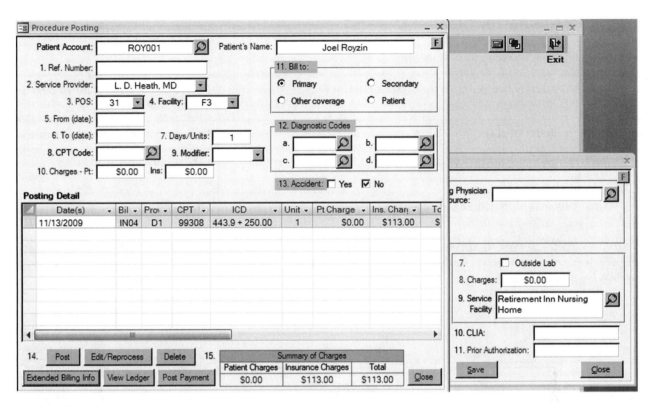

Figure WB6-50 *(Delmar/Cengage Learning)*

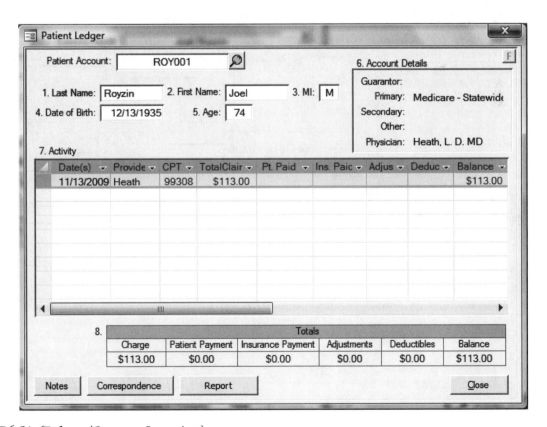

Figure WB6-51 *(Delmar/Cengage Learning)*

Nursing Home Patient Isabel Durand

Before entering data, answer the following:

A.	What is the reference number and date of service?	Reference #0020, Date of Service: 11/13/2009
B.	At which facility did the physician provide services?	Retirement Inn Nursing Home
C.	Which diagnostic and procedure codes will be used to enter procedures?	CPT 99307 and ICD 708.9
D.	Which physician provided the service(s)?	Dr. Heath

You are now ready to post the procedures in MOSS. (Hint: Check the Extended Billing to be certain the facility where services were provided is indicated, since all services were done outside the office.) Check your work with Figures WB6-52 and WB6-53.

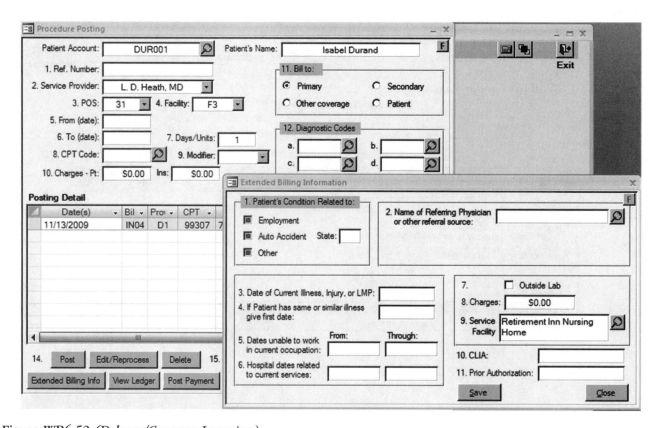

Figure WB6-52 *(Delmar/Cengage Learning)*

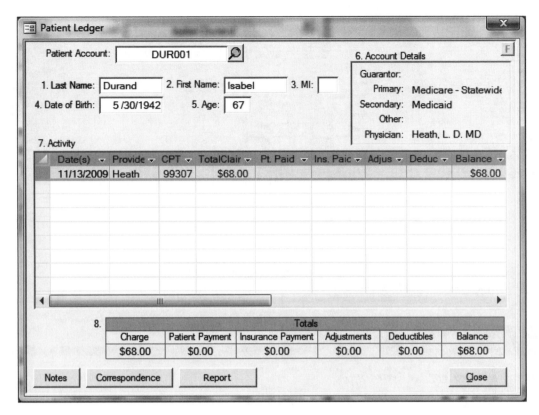

Figure WB6-53 *(Delmar/Cengage Learning)*

ER Patient Dennis Johnsen

Before entering data, answer the following:

A.	What is the reference number and date of service?	Reference #0021, Date of Service: 11/09/2009
B.	At which facility did the physician provide services?	Community General Hospital
C.	Which diagnostic and procedure codes will be used to enter procedures?	CPT 99282 and ICD 682.9
D.	Which physician provided the service(s)?	Dr. Heath

You are now ready to post the procedures in MOSS. (Hint: Check the Extended Billing to be certain the facility where services were provided is indicated, since all services were done outside the office.) Check your work with Figures WB6-54 and WB6-55.

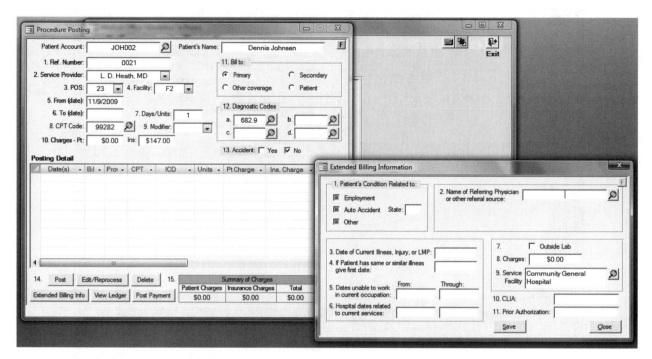

Figure WB6-54 *(Delmar/Cengage Learning)*

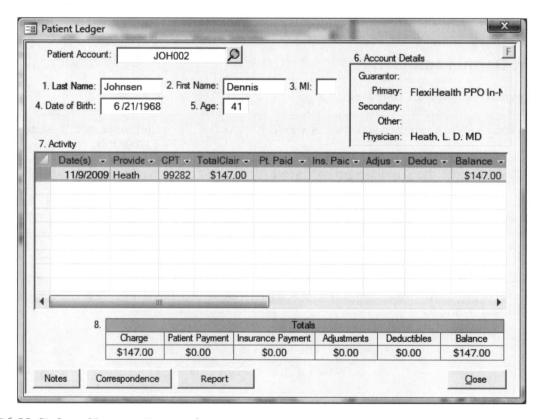

Figure WB6-55 *(Delmar/Cengage Learning)*

ER Patient William Bernardo

Before entering data, answer the following:

A.	What is the reference number and date of service?	Reference #0022, Date of Service: 11/09/2009
B.	At which facility did the physician provide services?	Community General Hospital
C.	Which diagnostic and procedure codes will be used to enter procedures?	CPT 99282 and ICD 496, 428.0
D.	Which physician provided the service(s)?	Dr. Heath

You are now ready to post the procedures in MOSS. (Hint: Check the Extended Billing to be certain the facility where services were provided is indicated, since all services were done outside the office.) Check your work with Figures WB6-56 and WB6-57.

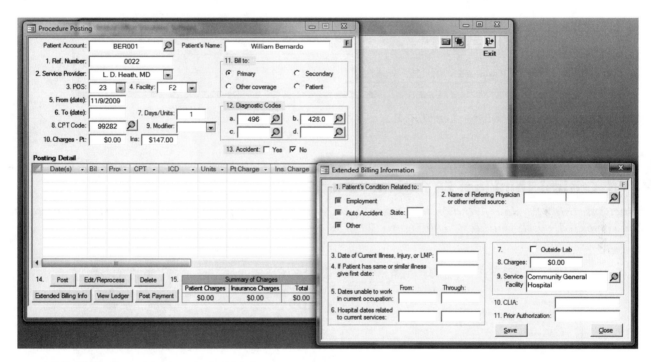

Figure WB6-56 *(Delmar/Cengage Learning)*

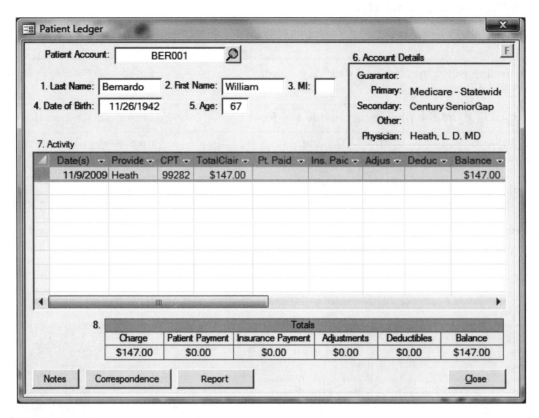

Figure WB6-57 *(Delmar/Cengage Learning)*

Critical Thinking: ER Patient Janet Souza

Instructions: Using the data found on the Outside Services Log, post the procedure to Patient Souza's account. When completed, check your work with Figures WB6-58 and WB6-59.

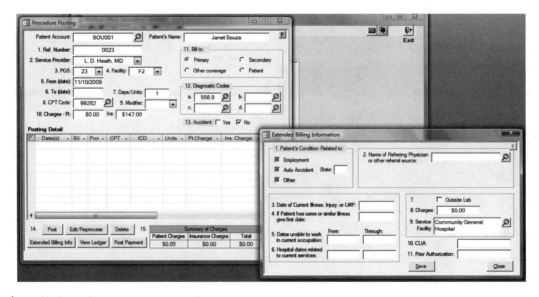

Figure WB6-58 *(Delmar/Cengage Learning)*

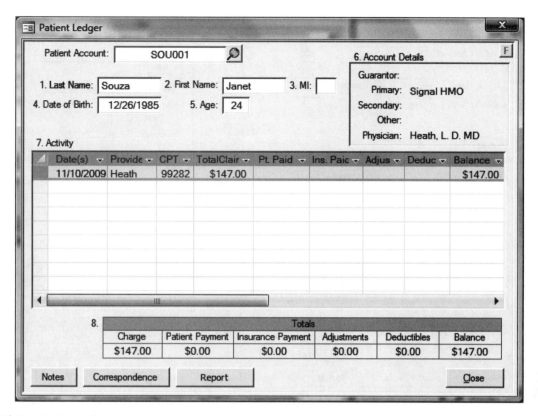

Figure WB6-59 *(Delmar/Cengage Learning)*

Critical Thinking: Hospital Patient Karen Ross

Instructions: Using the data found on the Outside Services Log, post the procedure to Patient Ross's account. When completed, check your work with Figures WB6-60 and WB6-61.

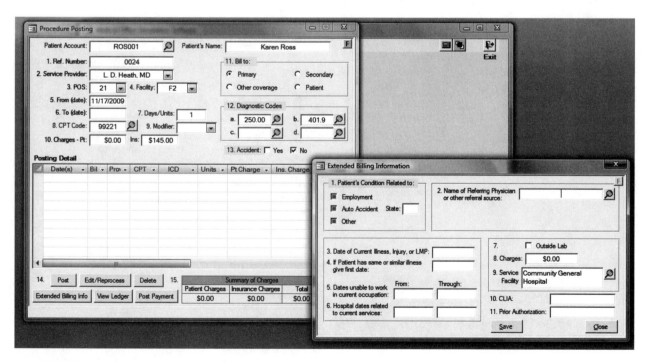

Figure WB6-60 *(Delmar/Cengage Learning)*

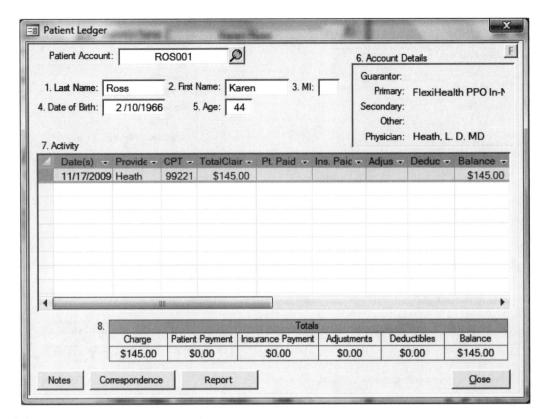

Figure WB6-61 *(Delmar/Cengage Learning)*

Critical Thinking: Hospital Patient Sean McKay

Instructions: Using the data found on the Outside Services Log, post the procedure to Patient McKay's account. When completed, check your work with Figures WB6-62 and WB6-63.

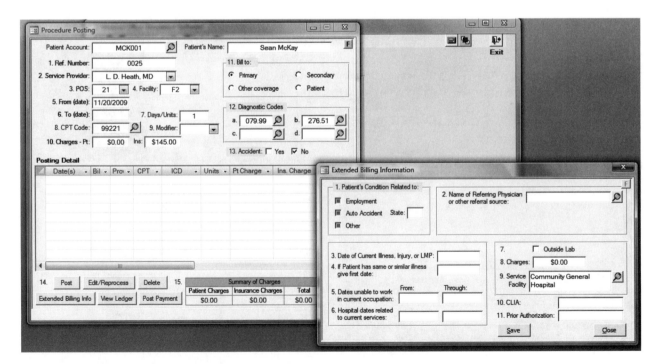

Figure WB6-62 *(Delmar/Cengage Learning)*

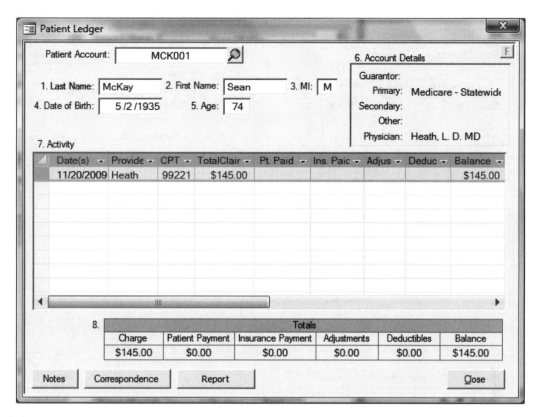

Figure WB6-63 *(Delmar/Cengage Learning)*

Critical Thinking: Hospital Patient Mark Hedensten

Instructions: Using the data found on the Outside Services Log, post the procedure to Patient Hedensten's account. When completed, check your work with Figures WB6-64 and WB6-65.

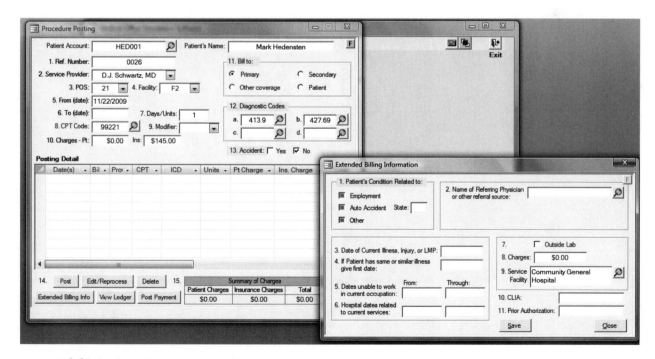

Figure WB6-64 *(Delmar/Cengage Learning)*

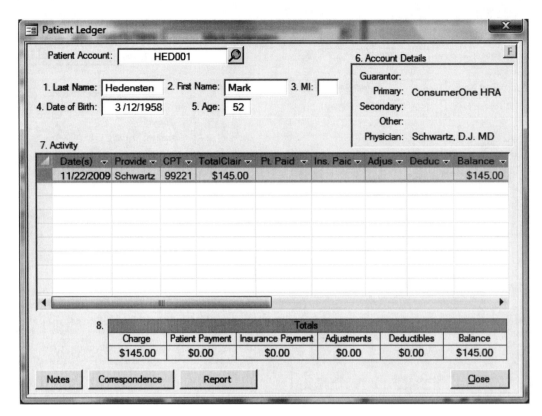

Figure WB6-65 *(Delmar/Cengage Learning)*

UNIT **7**

Insurance Billing Routines

BUILDING SKILLS 7-1: REVIEWING THE CLAIMS PREPARATION WINDOW IN MOSS

Instructions: Refer to Figure WB7-1 and describe the function of each of the following components of the Claims Preparation window in MOSS.

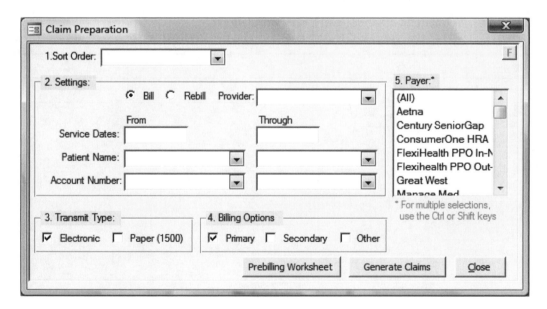

Figure WB7-1 *(Delmar/Cengage Learning)*

A. Field 1, Sort Order: _____

_____

_____

_____

B. Field 2, Settings: _____

_____

_____

_____

C. Field 3, Transmit Type: _____

_____

_____

_____

D. Field 4, Billing Options: _____

_____

_____

_____

E. Field 5, Payer: _____

_____

_____

_____

F. Command buttons: Prebilling Worksheet and Generate Claims: _____

_____

_____

_____

BUILDING SKILLS 7-2: PREPARING PAPER CLAIM FORMS FOR CONSUMERONE HRA PATIENTS

Instructions: Using the Claim Preparation screen in the Insurance Billing area of MOSS, complete the following tasks:

A. Prepare paper claims to be sent for patients with ConsumerONE HRA coverage for services performed by both Drs. Heath and Schwartz.

B. Use date range October 20 through November 30, 2009.

C. View a prebilling worksheet before submitting claims. Check your work with Figures WB7-2 and WB7-3 before proceeding. Correct any errors before proceeding by going back to Procedure Posting, if applicable. If ready for billing, proceed to Step D.

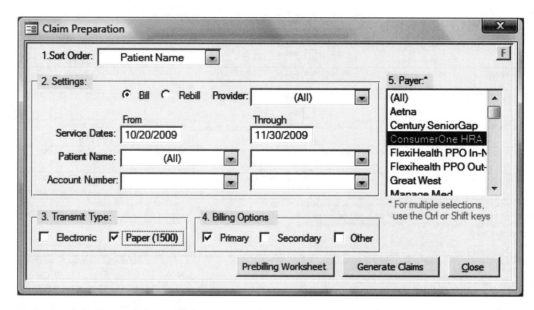

Figure WB7-2 *(Delmar/Cengage Learning)*

INSURANCE PREBILLING WORKSHEET
Student1

Dates of Service	Diag Code	Proc Code	POS	Units	Dr	As	Bill Amt	Receipts	Net
ConsumerOne HRA									
Bradley, Aimee									
10/22/2009	463	87081	11	1.00	D2	Y	$16.00	$0.00	$16.00
10/22/2009	463	99214	11	1.00	D2	Y	$180.00	$0.00	$180.00
					Totals		$196.00	$0.00	$196.00
Hedensten, Mark									
11/22/2009	413.9	99221	21	1.00	D2	Y	$145.00	$0.00	$145.00
					Totals		$145.00	$0.00	$145.00
Rizzo, Tina									
10/22/2009	477.9	36415	11	1.00	D1	Y	$18.00	$18.00	$0.00
10/22/2009	477.9	85031	11	1.00	D1	Y	$11.00	$11.00	$0.00
10/22/2009	477.9	99214	11	1.00	D1	Y	$180.00	$180.00	$0.00
					Totals		$209.00	$209.00	$0.00
Sheridan, Wynona									
10/27/2009	558.9	99203	11	1.00	D1	Y	$200.00	$200.00	$0.00
					Totals		$200.00	$200.00	$0.00
		TOTAL TO BE BILLED FOR ConsumerOne HRA							$341.00
Grand Total					Grand Total				$341.00

Figure WB7-3 *(Delmar/Cengage Learning)*

D. Close the prebilling worksheet and return to the Claims Preparation screen. Click on the *Generate Claims* button. Check the four claim forms that were printed with Figures WB7-4, WB7-5, WB7-6, and WB7-7.

1500	TEST VERSION - NOT FOR OFFICIAL USE

HEALTH INSURANCE CLAIM FORM
APPROVED BY NATIONAL UNIFORM CLAIM COMMITTEE 08/05

ConsumerOne HRA
1230 Main St.
Missoula, MT 08896

Student No: Student1

☐☐☐ PICA   PICA ☐☐☐

1. MEDICARE MEDICAID TRICARE CHAMPUS CHAMPVA GROUP HEALTH PLAN FECA BLK LUNG OTHER	1a. INSURED'S I.D. NUMBER (FOR PROGRAM IN ITEM 1)
☐(Medicare #) ☐(Medicaid #) ☐(Sponsor's SSN) ☐(Member ID 🅇(SSN or ID) ☐(SSN) ☐(ID)	999221438-02

2. PATIENT'S NAME (Last Name, First Name, Middle Initial)	3. PATIENT'S BIRTHDATE SEX	4. INSURED'S NAME (Last Name, First Name, Middle Initial)
BRADLEY AIMEE R	10 28 1990 M ☐ F 🅇	BRADLEY GERALDINE A

5. PATIENT'S ADDRESS (No., Street)	6. PATIENT'S RELATIONSHIP TO INSURED	7. INSURED'S ADDRESS (No., Street)
5133 SOUTH STREET	Self ☐ Spouse ☐ Child 🅇 Other ☐	5133 SOUTH STREET

CITY	STATE	8. PATIENT STATUS	CITY	STATE
DOUGLASVILLE	NY	Single 🅇 Married ☐ Other ☐	DOUGLASVILLE	NY

ZIP CODE	TELEPHONE (include Area Code)		ZIP CODE	TELEPHONE (include Area Code)
01234	(123) 457-1446	Employed ☐ Full-Time Student 🅇 Part-Time Student ☐	01234	(123) 457-1446

9. OTHER INSURED'S NAME (Last Name, First Name, Mid. Initial)	10. IS PATIENT'S CONDITION RELATED TO:	11. INSURED'S POLICY GROUP OR FECA NUMBER
		MIS015
a. OTHER INSURED'S POLICY OR GROUP NUMBER	a. EMPLOYMENT (CURRENT OR PREVIOUS) ☐YES 🅇NO	a. INSURED'S DATE OF BIRTH SEX 02 20 1969 M ☐ F 🅇
b. OTHER INSURED'S BIRTHDATE SEX M ☐ F ☐	b. AUTO ACCIDENT? PLACE (State) ☐YES 🅇NO	b. EMPLOYER NAME OR SCHOOL NAME MIDWAY INVESTMENTS
c. EMPLOYER NAME OR SCHOOL NAME	c. OTHER ACCIDENT? ☐YES 🅇NO	c. INSURANCE PLAN NAME OR PROGRAM NAME CONSUMERONE HRA
d. INSURANCE PLAN NAME OR PROGRAM NAME	10d. RESERVED FOR LOCAL USE	d. IS THERE ANOTHER HEALTH BENEFIT PLAN? ☐YES 🅇NO If yes, return to and complete 9 a-d.

READ BACK OF FORM BEFORE COMPLETING & SIGNING THIS FORM.

12. PATIENT'S OR AUTHORIZED PERSONS'S SIGNATURE I authorize the release of any medical or other info necessary to process this claim. I also request payment of government benefits either to myself or the party who accepts assignment below.

SIGNED ___ SIGNATURE ON FILE ___ DATE ___ 10222009

13. PATIENT'S OR AUTHORIZED PERSONS'S SIGNATURE I authorize payment of medical benefits to the undersigned physician or supplier for services described below.

SIGNED ___ SIGNATURE ON FILE ___

14. DATE OF CURRENT: ◄ ILLNESS (First symptom) OR INJURY (Accident) OR PREGRANCY (LMP)	15. IF PATIENT HAS HAD SAME ILLNESS, GIVE FIRST DATE	16. DATES PATIENT UNABLE TO WORK IN CURRENT OCCUPATION FROM ___ TO ___
17. NAME OF REFERRING PROVIDER OR OTHER SOURCE	17a ___ 17b NPI ___	18. HOSPITALIZATION DATES RELATED TO CURRENT SERVICES FROM ___ TO ___
19. RESERVED FOR LOCAL USE		20. OUTSIDE LAB? ☐YES 🅇NO $ CHARGES

21. DIAGNOSIS OR NATURE OF ILLNESS OR INJURY (RELATE ITEMS 1, 2, 3 OR 4 TO ITEM 24E BY LINE

1. | 463   3. | ___
2. | 462   4. | ___

22. MEDICAID SUBMISSION CODE ___ ORIGINAL REF. NO. ___

23. PRIOR AUTHORIZATION NUMBER ___

24. A DATE(S) OF SERVICE From MM DD YY	To MM DD YY	B. Place of Service	C. EMG	D. PROCEDURES, SERVICES OR SUPPLIES (Explain Unusual Circumstances) CPT/HCPCS	MODIFIER	E. DIAGNOSIS POINTER	F. $ CHARGES	G. DAYS OR UNITS	H. EPSDT Famly Plan	I. ID. QUAL	J. RENDERING PROVIDER ID#
1 10 22 2009		11		99214		1 2	180 00	1		NPI	999502
2 10 22 2009		11		87081		2	16 00	1		NPI	999502
3										NPI	
4										NPI	
5										NPI	
6										NPI	

25. FEDERAL TAX I.D. NUMBER SSN EIN	26. PATIENT'S ACCOUNT NO	27. ACCEPT ASSIGNMENT?	28. TOTAL CHARGE	29. AMOUNT PAID	30. BALANCE DUE
00-1234560 ☐ 🅇	BRA001	🅇YES ☐NO	$ 196 00	$	$

31. SIGNATURE OF PHYSICIAN OR SUPPLIER INCLUDING DEGREES OR CREDENTIALS (I certify that the statements on the reverse apply to this bill and are made a part thereof.) 10222009 SIGNED D.J. SCHWARTZ, MD DAT	32. SERVICE FACILITY LOCATION INFORMATION DOUGLASVILLE MEDICINE ASSOCIATES 5076 BRAND BLVD., SUITE 401 DOUGLASVILLE, NY 01234 a. 9995020212 b.	33. BILLING PROVIDER INFO PH # (123) 456-7892 DOUGLASVILLE MEDICINE ASSOCIATES 5076 BRAND BLVD., SUITE 401 DOUGLASVILLE, NY 01234 a. 9995020212 b.

NUCC Instruction Manual available at: www.nucc.org   OMB APPROVAL PENDING

Figure WB7-4 *(Courtesy of the Centers for Medicare & Medicaid Services.)*

1500	TEST VERSION - NOT FOR OFFICIAL USE

HEALTH INSURANCE CLAIM FORM
APPROVED BY NATIONAL UNIFORM CLAIM COMMITTEE 08/05

ConsumerOne HRA
1230 Main St.
Missoula, MT 08896

Student No: Student1

☐☐☐ PICA
PICA ☐☐☐

1. MEDICARE ☐ (Medicare #)	MEDICAID ☐ (Medicaid #)	TRICARE CHAMPUS ☐ (Sponsor's SSN)	CHAMPVA ☐ (Member ID	GROUP HEALTH PLAN ☒ (SSN or ID)	FECA BLK LUNG ☐ (SSN)	OTHER ☐ (ID)	1a. INSURED'S I.D. NUMBER (FOR PROGRAM IN ITEM 1) 999653218-02

2. PATIENT'S NAME (Last Name, First Name, Middle Initial) RIZZO TINA L	3. PATIENT'S BIRTHDATE 01 | 18 | 1994 SEX M ☐ F ☒	4. INSURED'S NAME (Last Name, First Name, Middle Initial) RIZZO ANTHONY R

5. PATIENT'S ADDRESS (No., Street) 4936 COLUMBINE STREET	6. PATIENT'S RELATIONSHIP TO INSURED Self ☐ Spouse ☐ Child ☒ Other ☐	7. INSURED'S ADDRESS (No., Street) 4936 COLUMBINE STREET
CITY DOUGLASVILLE	STATE NY	8. PATIENT STATUS Single ☒ Married ☐ Other ☐	CITY DOUGLASVILLE	STATE NY
ZIP CODE 01234	TELEPHONE (include Area Code) (123) 457-2001	Employed ☐ Full-Time Student ☐ Part-Time Student ☒	ZIP CODE 01234	TELEPHONE (include Area Code) (123) 457-2001

9. OTHER INSURED'S NAME (Last Name, First Name, Mid. Initial)	10. IS PATIENT'S CONDITION RELATED TO:	11. INSURED'S POLICY GROUP OR FECA NUMBER MIS015
a. OTHER INSURED'S POLICY OR GROUP NUMBER	a. EMPLOYMENT (CURRENT OR PREVIOUS) ☐ YES ☒ NO	a. INSURED'S DATE OF BIRTH 06 | 24 | 1972 SEX M ☒ F ☐
b. OTHER INSURED'S BIRTHDATE SEX M ☐ F ☐	b. AUTO ACCIDENT? ☐ YES ☒ NO PLACE (State)	b. EMPLOYER NAME OR SCHOOL NAME MIDWAY INVESTMENTS
c. EMPLOYER NAME OR SCHOOL NAME	c. OTHER ACCIDENT? ☐ YES ☒ NO	c. INSURANCE PLAN NAME OR PROGRAM NAME CONSUMERONE HRA
d. INSURANCE PLAN NAME OR PROGRAM NAME	10d. RESERVED FOR LOCAL USE	d. IS THERE ANOTHER HEALTH BENEFIT PLAN ☐ YES ☒ NO If yes, return to and complete 9 a-d.

READ BACK OF FORM BEFORE COMPLETING & SIGNING THIS FORM.
12. PATIENT'S OR AUTHORIZED PERSON'S SIGNATURE I authorize the release of any medical or other info necessary to process this claim. I also request payment of government benefits either to myself or the party who accepts assignment below.

SIGNED ___ SIGNATURE ON FILE ___ DATE ___ 10222009 ___

13. PATIENT'S OR AUTHORIZED PERSON'S SIGNATURE I authorize payment of medical benefits to the undersigned physician or supplier for services described below.

SIGNED ___ SIGNATURE ON FILE ___

14. DATE OF CURRENT: ILLNESS (First symptom) OR INJURY (Accident) OR PREGNANCY (LMP)	15. IF PATIENT HAS HAD SAME ILLNESS, GIVE FIRST DATE	16. DATES PATIENT UNABLE TO WORK IN CURRENT OCCUPATION FROM ___ TO ___
17. NAME OF REFERRING PROVIDER OR OTHER SOURCE	17a. 17b. NPI	18. HOSPITALIZATION DATES RELATED TO CURRENT SERVICES FROM ___ TO ___
19. RESERVED FOR LOCAL USE		20. OUTSIDE LAB? ☐ YES ☒ NO $ CHARGES

21. DIAGNOSIS OR NATURE OF ILLNESS OR INJURY (RELATE ITEMS 1, 2, 3 OR 4 TO ITEM 24E BY LINE)
1. 477.9
2. 782.1
3. |___
4. |___

22. MEDICAID SUBMISSION CODE ___ ORIGINAL REF. NO. ___
23. PRIOR AUTHORIZATION NUMBER

24. A. DATE(S) OF SERVICE From MM DD YY — To MM DD YY	B. Place of Service	C. EMG	D. PROCEDURES, SERVICES OR SUPPLIES (Explain Unusual Circumstances) CPT/HCPCS — MODIFIER	E. DIAGNOSIS POINTER	F. $ CHARGES	G. DAYS OR UNITS	H. EPSDT Family Plan	I. ID. QUAL	J. RENDERING PROVIDER ID#
1	10 22 2009	11		99214	1 2	180 00	1		NPI	999501
2	10 22 2009	11		85031	1 2	11 00	1		NPI	999501
3	10 22 2009	11		36415	2	18 00	1		NPI	999501
4									NPI	
5									NPI	
6									NPI	

25. FEDERAL TAX I.D. NUMBER SSN EIN 00-1234560 ☐ ☒	26. PATIENT'S ACCOUNT NO. RIZ001	27. ACCEPT ASSIGNMENT? ☒ YES ☐ NO	28. TOTAL CHARGE $ 209 00	29. AMOUNT PAID $	30. BALANCE DUE $

31. SIGNATURE OF PHYSICIAN OR SUPPLIER INCLUDING DEGREES OR CREDENTIALS (I certify that the statements on the reverse apply to this bill and are made a part thereof.) 10222009 SIGNED L. D. HEATH, MD DAT	32. SERVICE FACILITY LOCATION INFORMATION DOUGLASVILLE MEDICINE ASSOCIATES 5076 BRAND BLVD., SUITE 401 DOUGLASVILLE, NY 01234 a. 9995010111 b.	33. BILLING PROVIDER INFO PH # (123) 456-7890 DOUGLASVILLE MEDICINE ASSOCIATES 5076 BRAND BLVD., SUITE 401 DOUGLASVILLE, NY 01234 a. 9995010111 b.

NUCC Instruction Manual available at: www.nucc.org

OMB APPROVAL PENDING

Figure WB7-5 *(Courtesy of the Centers for Medicare & Medicaid Services.)*

1500	TEST VERSION - NOT FOR OFFICIAL USE

HEALTH INSURANCE CLAIM FORM
APPROVED BY NATIONAL UNIFORM CLAIM COMMITTEE 08/05

ConsumerOne HRA
1230 Main St.
Missoula, MT 08896

Student No: **Student1**

☐☐☐ PICA   PICA ☐☐☐

1. MEDICARE ☐(Medicare #) MEDICAID ☐(Medicaid #) TRICARE CHAMPUS ☐(Sponsor's SSN) CHAMPVA ☐(Member ID) GROUP HEALTH PLAN ☒(SSN or ID) FECA BLK LUNG ☐(SSN) OTHER ☐(ID)	1a. INSURED'S I.D. NUMBER (FOR PROGRAM IN ITEM 1) 999320169

2. PATIENT'S NAME (Last Name, First Name, Middle Initial) SHERIDAN WYNONA	3. PATIENT'S BIRTHDATE 06 | 05 | 1984 SEX M☐ F☒	4. INSURED'S NAME (Last Name, First Name, Middle Initial) SHERIDAN WYNONA

5. PATIENT'S ADDRESS (No., Street) 12390 MARBLE WAY	6. PATIENT'S RELATIONSHIP TO INSURED Self ☒ Spouse ☐ Child ☐ Other ☐	7. INSURED'S ADDRESS (No., Street) SAME

CITY DOUGLASVILLE	STATE NY	8. PATIENT STATUS Single ☒ Married ☐ Other ☐	CITY	STATE

ZIP CODE 01234	TELEPHONE (include Area Code) (123) 970-6123	Employed ☒ Full-Time Student ☐ Part-Time Student ☐	ZIP CODE	TELEPHONE (include Area Code)

9. OTHER INSURED'S NAME (Last Name, First Name, Mid. Initial)	10. IS PATIENT'S CONDITION RELATED TO:	11. INSURED'S POLICY GROUP OR FECA NUMBER MI5015

a. OTHER INSURED'S POLICY OR GROUP NUMBER	a. EMPLOYMENT (CURRENT OR PREVIOUS) ☐YES ☒NO	a. INSURED'S DATE OF BIRTH SEX M☐ F☐

b. OTHER INSURED'S BIRTHDATE SEX M☐ F☐	b. AUTO ACCIDENT? ☐YES ☒NO PLACE (State)	b. EMPLOYER NAME OR SCHOOL NAME MIDWAY INVESTMENTS

c. EMPLOYER NAME OR SCHOOL NAME	c. OTHER ACCIDENT? ☐YES ☒NO	c. INSURANCE PLAN NAME OR PROGRAM NAME CONSUMERONE HRA

d. INSURANCE PLAN NAME OR PROGRAM NAME	10d. RESERVED FOR LOCAL USE	d. IS THERE ANOTHER HEALTH BENEFIT PLAN ☐ YES ☒ NO *If yes, return to and complete 9 a-d.*

READ BACK OF FORM BEFORE COMPLETING & SIGNING THIS FORM.
12. PATIENT'S OR AUTHORIZED PERSONS'S SIGNATURE I authorize the release of any medical or other info necessary to process this claim. I also request payment of government benefits either to myself or the party who accepts assignment below.

SIGNED _SIGNATURE ON FILE_   DATE _10272009_

13. PATIENT'S OR AUTHORIZED PERSONS'S SIGNATURE I authorize payment of medical benefits to the undersigned physician or supplier for services described below.

SIGNED _SIGNATURE ON FILE_

14. DATE OF CURRENT: ◄ ILLNESS (First symptom) OR INJURY (Accident) OR PREGRANCY (LMP)	15. IF PATIENT HAS HAD SAME ILLNESS, GIVE FIRST DATE	16. DATES PATIENT UNABLE TO WORK IN CURRENT OCCUPATION FROM TO

17. NAME OF REFERRING PROVIDER OR OTHER SOURCE	17a 17b NPI	18. HOSPITALIZATION DATES RELATED TO CURRENT SERVICES FROM TO

19. RESERVED FOR LOCAL USE	20. OUTSIDE LAB? ☐YES ☒NO $ CHARGES

21. DIAGNOSIS OR NATURE OF ILLNESS OR INJURY (RELATE ITEMS 1, 2, 3 OR 4 TO ITEM 24E BY LINE) 1. |558.9___ 3. |_____ 2. |_____ 4. |_____	22. MEDICAID SUBMISSION CODE ORIGINAL REF. NO. 23. PRIOR AUTHORIZATION NUMBER

24. A	DATE(S) OF SERVICE From	To	B. Place of Service	C. EMG	D. PROCEDURES, SERVICES OR SUPPLIES (Explain Unusual Circumstances) CPT/HCPCS MODIFIER	E. DIAGNOSIS POINTER	F. $ CHARGES	G. DAYS OR UNITS	H. EPSDT Famly Plan	I. ID. QUAL	J. RENDERING PROVIDER ID#
1	10 27 2009		11		99203	1	200 00	1		NPI	999501
2										NPI	
3										NPI	
4										NPI	
5										NPI	
6										NPI	

25. FEDERAL TAX I.D. NUMBER SSN EIN 00-1234560 ☐ ☒	26. PATIENT'S ACCOUNT NO SHE002	27. ACCEPT ASSIGNMENT? ☒YES ☐NO	28. TOTAL CHARGE $ 200 00	29. AMOUNT PAID $	30. BALANCE DUE $

31. SIGNATURE OF PHYSICIAN OR SUPPLIER INCLUDING DEGREES OR CREDENTIALS (I certify that the statements on the reverse apply to this bill and are made a part thereof.) 10272009 SIGNED L. D. HEATH, MD DAT	32. SERVICE FACILITY LOCATION INFORMATION DOUGLASVILLE MEDICINE ASSOCIATES 5076 BRAND BLVD., SUITE 401 DOUGLASVILLE, NY 01234 a. 9995010111 b.	33. BILLING PROVIDER INFO PH # (123) 456-7890 DOUGLASVILLE MEDICINE ASSOCIATES 5076 BRAND BLVD., SUITE 401 DOUGLASVILLE, NY 01234 a. 9995010111 b.

NUCC Instruction Manual available at: www.nucc.org   OMB APPROVAL PENDING

Figure WB7-6 *(Courtesy of the Centers for Medicare & Medicaid Services.)*

1500	TEST VERSION - NOT FOR OFFICIAL USE		

HEALTH INSURANCE CLAIM FORM
APPROVED BY NATIONAL UNIFORM CLAIM COMMITTEE 08/05

ConsumerOne HRA
1230 Main St.
Missoula, MT 08896

Student No: Student1

PICA [ ][ ][ ] PICA [ ][ ][ ]

1. MEDICARE MEDICAID TRICARE CHAMPUS CHAMPVA GROUP HEALTH PLAN FECA BLK LUNG OTHER	1a. INSURED'S I.D. NUMBER (FOR PROGRAM IN ITEM 1)
[ ](Medicare #) [ ](Medicaid #) [ ](Sponsor's SSN) [ ](Member ID [X](SSN or ID) [ ](SSN) [ ](ID)	999541163

2. PATIENT'S NAME (Last Name, First Name, Middle Initial)	3. PATIENT'S BIRTHDATE SEX	4. INSURED'S NAME (Last Name, First Name, Middle Initial)
HEDENSTEN MARK	03 | 12 | 1958 M [X] F [ ]	HEDENSTEN MARK

5. PATIENT'S ADDRESS (No., Street)	6. PATIENT'S RELATIONSHIP TO INSURED	7. INSURED'S ADDRESS (No., Street)
12341 SLATE COURT	Self [X] Spouse [ ] Child [ ] Other [ ]	SAME

CITY STATE	8. PATIENT STATUS	CITY STATE
DOUGLASVILLE NY	Single [ ] Married [X] Other [ ]	

ZIP CODE	TELEPHONE (include Area Code)		ZIP CODE	TELEPHONE (include Area Code)
01235	(123) 466-1120	Employed [X] Full-Time Student [ ] Part-Time Student [ ]		

9. OTHER INSURED'S NAME (Last Name, First Name, Mid. Initial)	10. IS PATIENT'S CONDITION RELATED TO:	11. INSURED'S POLICY GROUP OR FECA NUMBER
		CME89116
a. OTHER INSURED'S POLICY OR GROUP NUMBER	a. EMPLOYMENT (CURRENT OR PREVIOUS) [ ]YES [X]NO	a. INSURED'S DATE OF BIRTH SEX M [ ] F [ ]
b. OTHER INSURED'S BIRTHDATE SEX M [ ] F [ ]	b. AUTO ACCIDENT? PLACE (State) [ ]YES [X]NO	b. EMPLOYER NAME OR SCHOOL NAME CONCEPTS MEDIA, LLC
c. EMPLOYER NAME OR SCHOOL NAME	c. OTHER ACCIDENT? [ ]YES [X]NO	c. INSURANCE PLAN NAME OR PROGRAM NAME CONSUMERONE HRA
d. INSURANCE PLAN NAME OR PROGRAM NAME	10d. RESERVED FOR LOCAL USE	d. IS THERE ANOTHER HEALTH BENEFIT PLAN [ ]YES [X]NO If yes, return to and complete 9 a-d.

READ BACK OF FORM BEFORE COMPLETING & SIGNING THIS FORM.

12. PATIENT'S OR AUTHORIZED PERSONS'S SIGNATURE I authorize the release of any medical or other info necessary to process this claim. I also request payment of government benefits either to myself or the party who accepts assignment below.

SIGNED ___ SIGNATURE ON FILE ___   DATE ___ 11222009 ___

13. PATIENT'S OR AUTHORIZED PERSONS'S SIGNATURE I authorize payment of medical benefits to the undersigned physician or supplier for services described below.

SIGNED ___ SIGNATURE ON FILE ___

14. DATE OF CURRENT: ◄ ILLNESS (First symptom) OR INJURY (Accident) OR PREGRANCY (LMP)	15. IF PATIENT HAS HAD SAME ILLNESS, GIVE FIRST DATE	16. DATES PATIENT UNABLE TO WORK IN CURRENT OCCUPATION FROM ___ TO ___
17. NAME OF REFERRING PROVIDER OR OTHER SOURCE	17a 17b NPI	18. HOSPITALIZATION DATES RELATED TO CURRENT SERVICES FROM ___ TO ___
19. RESERVED FOR LOCAL USE		20. OUTSIDE LAB? $ CHARGES [ ]YES [X]NO

21. DIAGNOSIS OR NATURE OF ILLNESS OR INJURY (RELATE ITEMS 1, 2, 3 OR 4 TO ITEM 24E BY LINE)	22. MEDICAID SUBMISSION CODE ORIGINAL REF. NO.
1. | 413.9 3. | ___ 2. | 427.69 4. | ___	23. PRIOR AUTHORIZATION NUMBER

24. A DATE(S) OF SERVICE From — To MM DD YY MM DD YY	B. Place of Service	C. EMG	D. PROCEDURES, SERVICES OR SUPPLIES (Explain Unusual Circumstances) CPT/HCPCS MODIFIER	E. DIAGNOSIS POINTER	F. $ CHARGES	G. DAYS OR UNITS	H. EPSDT Family Plan	I. ID. QUAL	J. RENDERING PROVIDER ID#
1 11 22 2009	21		99221	1 2	145 | 00	1		NPI	999502
2								NPI	
3								NPI	
4								NPI	
5								NPI	
6								NPI	

25. FEDERAL TAX I.D. NUMBER SSN EIN	26. PATIENT'S ACCOUNT NO	27. ACCEPT ASSIGNMENT?	28. TOTAL CHARGE	29. AMOUNT PAID	30. BALANCE DUE
00-1234560 [ ] [X]	HED001	[X]YES [ ]NO	$ 145 00	$	$

31. SIGNATURE OF PHYSICIAN OR SUPPLIER INCLUDING DEGREES OR CREDENTIALS (I certify that the statements on the reverse apply to this bill and are made a part thereof.) 11222009 SIGNED D.J. SCHWARTZ, MD DAT	32. SERVICE FACILITY LOCATION INFORMATION COMMUNITY GENERAL HOSPITAL 4000 BRAND BLVD. DOUGLASVILLE, NY 01234 a. 9997794511 b.	33. BILLING PROVIDER INFO PH # (123) 456-7892 DOUGLASVILLE MEDICINE ASSOCIATES 5076 BRAND BLVD., SUITE 401 DOUGLASVILLE, NY 01234 a. 9995020212 b.

NUCC Instruction Manual available at: www.nucc.org   OMB APPROVAL PENDING

Figure WB7-7 *(Courtesy of the Centers for Medicare & Medicaid Services.)*

E. In an actual medical office, the four claim forms would be mailed to the address for the insurance carrier that appears at the top of each CMS-1500 form. If requested, your instructor may collect these insurance claim forms.

BUILDING SKILLS 7-3: PREPARING ELECTRONIC CLAIMS FOR FLEXIHEALTH PPO IN-NETWORK PATIENTS

Instructions: Using the Claim Preparation screen in the Insurance Billing area of MOSS, complete the following tasks:

A. Prepare electronic claims to be sent for patients with FlexiHealth PPO In-Network coverage for services performed by both Drs. Heath and Schwartz.

B. Use date range October 20 through November 30, 2009.

C. View a prebilling worksheet before submitting claims. Check your work with Figures WB7-8 and WB7-9 before proceeding.

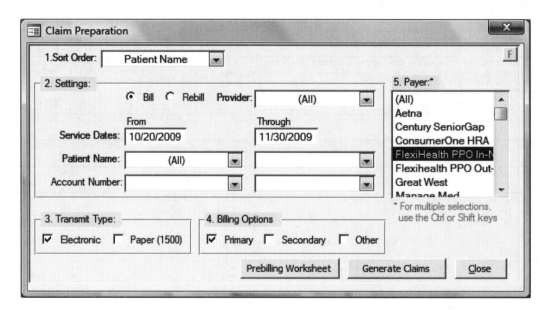

Figure WB7-8 *(Delmar/Cengage Learning)*

INSURANCE PREBILLING WORKSHEET
Student1

Dates of Service	Diag Code	Proc Code	POS	Units	Dr	As	Bill Amt	Receipts	Net
FlexiHealth PPO In-Network									
Barryroe, Caitlin									
10/23/2009	599.0	81000	11	1.00	D1	Y	$12.00	$0.00	$12.00
10/23/2009	599.0	80053	11	1.00	D1	Y	$47.00	$0.00	$47.00
10/23/2009	599.0	99214	11	1.00	D1	Y	$180.00	$20.00	$160.00
						Totals	$239.00	$20.00	$219.00
Johnsen, Dennis									
11/9/2009	682.9	99282	23	1.00	D1	Y	$147.00	$0.00	$147.00
						Totals	$147.00	$0.00	$147.00
Jouharian, Siran									
11/12/2009	780.4	99282	23	1.00	D1	Y	$147.00	$0.00	$147.00
						Totals	$147.00	$0.00	$147.00
Ross, Karen									
11/17/2009	250.00	99221	21	1.00	D1	Y	$145.00	$0.00	$145.00
						Totals	$145.00	$0.00	$145.00
Shuman, Alan									
10/22/2009	496	90772	11	1.00	D1	Y	$81.00	$0.00	$81.00
10/22/2009	496	90658	11	1.00	D1	Y	$22.00	$0.00	$22.00
10/22/2009	496	99215	11	1.00	D1	Y	$249.00	$20.00	$229.00
						Totals	$352.00	$20.00	$332.00
Wallace, Derek									
10/22/2009	599.0	99212	11	1.00	D1	Y	$80.00	$20.00	$60.00
						Totals	$80.00	$20.00	$60.00
			TOTAL TO BE BILLED FOR FlexiHealth PPO In-Network						$1,050.00
Grand Total			**Grand Total**						$1,050.00

Figure WB7-9 *(Delmar/Cengage Learning)*

D. Close the prebilling worksheet and return to the Claims Preparation screen. Click on the *Generate Claims* button.

E. Review the CMS-1500 forms for each patient. You may use the Patient Registration and/or Patient Ledger screens to check your work as it appears on the claim forms. Correct any errors before proceeding by clicking on the *Claim Prep* button to return to the Claims Preparation screen, and then *Close* in order to return to the areas of the software necessary to make corrections. If ready for billing, proceed to Step F.

F. Click on the *Transmit EMC* button to submit claims electronically.

G. When finished, click on *View* and then print the report for your records. (Hint: Close the report to return to the Transmission Status screen, and then click on *Print*.) Review your work with Figures WB7-10 and WB7-11. Follow your instructor's directions for turning in the report.

Claims Submission Report
Student1

FlexiHealth PPO In-Network

Patient Name
Caitlin Barryroe

Account No	BAR001	*DOS*	*Procedure*	*Charges*	*Result*
		10/23/2009	99214	$180.00	A
		10/23/2009	80053	$47.00	A
		10/23/2009	81000	$12.00	A
Patient Totals				$239.00	

Patient Name
Dennis Johnsen

Account No	JOH002	*DOS*	*Procedure*	*Charges*	*Result*
		11/9/2009	99282	$147.00	A
Patient Totals				$147.00	

Patient Name
Siran Jouharian

Account No	JOU001	*DOS*	*Procedure*	*Charges*	*Result*
		11/12/2009	99282	$147.00	A
Patient Totals				$147.00	

Patient Name
Karen Ross

Account No	ROS001	*DOS*	*Procedure*	*Charges*	*Result*
		11/17/2009	99221	$145.00	A
Patient Totals				$145.00	

Figure WB7-10 *(Delmar/Cengage Learning)*

Patient Name
Alan Shuman

Account No	SHU001	*DOS*	*Procedure*	*Charges*	*Result*
		10/22/2009	99215	$249.00	A
		10/22/2009	90658	$22.00	A
		10/22/2009	90772	$81.00	A
Patient Totals				$352.00	

Patient Name
Derek Wallace

Account No	WAL001	*DOS*	*Procedure*	*Charges*	*Result*
		10/22/2009	99212	$80.00	A
Patient Totals				$80.00	

Figure WB7-11 *(Delmar/Cengage Learning)*

BUILDING SKILLS 7-4: PREPARING ELECTRONIC CLAIMS FOR FLEXIHEALTH PPO OUT-OF-NETWORK PATIENTS

Instructions: Using the Claim Preparation screen in the Insurance Billing area of MOSS, complete the following tasks:

A. Prepare electronic claims to be sent for patients with FlexiHealth PPO Out-of-Network coverage for services performed by both Drs. Heath and Schwartz.

B. Use date range October 20 through November 30, 2009.

C. View a prebilling worksheet before submitting claims. Check your work with Figures WB7-12 and WB7-13 before proceeding.

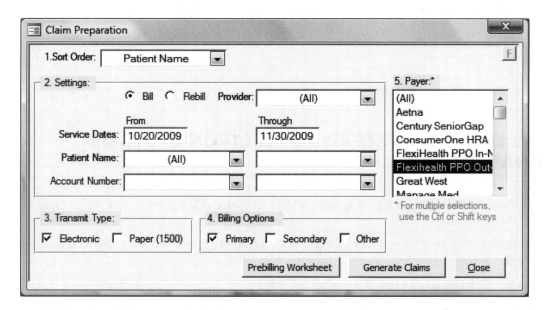

Figure WB7-12 *(Delmar/Cengage Learning)*

Dates of Service	Diag Code	Proc Code	POS	Units	Dr	As	Bill Amt	Receipts	Net
INSURANCE PREBILLING WORKSHEET									
Student1									
Flexihealth PPO Out-of-Netwo									
Engleman, Harold									
10/22/2009	530.81	99205	11	1.00	D2	N	$358.00	$0.00	$358.00
					Totals		$358.00	$0.00	$358.00
			TOTAL TO BE BILLED FOR Flexihealth PPO Out-of-Network						$358.00
Grand Total			**Grand Total**						$358.00

Figure WB7-13 *(Delmar/Cengage Learning)*

D. Close the prebilling worksheet and return to the Claims Preparation screen. Click on the *Generate Claims* button.

E. Review the CMS-1500 form. You may use the Patient Registration and/or Patient Ledger screen to check your work as it appears on the claim form. Correct any errors before proceeding by clicking on the *Claim Prep* button to return to the Claims Preparation screen, and then *Close* in order to return to the areas of the software necessary to make corrections. If ready for billing, proceed to Step F.

F. Click on the *Transmit EMC* button to submit claims electronically.

G. When finished, click on *View* and then print the report for your records. (Hint: Close the report to return to the Transmission Status screen, and then click on *Print*.) Review your work with Figure WB7-14. Follow your instructor's directions for turning in the report.

Claims Submission Report
Student1

Flexihealth PPO Out-of-Network

Patient Name
Harold Engleman

Account No	ENG001	*DOS*	*Procedure*	*Charges*	*Result*
		10/22/2009	99205	$358.00	A
Patient Totals				$358.00	

Figure WB7-14 *(Delmar/Cengage Learning)*

BUILDING SKILLS 7-5: PREPARING ELECTRONIC CLAIMS FOR SIGNAL HMO PATIENTS

Instructions: Using the Claim Preparation screen in the Insurance Billing area of MOSS, complete the following tasks:

A. Prepare electronic claims to be sent for patients with Signal HMO coverage for services performed by both Drs. Heath and Schwartz.

B. Use date range October 20 through November 30, 2009.

C. View a prebilling worksheet before submitting claims. Check your work with Figures WB7-15 and WB7-16 before proceeding.

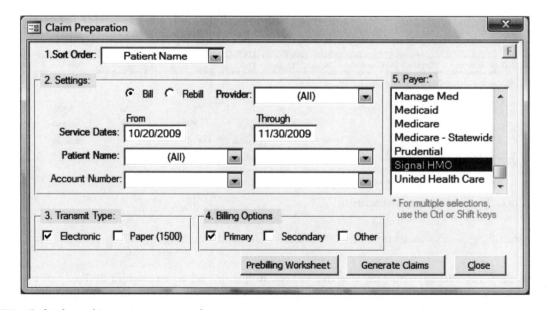

Figure WB7-15 *(Delmar/Cengage Learning)*

INSURANCE PREBILLING WORKSHEET
Student1

Dates of Service	Diag Code	Proc Code	POS	Units	Dr	As	Bill Amt	Receipts	Net
Signal HMO									
Camille, Emery									
10/22/2009	382.9	85031	11	1.00	D2	Y	$11.00	$0.00	$11.00
10/22/2009	382.9	99213	11	1.00	D2	Y	$111.00	$10.00	$101.00
					Totals		$122.00	$10.00	$112.00
Souza, Janet									
11/10/2009	558.9	99282	23	1.00	D1	Y	$147.00	$0.00	$147.00
					Totals		$147.00	$0.00	$147.00
Trimble, Devon									
10/20/2009	250.00	81002	11	1.00	D1	Y	$9.00	$0.00	$9.00
10/20/2009	250.00	80053	11	1.00	D1	Y	$47.00	$0.00	$47.00
10/20/2009	250.00	99204	11	1.00	D1	Y	$283.00	$10.00	$273.00
					Totals		$339.00	$10.00	$329.00
Yamagata, Naomi									
10/22/2009	493.90	99214	11	1.00	D2	Y	$180.00	$10.00	$170.00
					Totals		$180.00	$10.00	$170.00
TOTAL TO BE BILLED FOR Signal HMO									$758.00
Grand Total					*Grand Total*				$758.00

Figure WB7-16 *(Delmar/Cengage Learning)*

D. Close the prebilling worksheet and return to the Claims Preparation screen. Click on the *Generate Claims* button.

E. Review the CMS-1500 forms. You may use the Patient Registration and/or Patient Ledger screen to check your work as it appears on the claim forms. Correct any errors before proceeding by clicking on the *Claim Prep* button to return to the Claims Preparation screen, and then *Close* in order to return to the areas of the software necessary to make corrections. If ready for billing, proceed to Step F.

F. Click on the *Transmit EMC* button to submit claims electronically.

G. When finished, click on *View* and then print the report for your records. (Hint: Close the report to return to the Transmission Status screen, and then click on *Print*.) Review your work with Figure WB7-17. Follow your instructor's directions for turning in the report.

Claims Submission Report
Student1

Signal HMO

Patient Name
Emery Camille

Account No CAM001	*DOS*	*Procedure*	*Charges*	*Result*
	10/22/2009	99213	$111.00	A
	10/22/2009	85031	$11.00	A
Patient Totals			$122.00	

Patient Name
Janet Souza

Account No SOU001	*DOS*	*Procedure*	*Charges*	*Result*
	11/10/2009	99282	$147.00	A
Patient Totals			$147.00	

Patient Name
Devon Trimble

Account No TRI001	*DOS*	*Procedure*	*Charges*	*Result*
	10/20/2009	99204	$283.00	A
	10/20/2009	80053	$47.00	A
	10/20/2009	81002	$9.00	A
Patient Totals			$339.00	

Patient Name
Naomi Yamagata

Account No YAM001	*DOS*	*Procedure*	*Charges*	*Result*
	10/22/2009	99214	$180.00	A
Patient Totals			$180.00	

Figure WB7-17 *(Delmar/Cengage Learning)*

BUILDING SKILLS 7-6: PREPARING ELECTRONIC CLAIMS FOR MEDICARE STATEWIDE PATIENTS

Instructions: Using the Claim Preparation screen in the Insurance Billing area of MOSS, complete the following tasks:

A. Prepare electronic claims to be sent for patients with Medicare Statewide coverage for services performed by both Drs. Heath and Schwartz.

B. Use date range October 20 through November 30, 2009.

C. View a prebilling worksheet before submitting claims. Check your work with Figures WB7-18 and WB7-19 before proceeding.

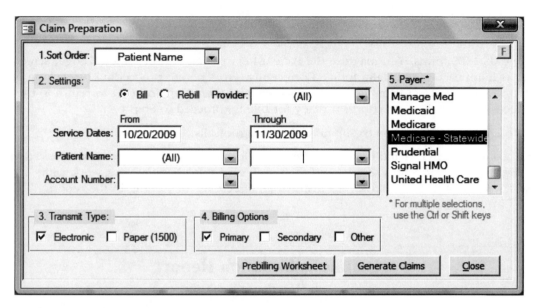

Figure WB7-18 *(Delmar/Cengage Learning)*

INSURANCE PREBILLING WORKSHEET
Student1

Dates of Service	Diag Code	Proc Code	POS	Units	Dr	As	Bill Amt	Receipts	Net
Medicare - Statewide Corp.									
Bernardo, William									
11/9/2009	496	99282	23	1.00	D1	Y	$147.00	$0.00	$147.00
						Totals	$147.00	$0.00	$147.00
Durand, Isabel									
11/13/2009	708.9	99307	32	1.00	D1	Y	$68.00	$0.00	$68.00
						Totals	$68.00	$0.00	$68.00
Hartsfeld, Deanna									
10/22/2009	272.0	80053	11	1.00	D1	Y	$47.00	$0.00	$47.00
10/22/2009	272.0	99214	11	1.00	D1	Y	$180.00	$0.00	$180.00
						Totals	$227.00	$0.00	$227.00
Herbert, Nancy									
10/22/2009	496	85014	11	1.00	D1	Y	$7.00	$0.00	$7.00
10/22/2009	496	80053	11	1.00	D1	Y	$47.00	$0.00	$47.00
10/22/2009	496	99215	11	1.00	D1	Y	$249.00	$0.00	$249.00
						Totals	$303.00	$0.00	$303.00
McKay, Sean									
11/20/2009	079.99	99221	21	1.00	D1	Y	$145.00	$0.00	$145.00
						Totals	$145.00	$0.00	$145.00
Royzin, Joel									
11/13/2009	443.9	99308	32	1.00	D1	Y	$113.00	$0.00	$113.00
						Totals	$113.00	$0.00	$113.00
		TOTAL TO BE BILLED FOR Medicare - Statewide Corp.							$1,003.00
Grand Total			**Grand Total**						**$1,003.00**

Figure WB7-19 *(Delmar/Cengage Learning)*

D. Close the prebilling worksheet and return to the Claims Preparation screen. Click on the *Generate Claims* button.

E. Review the CMS-1500 forms. You may use the Patient Registration and/or Patient Ledger screen to check your work as it appears on the claim forms. Correct any errors before proceeding by clicking on the *Claim Prep* button to return to the Claims Preparation screen, and then *Close* in order to return to the areas of the software necessary to make corrections. If ready for billing, proceed to Step F.

F. Click on the *Transmit EMC* button to submit claims electronically.

G. When finished, click on *View* and then print the report for your records. (Hint: Close the report to return to the Transmission Status screen, and then click on *Print*.) Review your work with Figures WB7-20 and WB7-21. Follow your instructor's directions for turning in the report.

Claims Submission Report
Student1

Medicare - Statewide Corp.

Patient Name
William Bernardo

Account No BER001	*DOS*	*Procedure*	*Charges*	*Result*
	11/9/2009	99282	$147.00	A
Patient Totals			$147.00	

Patient Name
Isabel Durand

Account No DUR001	*DOS*	*Procedure*	*Charges*	*Result*
	11/13/2009	99307	$68.00	A
Patient Totals			$68.00	

Patient Name
Deanna Hartsfeld

Account No HAR001	*DOS*	*Procedure*	*Charges*	*Result*
	10/22/2009	99214	$180.00	A
	10/22/2009	80053	$47.00	A
Patient Totals			$227.00	

Patient Name
Nancy Herbert

Account No HER001	*DOS*	*Procedure*	*Charges*	*Result*
	10/22/2009	99215	$249.00	A
	10/22/2009	80053	$47.00	A
	10/22/2009	85014	$7.00	A
Patient Totals			$303.00	

Figure WB7-20 *(Delmar/Cengage Learning)*

Patient Name					
Sean McKay					
Account No	MCK001	*DOS*	*Procedure*	*Charges*	*Result*
		11/20/2009	99221	$145.00	A
Patient Totals				$145.00	
Patient Name					
Joel Royzin					
Account No	ROY001	*DOS*	*Procedure*	*Charges*	*Result*
		11/13/2009	99308	$113.00	A
Patient Totals				$113.00	

Figure WB7-21 *(Delmar/Cengage Learning)*

U N I T **8**

Posting Payments and Secondary Insurance Billing

BUILDING SKILLS 8-1: REVIEWING THE COMPONENTS OF A REMITTANCE ADVICE (RA) OR EXPLANATION OF BENEFITS (EOB)

1. Remittance Advices (RAs) and Explanation of Benefits (EOBs) from various insurance carriers may look different from each other, but they have several basic components in common. Discuss these basic components common to most RAs and EOBs, no matter which insurance carrier has issued them with a payment.

   _____

   _____

   _____

   _____

   _____

2. Traditionally, insurance carriers would issue a paper check for one or several patients, accompanied by an RA or EOB. Explain a newer system and technology called EPS.

   _____

   _____

   _____

   _____

   _____

3. Why is it important for a staff member to be accurate when posting payments from insurance carriers to patient accounts?

   _____

   _____

   _____

   _____

   _____

BUILDING SKILLS 8-2: POSTING PAYMENTS FROM HRA PLANS

Instructions: Refer to the ConsumerONE HRA Service Detail EOB shown on Source Document WB8-1 in the back of the workbook. For each of the patients below, post payments, adjustments, and other applicable details as required.

Patient Aimee Bradley

1. Go to Posting Payments from the Main Menu in MOSS and open the Posting screen for Patient Bradley as shown in Figure WB8-1.

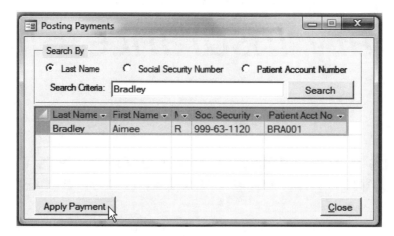

Figure WB8-1 *(Delmar/Cengage Learning)*

2. Read the EOB from ConsumerONE and answer the following questions regarding Patient Bradley's services.

 Cover the answers using the tear-off bookmark from the cover of your textbook. Check your work before entering data into MOSS to be sure you have correctly interpreted the source documents.

A.	How much did the health insurance plan allow for each procedure?	$168.70 and $11.00
B.	How much did the health insurance plan disallow for each procedure? How will these disallowed amounts be posted on the patient account?	$11.30 and $5.00. These will be posted as adjustments on the patient account.
C.	How much did the health insurance plan pay on each procedure, and at which level?	$168.00 and $11.00 at Level 1.

3. Post the payments using the Claim Number as the reference. The posting date is 12/1/2009. Check your work with Figures WB8-2 and WB8-3.

4. When both payments have been posted, click on the *View Ledger* button and check your work with Figure WB8-4.

5. Close all windows and return to the Patient Selection screen for Posting Payments.

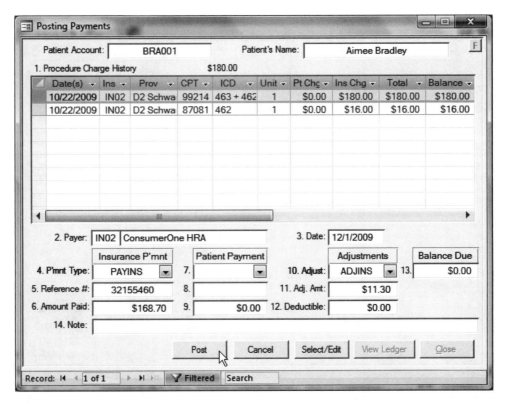

Figure WB8-2 *(Delmar/Cengage Learning)*

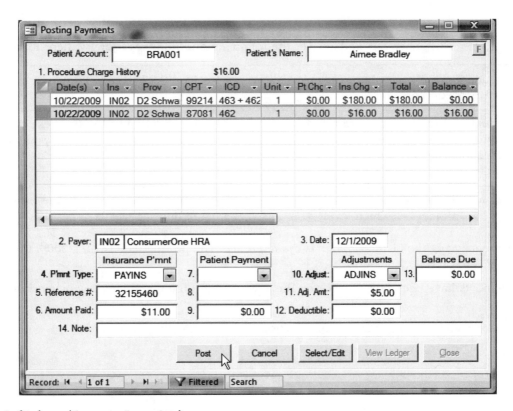

Figure WB8-3 *(Delmar/Cengage Learning)*

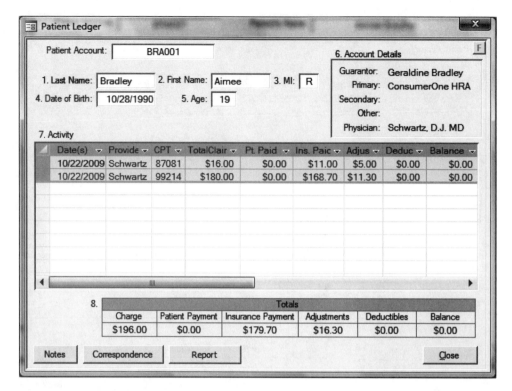

Figure WB8-4 *(Delmar/Cengage Learning)*

Patient Tina Rizzo

1. Open the Posting screen for Patient Rizzo.

2. Read the EOB from ConsumerONE and answer the following questions regarding Patient Rizzo's services.

A.	How much did the health insurance plan allow for each procedure?	$168.70, $9.00, and $5.00
B.	How much did the health insurance plan disallow for each procedure? How will these disallowed amounts be posted on the patient account?	$11.30, $2.00, and $13.00. These will be posted as adjustments on the patient account.
C.	How much did the health insurance plan pay on each procedure, and at which level?	$0.00. The patient is responsible for the entire amount due at Level 2.

3. Post the payments using the Claim Number as the reference. The posting date is 12/1/2009. Check your work with Figures WB8-5, WB8-6, and WB8-7.

4. When all payments have been posted, click on the *View Ledger* button and check your work with Figure WB8-8.

5. Close all windows and return to the Patient Selection screen for Posting Payments.

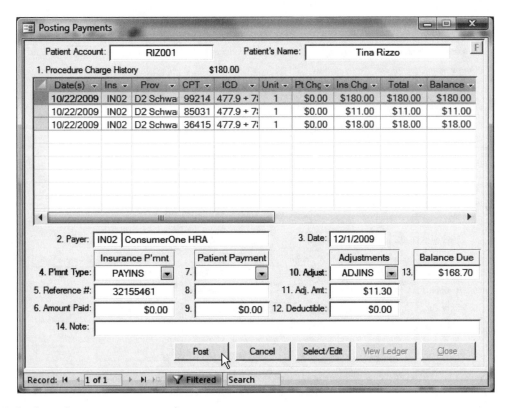

Figure WB8-5 *(Delmar/Cengage Learning)*

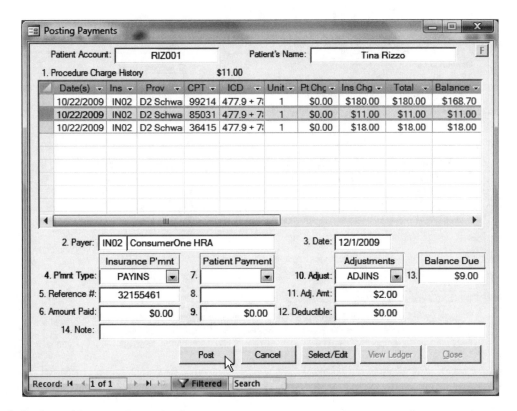

Figure WB8-6 *(Delmar/Cengage Learning)*

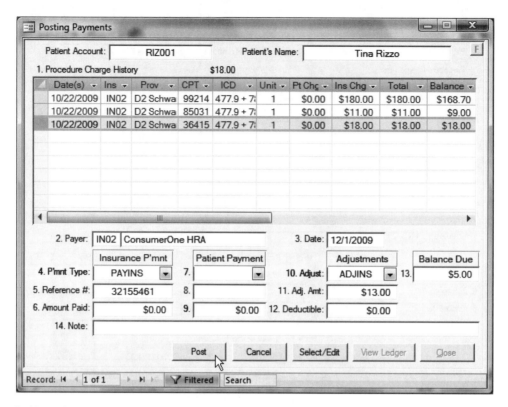

Figure WB8-7 *(Delmar/Cengage Learning)*

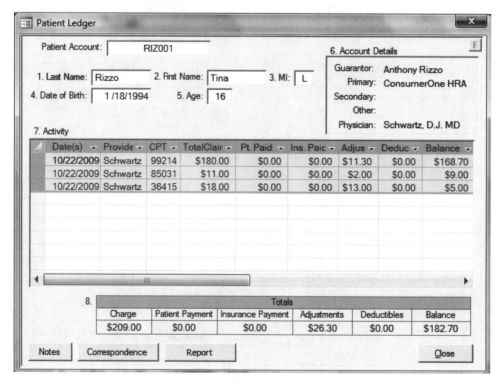

Figure WB8-8 *(Delmar/Cengage Learning)*

Critical Thinking: Patient Wynona Sheridan

1. Open the Posting screen for Patient Sheridan.

2. Read the EOB from ConsumerONE and post the payment, using date 12/01/2009 and the Claim Number as the reference.

3. Check your work with Figures WB8-9 and WB8-10.

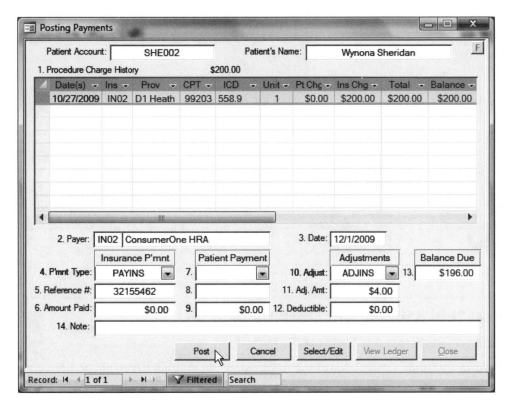

Figure WB8-9 *(Delmar/Cengage Learning)*

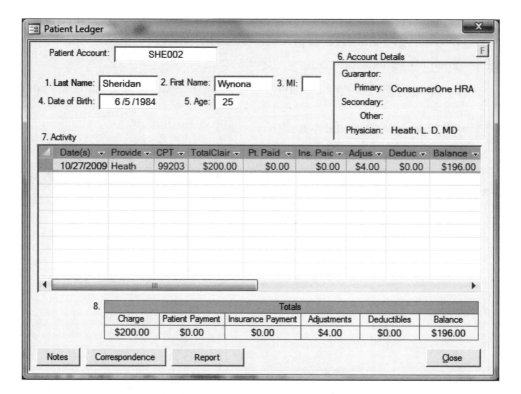

Figure WB8-10 *(Delmar/Cengage Learning)*

Critical Thinking: Patient Mark Hedensten

1. Open the Posting screen for Patient Hedensten.

2. Read the EOB from ConsumerONE and post the payment, using date 12/01/2009 and the Claim Number as the reference.

3. Check your work with Figures WB8-11 and WB8-12.

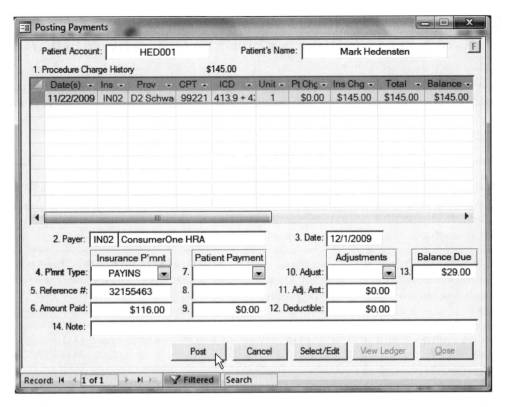

Figure WB8-11 *(Delmar/Cengage Learning)*

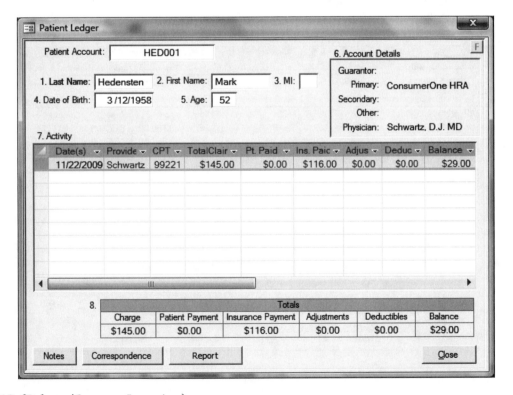

Figure WB8-12 *(Delmar/Cengage Learning)*

BUILDING SKILLS 8-3: POSTING PAYMENTS FROM FLEXIHEALTH PPO IN-NETWORK PLANS FOR SERVICES RENDERED IN THE MEDICAL OFFICE

Instructions: Refer to the FlexiHealth PPO In-Network EOB shown on Source Document WB8-2 in the back of the workbook. For each of the patients below, post payments, adjustments, and other applicable details as required.

Patient Caitlin Barryroe

1. Open the Posting screen for Patient Barryroe.

2. Read the EOB from FlexiHealth PPO and answer the following questions regarding Patient Barryroe's services.

A.	How much did the health insurance plan allow for each procedure?	$160.00, $32.00, and $9.00
B.	How much did the health insurance plan disallow for each procedure? How will these disallowed amounts be posted on the patient account?	$20.00, $15.00, and $3.00. These will be posted as adjustments on the patient account.
C.	How much did the health insurance plan pay on each procedure?	$140.00, $32.00, and $9.00.

3. Post the payments using the Reference Number on the EOB. The posting date is 12/1/2009. Check your work with Figures WB8-13, WB8-14, and WB8-15.

4. When all payments have been posted, click on the *View Ledger* button and check your work with Figure WB8-16.

5. Close all windows and return to the Patient Selection screen for Posting Payments.

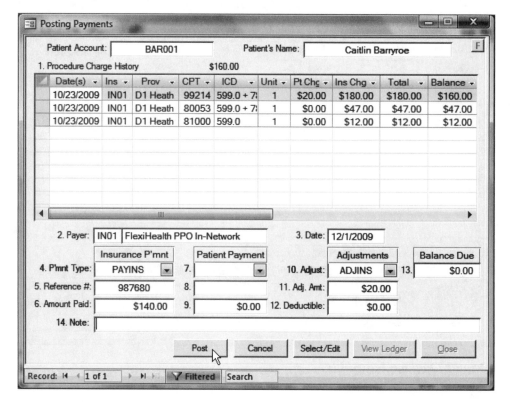

Figure WB8-13 *(Delmar/Cengage Learning)*

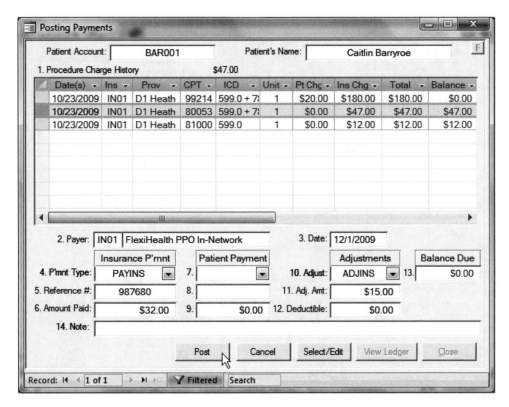

Figure WB8-14 *(Delmar/Cengage Learning)*

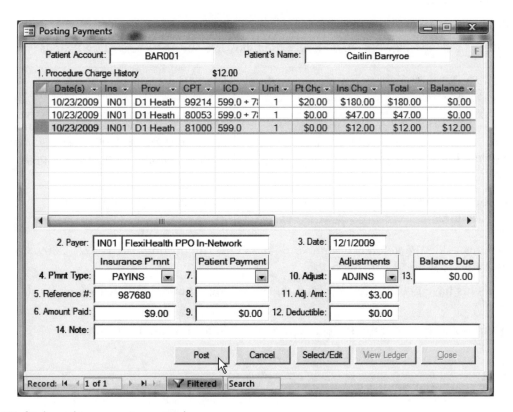

Figure WB8-15 *(Delmar/Cengage Learning)*

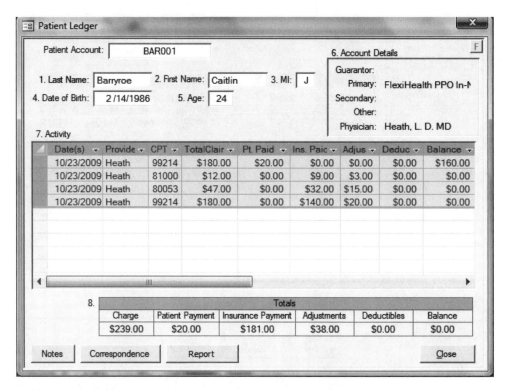

Figure WB8-16 *(Delmar/Cengage Learning)*

Patient Alan Shuman

1. Open the Posting screen for Patient Shuman.

2. Read the EOB from FlexiHealth PPO and answer the following questions regarding Patient Shuman's services.

A.	How much did the health insurance plan allow for each procedure?	$210.40, $22.00, and $71.00
B.	How much did the health insurance plan disallow for each procedure? How will these disallowed amounts be posted on the patient account?	$38.60, $0.00 (no discount, full amount approved) and $10.00. The discounts will be posted as adjustments on the patient account.
C.	How much did the health insurance plan pay on each procedure?	$190.40, $22.00, and $71.00

3. Post the payments using the Reference Number on the EOB. The posting date is 12/1/2009. Check your work with Figures WB8-17, WB8-18, and WB8-19.

4. When all payments have been posted, click on the *View Ledger* button and check your work with Figure WB8-20.

5. Close all windows and return to the Patient Selection screen for Posting Payments.

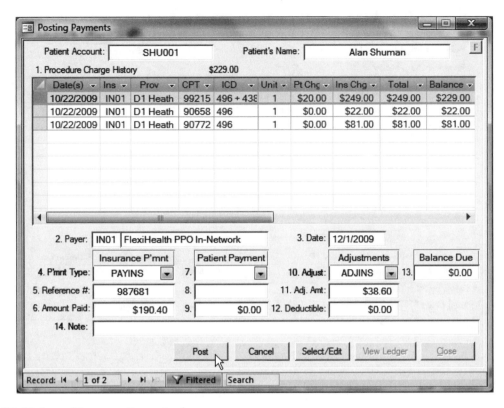

Figure WB8-17 *(Delmar/Cengage Learning)*

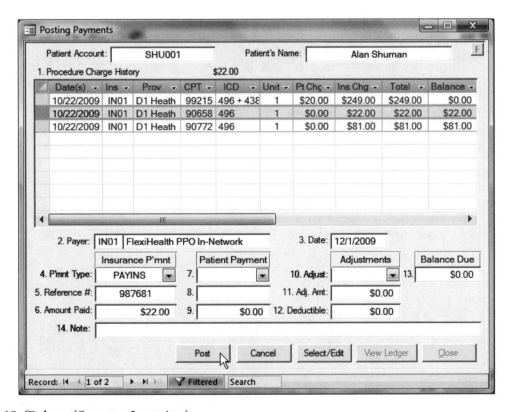

Figure WB8-18 *(Delmar/Cengage Learning)*

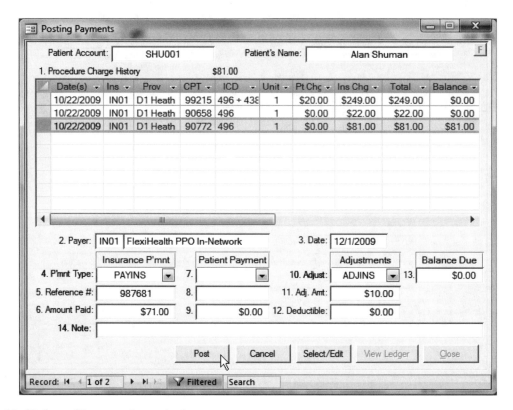

Figure WB8-19 *(Delmar/Cengage Learning)*

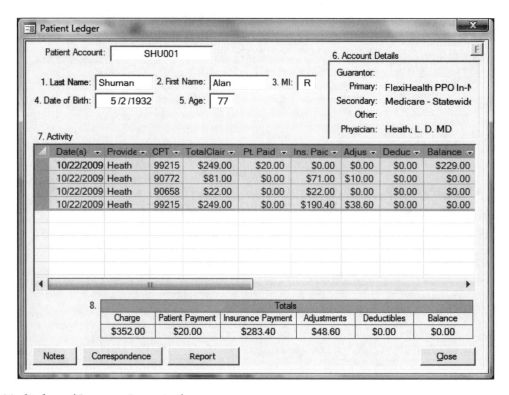

Figure WB8-20 *(Delmar/Cengage Learning)*

Critical Thinking: Patient Derek Wallace

1. Open the Posting screen for Patient Wallace.

2. Read the EOB from FlexiHealth PPO and post the payment, using date 12/01/2009 and the Reference Number as shown on the EOB.

3. Check your work with Figures WB8-21 and WB8-22.

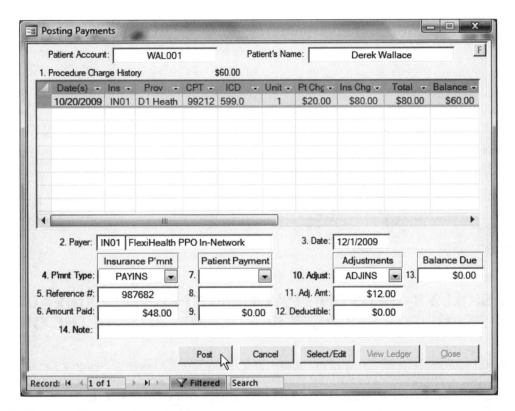

Figure WB8-21 *(Delmar/Cengage Learning)*

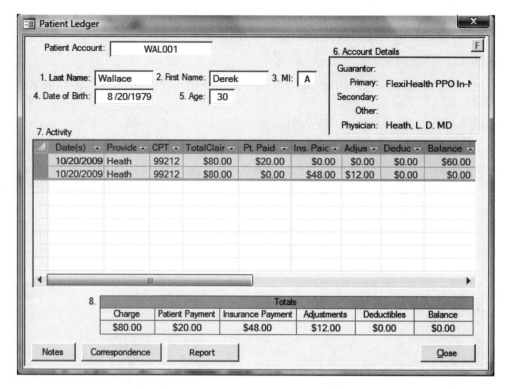

Figure WB8-22 *(Delmar/Cengage Learning)*

BUILDING SKILLS 8-4: POSTING PAYMENTS FROM FLEXIHEALTH PPO IN-NETWORK PLANS FOR SERVICES RENDERED OUTSIDE THE OFFICE

Instructions: It is common for health insurance plans to offer different coverage benefits for services rendered outside the physician's office, such as in hospitals, emergency rooms, or even facilities for diagnostic testing. These differences in benefits and what the patient may owe out-of-pocket can vary widely. Refer to the FlexiHealth PPO In-Network EOB shown on Source Document WB8-3 in the back of the workbook. For each of the patients below, post payments, adjustments, and other applicable details as shown for services that took place outside the office.

Patient Dennis Johnsen

1. Open the Posting screen for Patient Johnsen.

2. Read the EOB from FlexiHealth PPO and answer the following questions regarding Patient Johnsen's services.

A.	How much did the health insurance plan allow for the emergency room service?	$135.00
B.	How much did the health insurance plan disallow for the emergency room service? How will the disallowed amount be posted on the patient account?	$12.00. The discount will be posted as an adjustment on the patient account.
C.	How much did the health insurance plan pay on the emergency room service?	$0.00, the patient will need to pay $135.00, since that amount was applied to the deductible.

3. Post the adjustment and deductible as indicated on the EOB. The posting date is 12/1/2009. Check your work with Figures WB8-23 and the Patient Ledger on Figure WB8-24.

4. Close all windows and return to the Patient Selection screen for Posting Payments.

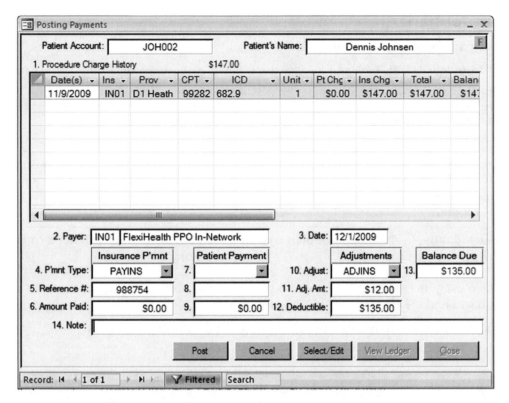

Figure WB8-23 *(Delmar/Cengage Learning)*

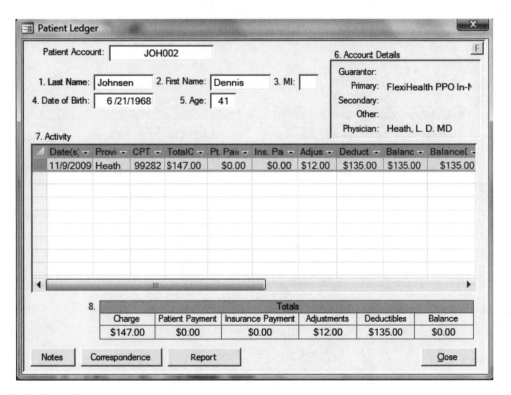

Figure WB8-24 *(Delmar/Cengage Learning)*

Patient Siran Jouharian

1. Open the Posting screen for Patient Jouharian.

2. Read the EOB from FlexiHealth PPO and answer the following questions regarding Patient Jouharian's services.

A.	How much did the health insurance plan allow for the emergency room service?	$135.00
B.	How much did the health insurance plan disallow for the emergency room service? How will the disallowed amount be posted on the patient account?	$12.00. The discount will be posted as adjustments on the patient account.
C.	How much did the health insurance plan pay on the emergency room service?	$108.00, the patient will need to pay $27.00 co-insurance.

3. Post the payment using the Reference Number on the EOB. The posting date is 12/1/2009. Check your work with Figure WB8-25 and the Patient Ledger in Figure WB8-26.

4. Close all windows and return to the Patient Selection screen for Posting Payments.

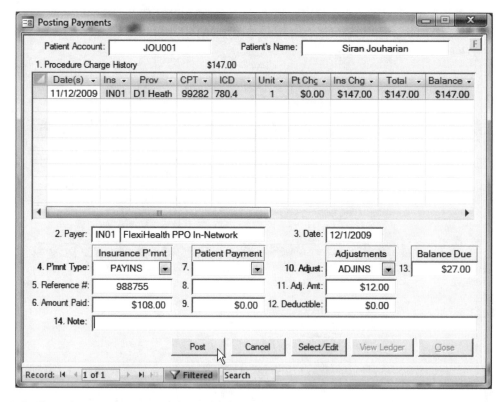

Figure WB8-25 *(Delmar/Cengage Learning)*

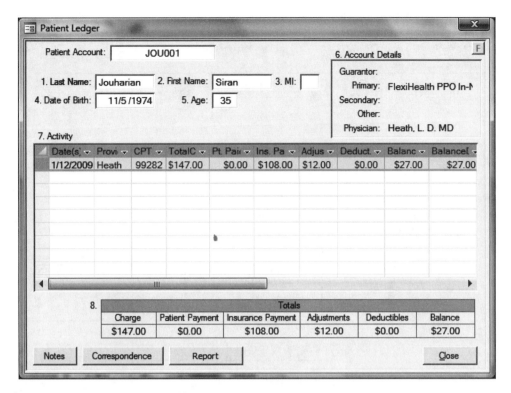

Figure WB8-26 *(Delmar/Cengage Learning)*

Critical Thinking: Patient Karen Ross

1. Open the Posting screen for Patient Ross.

2. Read the EOB from FlexiHealth PPO and post the details as indicated using the date 12/01/2009.

3. Check your work with Figures WB8-27 and WB8-28.

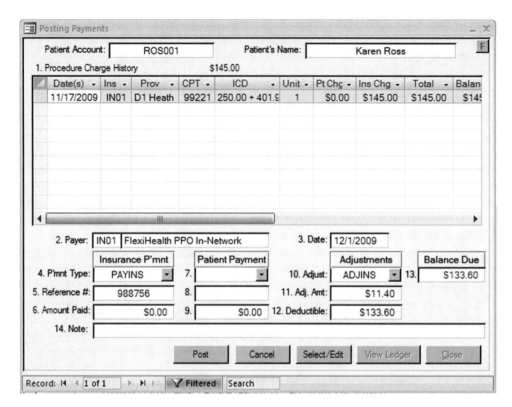

Figure WB8-27 *(Delmar/Cengage Learning)*

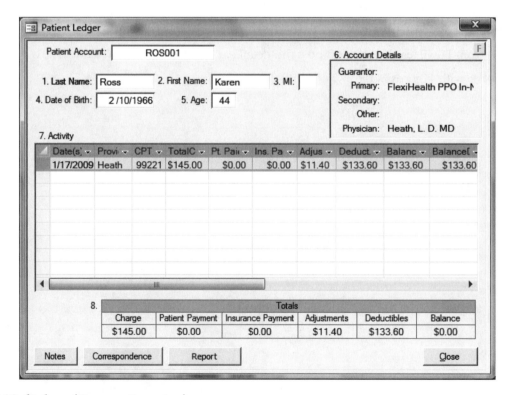

Figure WB8-28 *(Delmar/Cengage Learning)*

Critical Thinking: Patient Harold Engleman

1. Open the Posting screen for Patient Engleman.

 2. Refer to Source Document WB8-4 in the back of the workbook. Read the EOB from FlexiHealth PPO and answer the following questions.

A.	Which physician rendered services to the patient?	DJ Schwartz, MD
B.	Were the benefits in- or out-of-network?	Out-of-network, Dr. Schwartz does not participate.
C.	How much was allowed by the insurance plan?	$326.00 was allowed by the plan.
D.	How much was paid by the insurance plan?	$260.80 was paid by the insurance plan.
E.	How much will the patient pay, and why?	$97.20 is the patient responsibility. Code B indicates that the patient is responsible for the noncovered amount as well as the co-insurance ($32.00 + $65.20).

3. Post the payment using 12/01/2009 as the date and check your work with Figures WB8-29 and WB8-30. Use the note line if needed as a reminder of the posting details.

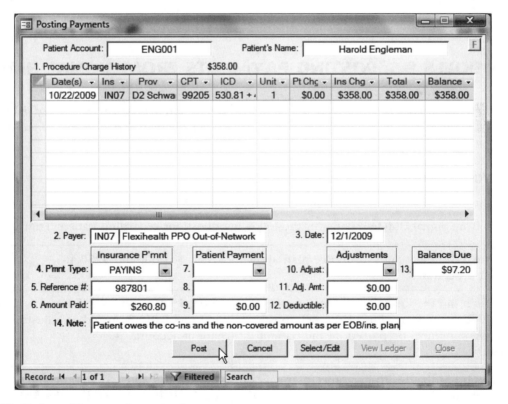

Figure WB8-29 *(Delmar/Cengage Learning)*

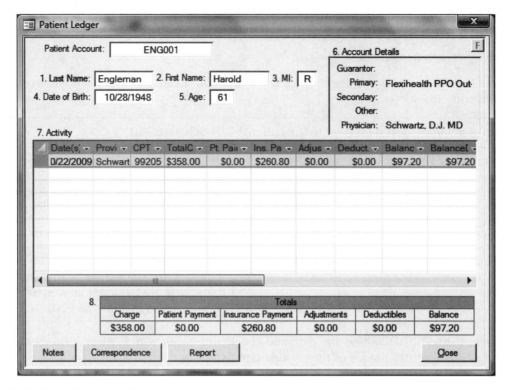

Figure WB8-30 *(Delmar/Cengage Learning)*

BUILDING SKILLS 8-5: POSTING PAYMENTS FROM SIGNAL HMO PLANS

Instructions: Refer to the Signal HMO EOB shown on Source Document WB8-5 in the back of the workbook. For each of the patients below, post payments, adjustments, and other applicable details as shown for services rendered.

Patient Devon Trimble

1. Open the Posting screen for Devon Trimble.

2. Read the EOB from Signal HMO and answer the following questions regarding Patient Trimble's services.

A.	How much did the health insurance plan allow for each procedure?	$7.97, $41.60, and $250.46
B.	How much did the health insurance plan disallow for each procedure? How will these disallowed amounts be posted on the patient account?	$1.03, $5.40, and $32.54. The disallowed amounts will be posted as adjustments on the patient account.
C.	How much did the health insurance plan pay on each procedure?	100% of the allowed amounts, $7.97, $41.60, and $240.46 ($250.46 less the $10.00 copay).

3. Post the payments and adjustments as indicated on the EOB. Use the posting date of 12/1/2009 and the Claim ID as the reference number. Check your work with Figures WB8-31, WB8-32, WB8-33, and WB8-34.

4. Close all windows and return to the Patient Selection screen for Posting Payments.

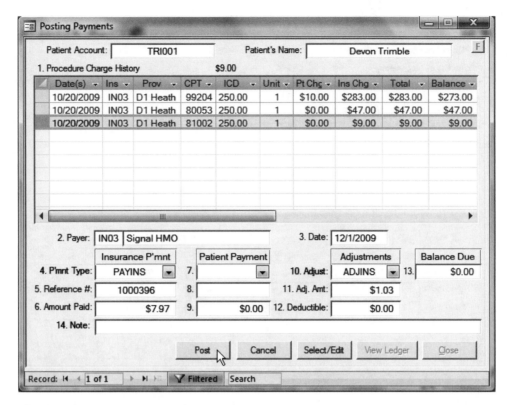

Figure WB8-31 *(Delmar/Cengage Learning)*

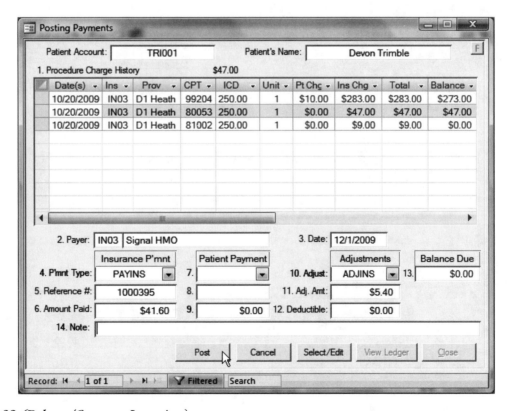

Figure WB8-32 *(Delmar/Cengage Learning)*

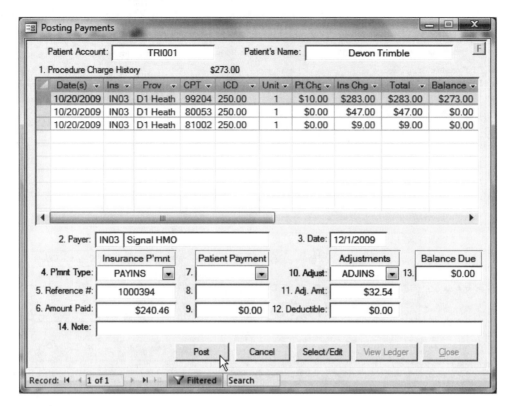

Figure WB8-33 *(Delmar/Cengage Learning)*

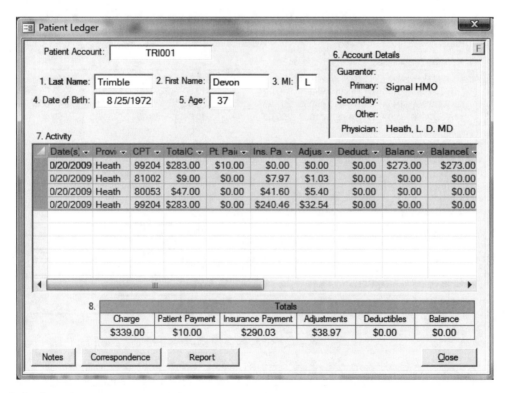

Figure WB8-34 *(Delmar/Cengage Learning)*

Patient Emery Camille

1. Open the Posting screen for Emery Camille.

2. Read the EOB from Signal HMO and answer the following questions regarding Patient Camille's services.

A.	How much did the health insurance plan allow for each procedure?	$9.74 and $98.24
B.	How much did the health insurance plan disallow for each procedure? How will these disallowed amounts be posted on the patient account?	$1.26 and $12.76. The disallowed amounts will be posted as adjustments on the patient account.
C.	How much did the health insurance plan pay on each procedure?	100% of the allowed amounts, $9.74 and $88.24 ($98.24 less the $10.00 patient copay).

3. Post the payments and adjustments as indicated on the EOB. Use the posting date of 12/1/2009 and the Claim ID as the reference number. Check your work with Figures WB8-35, WB8-36, and WB8-37.

4. Close all windows and return to the Patient Selection screen for Posting Payments.

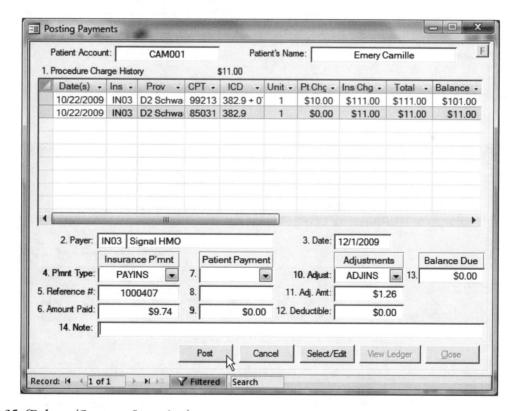

Figure WB8-35 *(Delmar/Cengage Learning)*

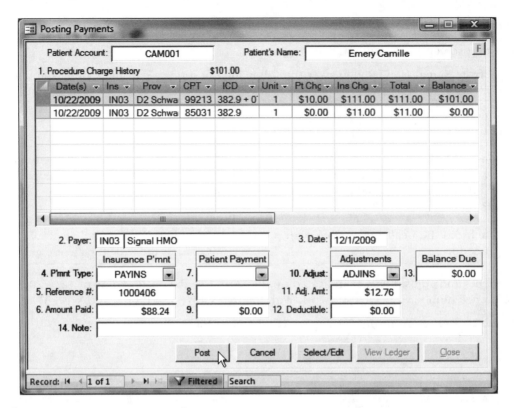

Figure WB8-36 *(Delmar/Cengage Learning)*

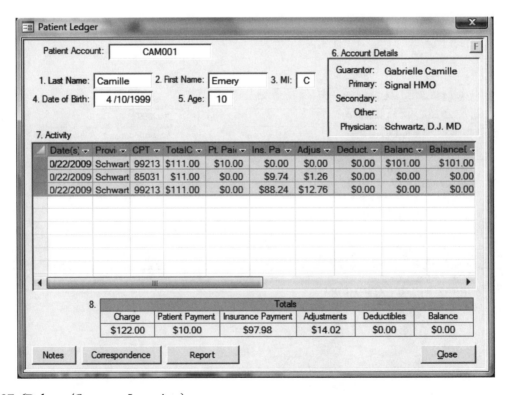

Figure WB8-37 *(Delmar/Cengage Learning)*

Critical Thinking: Patient Naomi Yamagata

1. Open the Posting screen for Patient Yamagata.

2. Read the EOB from Signal HMO (Source Document WB8-5) and post the payment, using date 12/01/2009 and the Claim Number as shown on the EOB.

3. Check your work with Figures WB8-38 and WB8-39.

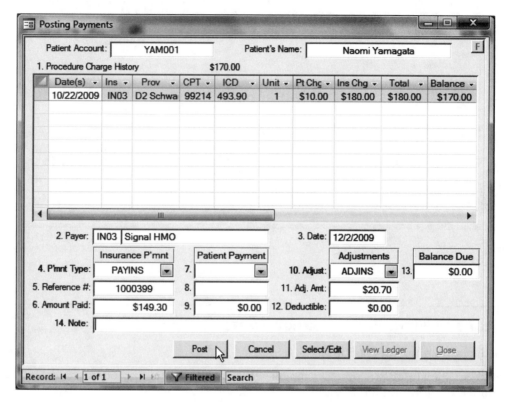

Figure WB8-38 *(Delmar/Cengage Learning)*

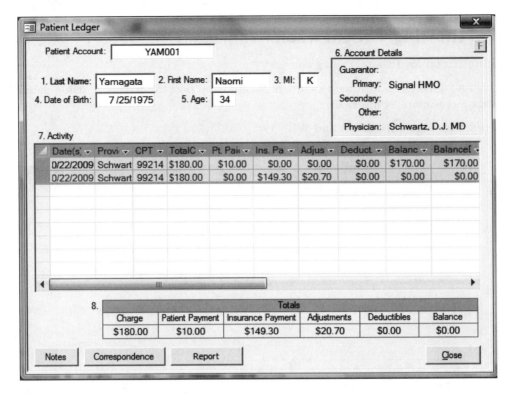

Figure WB8-39 *(Delmar/Cengage Learning)*

Critical Thinking: Patient Janet Souza

1. Open the Posting screen for Patient Souza.

2. Read the EOB from Signal HMO (Source Document WB8-5) and post the payment, using date 12/01/2009 and the Claim Number as shown on the EOB.

3. Check your work with Figures WB3-40 and WB3-41.

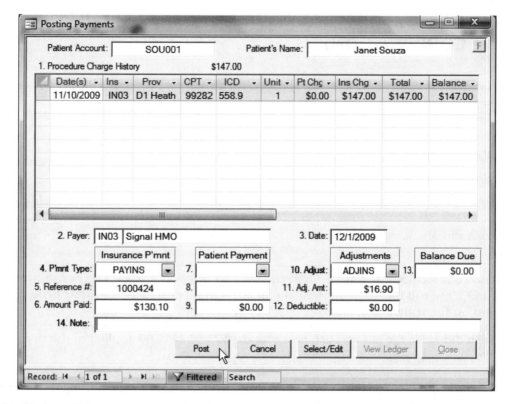

Figure WB8-40 *(Delmar/Cengage Learning)*

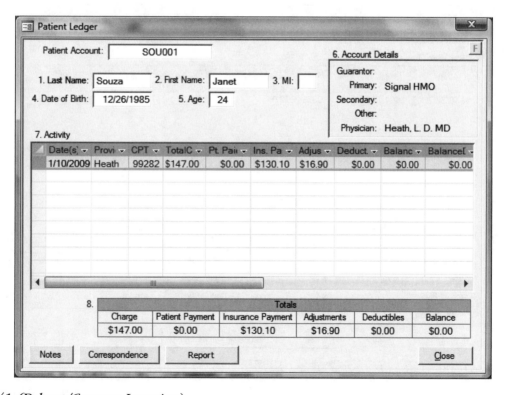

Figure WB8-41 *(Delmar/Cengage Learning)*

BUILDING SKILLS 8-6: POSTING PAYMENTS FROM MEDICARE (STATEWIDE CORPORATION)

Instructions: Refer to the Medicare Statewide Corporation RA shown on Source Document WB8-6 in the back of the workbook. For each of the patients below, post payments, adjustments, and other applicable details as shown for services rendered.

Patient Deanna Hartsfeld

1. Open the Posting screen for Patient Hartsfeld.

2. Read the RA from Medicare and answer the following questions regarding Patient Hartsfeld's services.

A.	How much did Medicare allow for each procedure?	$104.46 and $14.77
B.	How much did Medicare not allow for each procedure? How will these nonallowed amounts be posted on the patient account?	$75.54 and $32.23. The nonallowed amounts will be posted as adjustments on the patient account.
C.	How much did Medicare pay on each procedure?	$23.57 ($75.00 applied to the deductible) and $14.77.

3. Post the payments, deductible, and adjustments as indicated on the RA. Use the posting date of 12/1/2009 and the ICN as the reference number. Check your work with Figures WB8-42, WB8-43, and WB8-44.

4. Close all windows and return to the Patient Selection screen for Posting Payments.

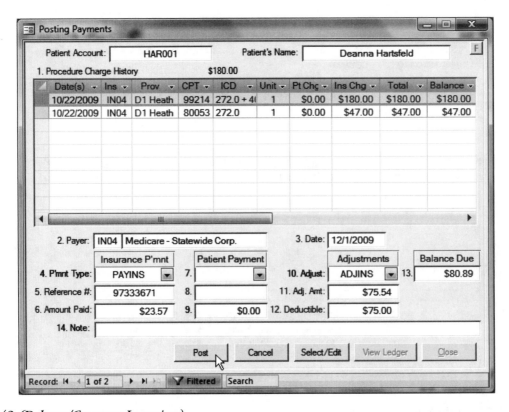

Figure WB8-42 *(Delmar/Cengage Learning)*

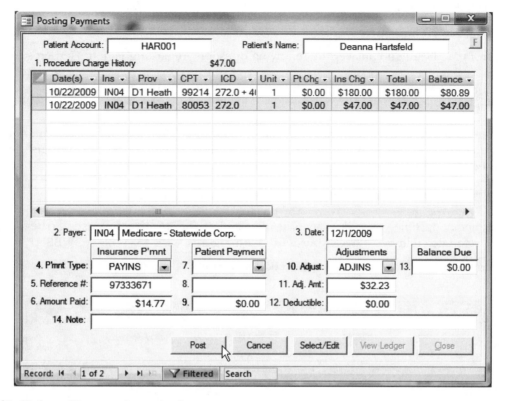

Figure WB8-43 *(Delmar/Cengage Learning)*

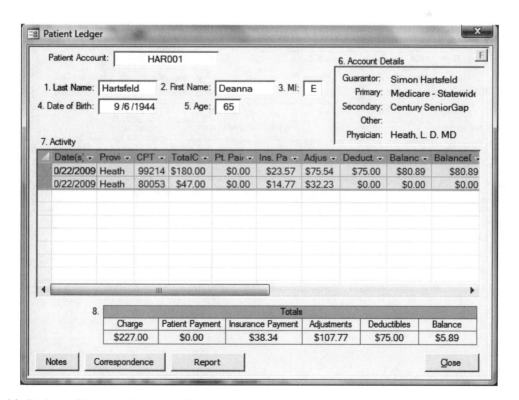

Figure WB8-44 *(Delmar/Cengage Learning)*

Patient Nancy Herbert

1. Open the Posting screen for Patient Herbert.

2. Read the RA from Medicare and answer the following questions regarding Patient Herbert's services.

A.	How much did Medicare allow for each procedure?	$140.31, $14.77, and $3.31.
B.	How much did Medicare not allow for each procedure? How will these nonallowed amounts be posted on the patient account?	$108.69, $32.23, and $3.69. The nonallowed amounts will be posted as adjustments on the patient account.
C.	How much did Medicare pay on each procedure?	$112.25, $14.77, and $3.31.

3. Post the payments, deductible, and adjustments as indicated on the RA. Use the posting date of 12/1/2009 and the ICN as the reference number. Check your work with Figures WB8-45, WB8-46, WB8-47, and WB8-48.

4. Close all windows and return to the Patient Selection screen for Posting Payments.

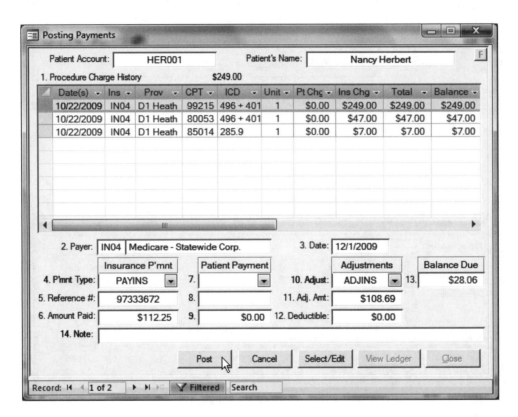

Figure WB8-45 *(Delmar/Cengage Learning)*

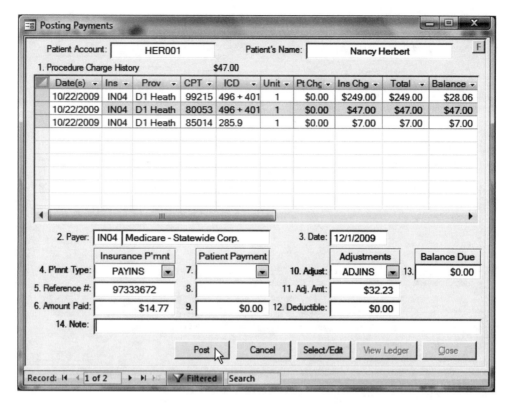

Figure WB8-46 *(Delmar/Cengage Learning)*

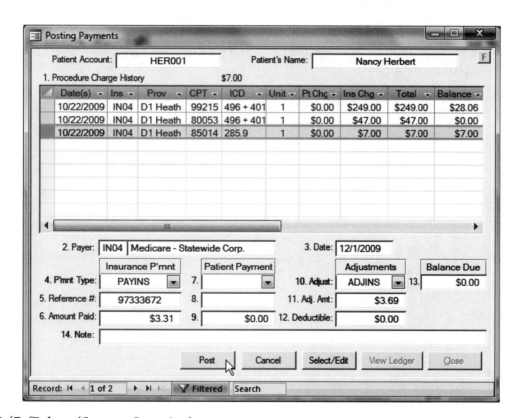

Figure WB8-47 *(Delmar/Cengage Learning)*

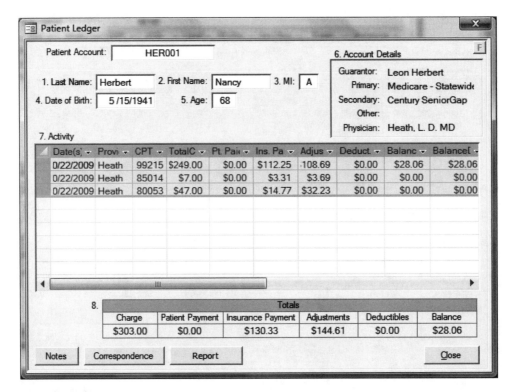

Figure WB8-48 *(Delmar/Cengage Learning)*

 Critical Thinking: Patient William Bernardo

1. Open the Posting screen for Patient Bernardo.

2. Read the RA from Medicare (Source Document WB8-7) and post the payment, using date 12/01/2009 and the ICN number as shown on the RA.

3. Check your work with Figures WB8-49 and WB8-50.

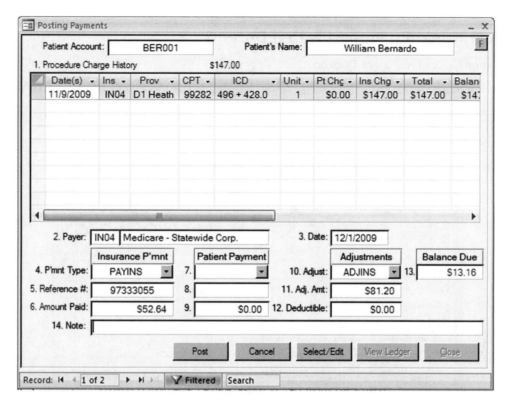

Figure WB8-49 *(Delmar/Cengage Learning)*

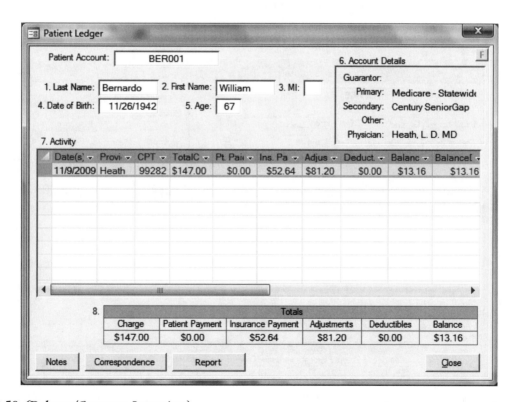

Figure WB8-50 *(Delmar/Cengage Learning)*

Critical Thinking: Patient Isabel Durand

1. Open the Posting screen for Patient Durand.

2. Read the RA from Medicare (Source Document WB8-7) and post the payment, using date 12/01/2009 and the ICN number as shown on the RA.

3. Check your work with Figures WB8-51 and WB8-52.

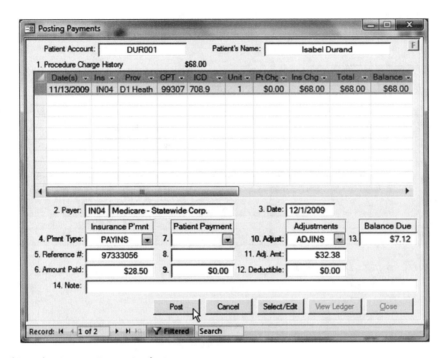

Figure WB8-51 *(Delmar/Cengage Learning)*

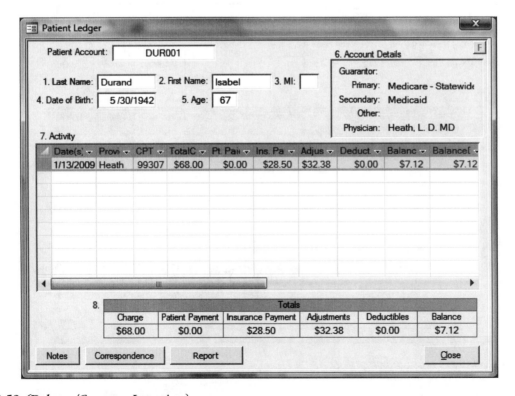

Figure WB8-52 *(Delmar/Cengage Learning)*

Critical Thinking: Patient Joel Royzin

1. Open the Posting screen for Patient Royzin.

2. Read the RA from Medicare (Source Document WB8-7) and post the payment, using date 12/01/2009 and the ICN number as shown on the RA.

3. Check your work with Figures WB8-53 and WB54.

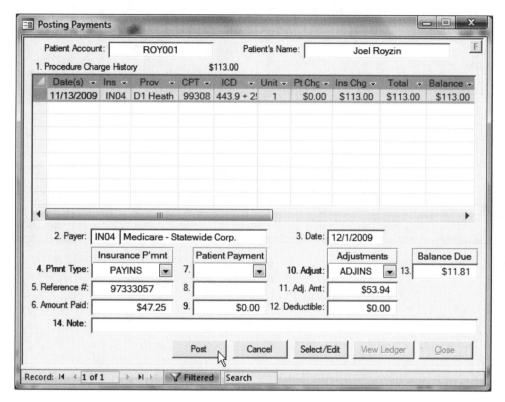

Figure WB8-53 *(Delmar/Cengage Learning)*

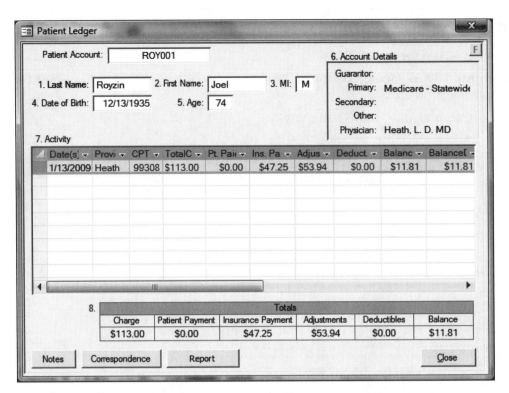

Figure WB8-54 *(Delmar/Cengage Learning)*

Critical Thinking: Patient Sean McKay

1. Open the Posting screen for Patient McKay.

2. Read the RA from Medicare (Source Document WB8-7) and post the payment, using date 12/01/2009 and the ICN number as shown on the RA.

3. Check your work with Figures WB8-55 and WB8-56.

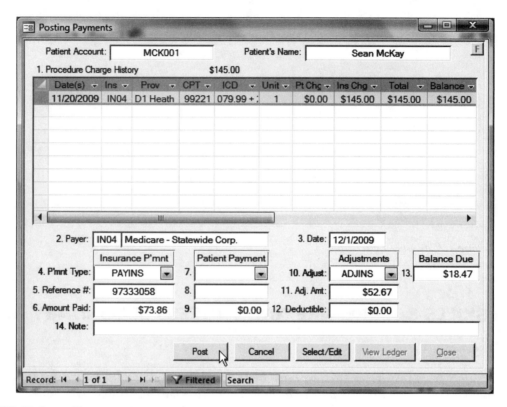

Figure WB8-55 *(Delmar/Cengage Learning)*

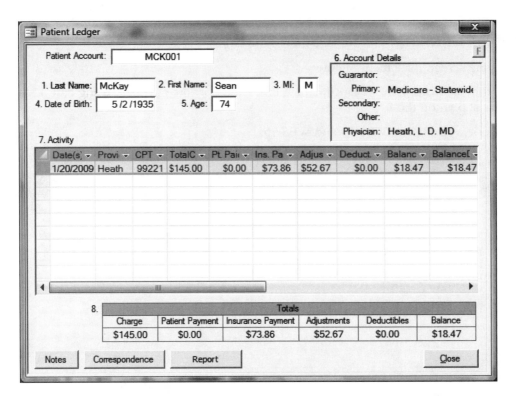

Figure WB8-56 *(Delmar/Cengage Learning)*

BUILDING SKILLS 8-7: PREPARE AND PROCESS SECONDARY MEDICAL CLAIMS

Instructions: Payments from insurance carriers have been posted on 12/01/2009 for claims submitted between 10/20/2009 through 11/30/2009. Prepare paper claim forms for the patients below who have secondary insurance plans as indicated.

William Bernardo – Century SeniorGap as Secondary Payer

1. Start MOSS and on the Main Menu, click on the *Insurance Billing* button. Select the following:
   A. Sort Order: Patient Name
   B. Provider: ALL
   C. Service Dates: 10/20/2009 through 11/30/2009
   D. Patient Number: Bernardo, William
   E. Transmit Type: Paper
   F. Billing Options: Check Secondary. Be sure the other two selections are unchecked.
   G. Payer: Century SeniorGap

2. Next, click on the *Prebilling Worksheet* button and check your screen with Figure WB8-57 before proceeding. Print the report by clicking on the *Printer* icon at the top left of the window. Close the window to return to the Claim Preparation window, and check your screen with Figure WB8-58.

3. Click on the *Generate Claims* button. After reviewing the CMS-1500 claim form for Patient Bernardo, click on the *Print Forms* button to print the claim for mailing. Compare your claim form to that in Figure WB8-59.

4. Attach the Prebilling Worksheet Report, Medicare Remittance Advice, and CMS-1500 claim form together and follow the directions of your instructor for turning in your work.

INSURANCE PREBILLING WORKSHEET
Student1

Century SeniorGap

Bernardo, William

Dates of Service	Diag Code	Proc Code	POS	Units	Dr	As	Bill Amt	Receipts	Net
11/9/2009	496	99282	23	1.00	D1	Y	$13.16	$0.00	$13.16
					Totals		$13.16	$0.00	$13.16
			TOTAL TO BE BILLED FOR Century SeniorGap						$13.16
Grand Total			*Grand Total*						$13.16

Figure WB8-57 *(Delmar/Cengage Learning)*

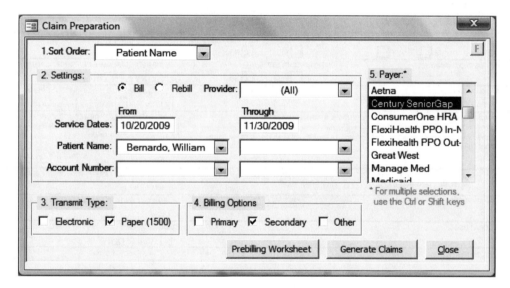

Figure WB8-58 *(Delmar/Cengage Learning)*

1500

TEST VERSION - NOT FOR OFFICIAL USE

HEALTH INSURANCE CLAIM FORM

APPROVED BY NATIONAL UNIFORM CLAIM COMMITTEE 08/05

Century SeniorGap
4500 Old Town Way
Lowville, NY 01453

<u>Student No: Student1</u>

| | PICA | | | | | | | | PICA | | |

1. MEDICARE	MEDICAID	TRICARE CHAMPUS	CHAMPVA	GROUP HEALTH PLAN	FECA BLK LUNG	OTHER	1a. INSURED'S I.D. NUMBER (FOR PROGRAM IN ITEM 1)
☐ (Medicare #)	☐ (Medicaid #)	☐ (Sponsor's SSN)	☐ (Member ID)	☒ (SSN or ID)	☐ (SSN)	☐ (ID)	999328652

2. PATIENT'S NAME (Last Name, First Name, Middle Initial)	3. PATIENT'S BIRTHDATE / SEX	4. INSURED'S NAME (Last Name, First Name, Middle Initial)
BERNARDO WILLIAM	11 | 26 | 1942 M ☒ F ☐	BERNARDO WILLIAM

5. PATIENT'S ADDRESS (No., Street)	6. PATIENT'S RELATIONSHIP TO INSURED	7. INSURED'S ADDRESS (No., Street)
13267 GRAVEL WAY	Self ☒ Spouse ☐ Child ☐ Other ☐	SAME

CITY	STATE	8. PATIENT STATUS	CITY	STATE
DOUGLASVILLE	NY	Single ☐ Married ☐ Other ☒		

ZIP CODE	TELEPHONE (include Area Code)		ZIP CODE	TELEPHONE (include Area Code)
01234	(123) 456-1129	Employed ☐ Full-Time Student ☐ Part-Time Student ☐		

9. OTHER INSURED'S NAME (Last Name, First Name, Mid. Initial)	10. IS PATIENT'S CONDITION RELATED TO:	11. INSURED'S POLICY GROUP OR FECA NUMBER
BERNARDO, WILLIAM		MG612

a. OTHER INSURED'S POLICY OR GROUP NUMBER	a. EMPLOYMENT (CURRENT OR PREVIOUS) ☐ YES ☒ NO	a. INSURED'S DATE OF BIRTH / SEX M ☐ F ☐

b. OTHER INSURED'S BIRTHDATE / SEX	b. AUTO ACCIDENT? PLACE (State) ☐ YES ☒ NO	b. EMPLOYER NAME OR SCHOOL NAME
11 | 26 | 1942 M ☐ F ☐		

c. EMPLOYER NAME OR SCHOOL NAME	c. OTHER ACCIDENT? ☐ YES ☒ NO	c. INSURANCE PLAN NAME OR PROGRAM NAME CENTURY SENIORGAP

d. INSURANCE PLAN NAME OR PROGRAM NAME MEDICARE - STATEWIDE CORP.	10d. RESERVED FOR LOCAL USE	d. IS THERE ANOTHER HEALTH BENEFIT PLAN ☒ YES ☐ NO If yes, return to and complete 9 a-d.

READ BACK OF FORM BEFORE COMPLETING & SIGNING THIS FORM.

12. PATIENT'S OR AUTHORIZED PERSONS'S SIGNATURE I authorize the release of any medical or other info necessary to process this claim. I also request payment of government benefits either to myself or the party who accepts assignment below.

SIGNED ___ SIGNATURE ON FILE ___ DATE ___ 11092009

13. PATIENT'S OR AUTHORIZED PERSONS'S SIGNATURE I authorize payment of medical benefits to the undersigned physician or supplier for services described below.

SIGNED ___ SIGNATURE ON FILE ___

14. DATE OF CURRENT: ◄ ILLNESS (First symptom) OR INJURY (Accident) OR PREGRACY (LMP)	15. IF PATIENT HAS HAD SAME ILLNESS, GIVE FIRST DATE	16. DATES PATIENT UNABLE TO WORK IN CURRENT OCCUPATION FROM TO

17. NAME OF REFERRING PROVIDER OR OTHER SOURCE	17a.	18. HOSPITALIZATION DATES RELATED TO CURRENT SERVICES
	17b NPI	FROM TO

19. RESERVED FOR LOCAL USE	20. OUTSIDE LAB? ☐ YES ☒ NO	$ CHARGES

21. DIAGNOSIS OR NATURE OF ILLNESS OR INJURY (RELATE ITEMS 1, 2, 3 OR 4 TO ITEM 24E BY LINE)	22. MEDICAID SUBMISSION CODE / ORIGINAL REF. NO.
1. 496 3.	23. PRIOR AUTHORIZATION NUMBER
2. 428.0 4.	

24. A. DATE(S) OF SERVICE From MM DD YY	To MM DD YY	B. Place of Service	C. EMG	D. PROCEDURES, SERVICES OR SUPPLIES (Explain Unusual Circumstances) CPT/HCPCS | MODIFIER	E. DIAGNOSIS POINTER	F. $ CHARGES	G. DAYS OR UNITS	H. EPSDT Family Plan	I. ID. QUAL	J. RENDERING PROVIDER ID#
1	11 09 2009		23		99282	1 2	13 16	1		NPI	999501
2										NPI	
3										NPI	
4										NPI	
5										NPI	
6										NPI	

25. FEDERAL TAX I.D. NUMBER SSN EIN	26. PATIENT'S ACCOUNT NO	27. ACCEPT ASSIGNMENT?	28. TOTAL CHARGE	29. AMOUNT PAID	30. BALANCE DUE
00-1234560 ☐ ☒	BER001	☒ YES ☐ NO	$ 13 16	$	$

31. SIGNATURE OF PHYSICIAN OR SUPPLIER INCLUDING DEGREES OR CREDENTIALS (I certify that the statements on the reverse apply to this bill and are made a part thereof.) 11092009 SIGNED L. D. HEATH, MD DAT	32. SERVICE FACILITY LOCATION INFORMATION COMMUNITY GENERAL HOSPITAL 4000 BRAND BLVD. DOUGLASVILLE, NY 01234 a. 9997794511 b.	33. BILLING PROVIDER INFO PH # (123) 456-7890 DOUGLASVILLE MEDICINE ASSOCIATES 5076 BRAND BLVD., SUITE 401 DOUGLASVILLE, NY 01234 a. 9995010111 b.

NUCC Instruction Manual available at: www.nucc.org

OMB APPROVAL PENDING

Figure WB8-59 *(Courtesy of the Centers for Medicare & Medicaid Services.)*

Deanna Hartsfeld – Century SeniorGap as Secondary Payer

1. Start MOSS and on the Main Menu, click on the *Insurance Billing* button. Select the following:
   A. Sort Order: Patient Name
   B. Provider: ALL
   C. Service Dates: 10/20/2009 through 11/30/2009
   D. Patient Number: Hartsfeld, Deanna
   E. Transmit Type: Paper
   F. Billing Options: Check Secondary. Be sure the other two selections are unchecked.
   G. Payer: Century SeniorGap

2. Next, click on the *Prebilling Worksheet* button and check your screen with Figure WB8-60 before proceeding. Print the report by clicking on the *Printer* icon at the top left of the window. Close the window to return to the Claim Preparation window, and check your screen with Figure WB8-61.

3. Click on the *Generate Claims* button. After reviewing the CMS-1500 claim form for Patient Hartsfeld, click on the *Print Forms* button to print the claim for mailing. Compare your claim form to that in Figure WB8-62.

4. Attach the Prebilling Worksheet Report, Medicare Remittance Advice, and CMS-1500 claim form together and follow the directions of your instructor for turning in your work.

INSURANCE PREBILLING WORKSHEET
Student1

Dates of Service	Diag Code	Proc Code	POS	Units	Dr	As	Bill Amt	Receipts	Net
Century SeniorGap									
Hartsfeld, Deanna									
10/22/2009	272.0	99214	11	1.00	D1	Y	$80.89	$0.00	$80.89
				Totals			$80.89	$0.00	$80.89
		TOTAL TO BE BILLED FOR Century SeniorGap							$80.89
Grand Total			**Grand Total**						$80.89

Figure WB8-60 *(Delmar/Cengage Learning)*

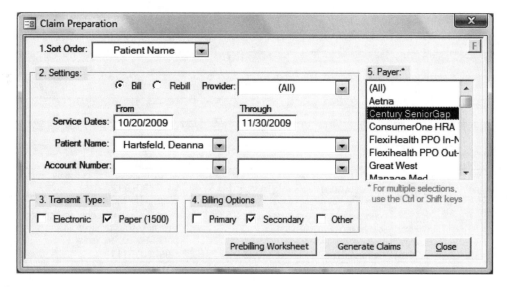

Figure WB8-61 *(Delmar/Cengage Learning)*

Figure WB8-62 *(Courtesy of the Centers for Medicare & Medicaid Services.)*

Critical Thinking: Nancy Herbert – Century SeniorGap as Secondary Payer

1. Prepare a paper claim form to bill the secondary insurance plan, Century SeniorGap, for services provided for Nancy Herbert on 10/22/2009.

2. Attach the Prebilling Worksheet Report, Medicare Remittance Advice, and CMS-1500 claim form together and follow the directions of your instructor for turning in your work.

3. Check your work with Figure WB8-63.

1500	**TEST VERSION - NOT FOR OFFICIAL USE**

HEALTH INSURANCE CLAIM FORM
APPROVED BY NATIONAL UNIFORM CLAIM COMMITTEE 08/05

Century SeniorGap
4500 Old Town Way
Lowville, NY 01453

☐☐☐ PICA   PICA ☐☐☐

1. MEDICARE ☐(Medicare #) MEDICAID ☐(Medicaid #) TRICARE CHAMPUS ☐(Sponsor's SSN) CHAMPVA ☐(Member ID) GROUP HEALTH PLAN ☒(SSN or ID) FECA BLK LUNG ☐(SSN) OTHER ☐(ID)	1a. INSURED'S I.D. NUMBER (FOR PROGRAM IN ITEM 1) 999181125

2. PATIENT'S NAME (Last Name, First Name, Middle Initial) HERBERT NANCY A	3. PATIENT'S BIRTHDATE 05 | 15 | 1941 SEX M ☐ F ☒	4. INSURED'S NAME (Last Name, First Name, Middle Initial) HERBERT NANCY A

5. PATIENT'S ADDRESS (No., Street) 9768 GOLDEN AVE	6. PATIENT'S RELATIONSHIP TO INSURED Self ☒ Spouse ☐ Child ☐ Other ☐	7. INSURED'S ADDRESS (No., Street) SAME
CITY DOUGLASVILLE / STATE NY	8. PATIENT STATUS Single ☐ Married ☒ Other ☐	CITY / STATE
ZIP CODE 01235 TELEPHONE (include Area Code) (123) 427-1133	Employed ☐ Full-Time Student ☐ Part-Time Student ☐	ZIP CODE TELEPHONE (include Area Code)

9. OTHER INSURED'S NAME (Last Name, First Name, Mid. Initial) HERBERT, NANCY A.	10. IS PATIENT'S CONDITION RELATED TO:	11. INSURED'S POLICY GROUP OR FECA NUMBER MG5133
a. OTHER INSURED'S POLICY OR GROUP NUMBER	a. EMPLOYMENT (CURRENT OR PREVIOUS) ☐YES ☒NO	a. INSURED'S DATE OF BIRTH SEX M ☐ F ☐
b. OTHER INSURED'S BIRTHDATE 05 15 1941 SEX M ☒ F ☐	b. AUTO ACCIDENT? ☐YES ☒NO PLACE (State)	b. EMPLOYER NAME OR SCHOOL NAME
c. EMPLOYER NAME OR SCHOOL NAME	c. OTHER ACCIDENT? ☐YES ☒NO	c. INSURANCE PLAN NAME OR PROGRAM NAME CENTURY SENIORGAP
d. INSURANCE PLAN NAME OR PROGRAM NAME MEDICARE - STATEWIDE CORP.	10d. RESERVED FOR LOCAL USE	d. IS THERE ANOTHER HEALTH BENEFIT PLAN ☒ YES ☐ NO If yes, return to and complete 9 a-d.

READ BACK OF FORM BEFORE COMPLETING & SIGNING THIS FORM.

12. PATIENT'S OR AUTHORIZED PERSONS'S SIGNATURE I authorize the release of any medical or other info necessary to process this claim. I also request payment of government benefits either to myself or the party who accepts assignment below. SIGNED _____ SIGNATURE ON FILE _____ DATE 10222009	13. PATIENT'S OR AUTHORIZED PERSONS'S SIGNATURE I authorize payment of medical benefits to the undersigned physician or supplier for services described below. SIGNED _____ SIGNATURE ON FILE _____

14. DATE OF CURRENT: ◄ ILLNESS (First symptom) OR INJURY (Accident) OR PREGRACY (LMP)	15. IF PATIENT HAS HAD SAME ILLNESS, GIVE FIRST DATE	16. DATES PATIENT UNABLE TO WORK IN CURRENT OCCUPATION FROM TO
17. NAME OF REFERRING PROVIDER OR OTHER SOURCE	17a. 17b. NPI	18. HOSPITALIZATION DATES RELATED TO CURRENT SERVICES FROM TO
19. RESERVED FOR LOCAL USE		20. OUTSIDE LAB? ☐YES ☒NO $ CHARGES

21. DIAGNOSIS OR NATURE OF ILLNESS OR INJURY (RELATE ITEMS 1, 2, 3 OR 4 TO ITEM 24E BY LINE 1. 496 3. 285.9 2. 401.9 4.	22. MEDICAID SUBMISSION CODE ORIGINAL REF. NO.
	23. PRIOR AUTHORIZATION NUMBER 01D0886230

24. A DATE(S) OF SERVICE			B. Place of Service	C. EMG	D. PROCEDURES, SERVICES OR SUPPLIES (Explain Unusual Circumstances) CPT/HCPCS MODIFIER	E. DIAGNOSIS POINTER	F. $ CHARGES	G. DAYS OR UNITS	H. EPSDT Family Plan	I. ID. QUAL	J. RENDERING PROVIDER ID#
From MM DD YY	To MM DD YY										
1	10 22 2009		11		99215	1 2 3	28 06	1		NPI	999501
2										NPI	
3										NPI	
4										NPI	
5										NPI	
6										NPI	

25. FEDERAL TAX I.D. NUMBER SSN EIN 00-1234560 ☐ ☒	26. PATIENT'S ACCOUNT NO HER001	27. ACCEPT ASSIGNMENT? ☒YES ☐NO	28. TOTAL CHARGE $ 28 06	29. AMOUNT PAID $	30. BALANCE DUE $

31. SIGNATURE OF PHYSICIAN OR SUPPLIER INCLUDING DEGREES OR CREDENTIALS (I certify that the statements on the reverse apply to this bill and are made a part thereof.) 10222009 SIGNED L. D. HEATH, MD DAT	32. SERVICE FACILITY LOCATION INFORMATION DOUGLASVILLE MEDICINE ASSOCIATES 5076 BRAND BLVD., SUITE 401 DOUGLASVILLE, NY 01234 a. 9995010111 b.	33. BILLING PROVIDER INFO PH # (123) 456-7890 DOUGLASVILLE MEDICINE ASSOCIATES 5076 BRAND BLVD., SUITE 401 DOUGLASVILLE, NY 01234 a. 9995010111 b.

NUCC Instruction Manual available at: www.nucc.org   OMB APPROVAL PENDING

Figure WB8-63 *(Courtesy of the Centers for Medicare & Medicaid Services.)*

BUILDING SKILLS 8-8: REVIEW OF COORDINATION OF BENEFITS (COB) RULES

1. A married couple, Sylvia and Michael, are each covered by large-group health plans through their employers. Sylvia has a Blue Cross/Blue Shield plan, and Michael has a Cigna PPO plan. In addition, they are dependents on each other's policies. When receiving medical services, which plan is primary for Sylvia? Which is primary for Michael? Explain your answer.

_____

_____

_____

_____

_____

2. George is still working and has a large-group health plan through his employer. He also was covered by Medicare after he turned 65 years of age. Which insurance is billed as primary for George's medical charges? Explain your answer.

_____

_____

_____

_____

_____

3. Paulina has a large-group health plan through her employer, and her husband, Jack, is a dependent on the plan. Jack has been retired for several years and has Original Medicare. Which plan is primary for Paulina when she receives medical services? Which is primary for Jack? Explain your answer.

_____

_____

_____

_____

_____

4. Joyce is 66 years old and has been working with the same company for 15 years part-time. Because of her part-time status, she is not entitled to benefits with her employer's group plan. She has Medicare coverage and opted for a Medicare Advantage Plan in her area. How will her medical services be billed?

_____

_____

_____

_____

_____

5. The Connor family consists of David and Cynthia, a married couple, and their three children, twins Becky and Beth and older brother Brandon. Both parents have medical insurance through their respective employers. Each spouse and children are dependents on both plans. If David was born on March 24, 1972, and Cynthia was born on January 16, 1975, which policy is primary for the children if one of them receives services? Which policy is primary for the parents if one of them receives services? Explain your answer.

_____

_____

_____

_____

_____

6. Ralph has Medicare and is working at a print shop with 18 employees. He has a group plan with this employer. Which insurance is primary for services? Explain your answer.

_____

_____

_____

_____

_____

7. Linda is involved in an automobile accident and requires medical services. She has Medicare, and the accident is covered under no-fault insurance as well. Which policy is primary for the medical services related to the automobile accident? Explain your answer.

_____

_____

_____

_____

_____

U N I T **9**

Patient Billing and Collections

BUILDING SKILLS 9-1: FINANCIAL DISCUSSIONS WITH PATIENTS REVIEW

1. Explain how using direct language to collect payments has a more or less successful outcome in obtaining money from patients at the time of service.

   _____

   _____

   _____

   _____

   _____

2. Discuss some alternatives that can be offered to a patient who is resistant to making a payment on a large balance due.

   _____

   _____

   _____

   _____

   _____

3. What kind of financial information should be discussed with new patients when scheduling appointments, or when they visit the office for the first time for service?

   _____

   _____

   _____

   _____

   _____

4. Which techniques can medical staff use to avoid an impersonal exchange, or giving the impression that ability to pay is more a priority than the patient's health concerns?

_____

_____

_____

_____

_____

5. Describe techniques medical staff can use to avoid or manage confrontations with angry patients.

_____

_____

_____

_____

_____

BUILDING SKILLS 9-2: ROLE-PLAY PRACTICE: FINANCIAL DISCUSSIONS WITH PATIENTS

Instructions: Practice the dialogue below for each case study with a classmate or study partner.

Case Study 1: Mr. Garner

Mr. Garner has returned to the front desk after visiting the doctor. He is ready to check out, but has a balance due on his account. Practice the dialogue below with a classmate or study partner.

Front-desk staff: Mr. Garner, the doctor has indicated that she would like to see you again in two weeks. Would you like to make that appointment today?

Patient: No, I'll have to check my calendar and call you back.

Front-desk staff: That would be fine. Our records show that you have a balance of $230.00 on your account for a deductible applied at the first of the year. Would you like to pay with a check or cash?

Patient: I'm not sure I have to pay that; I think my wife's insurance should pay for that.

Front-desk staff: It shows here that our billing staff billed the secondary insurance after payment was received; however, the payment was denied. Would you like to speak to our billing department?

Patient: No, I really need to get going; I have to go back to work right away.

Front-desk staff: Mr. Garner, we can accept a credit card payment today so that this balance is taken care of, and I can have the billing department follow up with you regarding your secondary insurance. Is that acceptable?

Patient: Ok, thank you. Please have them contact my wife so she can look into this.

Front-desk staff: I will prepare a message for them. Please give me your wife's contact information, and we will take care of this today. Thank you for your payment.

Case Study 2: Diane Valente

Diane Valente has arrived for her visit with the doctor. Her insurance plan has changed, and she now has a $50.00 copayment for each visit. Practice the dialogue below with a classmate or study partner.

Front-desk staff: Good morning (or afternoon), Diane! How are you today? Please sign in and I will be with you in a moment.

Patient: Hello! Thank you. I'm not feeling too well today, but I hope the doctor can do something about that.

Front-desk staff: Oh, I'm sorry to hear you're under the weather. Yes, hopefully the doctor will be able to help you today! Diane, has anything changed with your insurance, address, or phone number since you last visited us? Our records show that you previously had United Healthcare insurance. Is that still your plan?

Patient: Oh, thanks for reminding me. No, our insurance changed in January of this year. We now have a PPO through Anthem.

Front-desk staff: If you have your card today, I'd like to make a copy for our records.

Patient: Yes, I have it here. It's a new plan from my husband Jack's employer. They seem to change coverage all the time!

Front-desk staff: Thank you, Diane. I see on the card that you have a $50.00 copayment for office visits with the doctor. Will you be paying with a check or credit card today for that?

Patient: I can pay with a credit card.

Front-desk staff: Very well. Let me take your credit card, and I will return everything to you in a moment. Thank you for your payment.

Case Study 3: Hector Diaz

Hector Diaz is checking out after getting one of his special biweekly antibody injections. He has a balance due for co-insurance portions for the injections that have accumulated over the past several weeks. Practice the dialogue below with a classmate or study partner.

Front-desk staff: Hi, Hector. Before you leave today, I need to collect some co-insurance portions for your injections. We have received payments from your insurance company towards your injections, but the remainder of $450.00 is due for the patient cost-share portion. Will you be paying today with a check or credit card?

Patient: That is a lot of money. How come so much today?

Front-desk staff: Your insurance covers 80 percent of your injection costs, but because you come in every two weeks, the billing is done very often and close together as services are completed. That is the reason you tend to have amounts pending, and then due, as they get paid by the insurance. These accumulate over a short amount of time.

Patient: I see. Well, these injections sure are helping me, but that's more than I can pay at one time today.

Front-desk staff: We accept credit cards, if you'd like to use that method of payment. Are you able to pay the entire amount today with a credit card?

Patient: No, I don't think I can use my credit cards for medical bills right now. Since these injections are going to continue for a long time, can we do something else? I don't want to have large balances on the credit cards. I have a strict budget since I retired last year. It's been hard to make ends meet.

Front-desk staff: I can certainly suggest a payment plan so that you can make regular payments for these treatments directly to the medical office. I can have our billing department arrange that for you and prepare an agreement. If I could collect at least one-half, or $225.00 today, that would bring your account up to date and assist in setting up a plan. Can you pay with a check for that amount today?

Patient: Yes, let's do that, and I can set up a payment plan like you said.

Front-desk staff: Very well. Thank you for your payment of $225.00 today, and I will make sure the billing department contacts you to set up a payment plan for the balance, as well as future cost-share portions for your injections.

Patient: Thank you very much.

BUILDING SKILLS 9-3: GENERATE REPORTS FOR EVALUATING PATIENT ACCOUNTS

Instructions: Generate a report that provides data regarding insurance billing and payments. After printing the report, identify the patients from the Workbook exercises to prepare patient statements.

1. From the Main Menu in MOSS, click on the *Report Generation* button on the Main Menu.

2. The Reports Panel displays five different reports that come standard with MOSS. Select the Billing and Payment Report.

3. Next, enter the start date for the report. For this simulation, enter 10/20/2009. Next, enter an end date of 11/30/2009 for the report.

4. A report with the heading Billing & Payments opens. Be sure to maximize the window so the entire page can be viewed. There are several pages to this report. Print this report by clicking on the *Printer* icon at the top left corner of the window. Your own student number or log in name should appear at the top of the report for easy identification.

5. Using the hard copy of the report you just printed, locate and highlight the patients from the Workbook exercises. For each patient, note whether there is a balance due and the amount, a secondary insurance pending payment and the amount, or if there is a zero balance on the account. Use the Patient Ledger in MOSS to verify information as needed.

   (Hint: Workbook patients on this report are: Barryroe, Bernardo, Bradley, Camille, Durand, Engleman, Hartsfeld, Hedensten, Herbert, Johnsen, Jouharian, McKay, Rizzo, Ross, Royzin, Sheridan, Shuman, Souza, Trimble, Wallace, and Yamagata. Other patients appearing on this report are patients from the textbook exercises, or patients created by your instructor, and will be excluded from the following simulation exercises.)

6. Next, in preparation for creating patient statements, group the patients together by name as indicated below, and then suggest a dunning message to be added to statements:

   a. Patient accounts where Medicare has paid, and secondary insurance payment is still pending

   b. Patient accounts where Medicare has paid, and the patient owes a remainder balance

   c. Patient accounts where the primary private insurance has paid, and the patient owes a remainder balance

   d. Patient accounts where a deductible has been applied, and is now due from the patient

   e. Patient accounts with ConsumerONE HRA plans that owe a balance and reason

7. Follow the directions of your instructor for turning in or retaining your report and data results. Be sure to have the report ready for the next Building Skills exercise for preparing patient statements.

BUILDING SKILLS 9-4: PREPARE PATIENT STATEMENTS FOR MEDICARE PATIENTS WITH PENDING PAYMENTS FROM SECONDARY INSURANCE

Instructions: Using the Billing and Payments report from Building Skills 9-3 and data obtained from each of the Workbook patients, prepare patient statements with dunning messages. When completed, the statements are to be printed for mailing.

Patient Account: William Bernardo

1. From the Main Menu in MOSS, click on the *Patient Billing* button on the Main Menu. This opens the Patient Billing window, ready to input settings.

2. Select the following settings as shown in Figure WB9-1:

   a. Field 1, Remainder Statement. Click on this choice to produce statements that show only the remaining balances due.

b. Field 2, Provider. Drop down the selections and click on *All,* for all physicians.

c. Field 3, Settings. In the From/To fields for the service dates, enter 10/20/2009 through 11/30/2009.

d. Field 3, Settings. In the Patient Name field, drop down the selections and click on patient account *Bernardo*.

e. Field 4, Process Type. The Preview on Screen Selection should be checked.

f. There is no global message for Field 5. Proceed to Field 6, Account Dunning Message. Type in the dunning message you have prepared for this patient in Field 6.

g. Next, in Field 7, select *patient Bernardo* from the list so that the dunning message will be added to the statement.

h. Check your Patient Billing screen with Figure WB9-1 for accuracy.

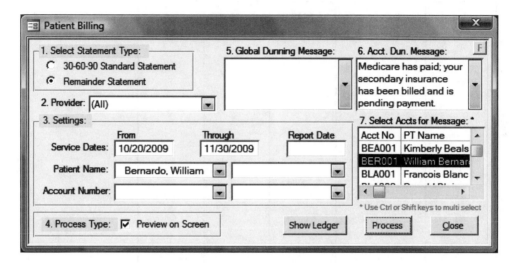

Figure WB9-1 *(Delmar/Cengage Learning)*

3. Click on the *Process* button to create the statement. Review the statement on the Preview screen and check for accuracy. Note the patient's name at the top of the statement and the statement information. Check the bottom of each statement and note the dunning message. Check your work with Figure WB9-2.

4. Next, print the statements for your records, or check if they are to be turned in to your instructor.

Douglasville Medicine Associates
5076 Brand Blvd., Suite 401
Douglasville, NY 01234
Ph: (123) 456-7890
Fax: (123) 456-7891
Email: admin@dfma.com
Website: www.dfma.com

REMAINDER STATEMENT

WILLIAM BERNARDO
13267 Gravel Way
Douglasville, NY 01234

Date:
Account No: BER001
Student No: Student1

Date	Patient	Procedure	Total Charges	Patient Co-Pay	Insurance Payment	Adjust-ments	Deduct-ibles	Current Balance
09-Nov-09	William Bernardo	99282	$147.00	$0.00	$52.64	$81.20	$0	$26.32
		Totals:	$147.00	$0.00	$52.64	$81.20	$0	$26.32

Please make checks payable to:
Douglasville Medicine Associates

BALANCE DUE	$26.32

Important Note:
Medicare has paid; your secondary insurance has been billed and is pending payment.

Figure WB9-2 *(Delmar/Cengage Learning)*

Patient Account: Isabel Durand

1. From the Main Menu in MOSS, click on the *Patient Billing* button on the Main Menu. This opens the Patient Billing window, ready to input settings.

2. Select the following settings as shown below:

   a. Field 1, Remainder Statement. Click on this choice to produce statements that show only the remaining balances due.

   b. Field 2, Provider. Drop down the selections and click on *All*, for all physicians.

   c. Field 3, Settings. In the From/To fields for the service dates, enter 10/20/2009 through 11/30/2009.

   d. Field 3, Settings. In the Patient Name field, drop down the selections and click on patient account *Durand*.

   e. Field 4, Process Type. The Preview on Screen Selection should be checked.

   f. There is no global message for Field 5. Proceed to Field 6, Account Dunning Message. Type in the dunning message you have prepared for this patient in Field 6.

   g. Next, in Field 7, select *patient Durand* from the list so that the dunning message will be added to the statement.

   h. Check your Patient Billing screen with Figure WB9-3 for accuracy.

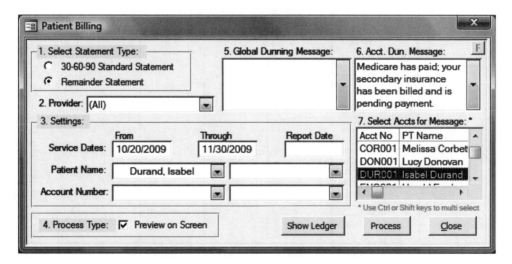

Figure WB9-3 *(Delmar/Cengage Learning)*

3. Click on the *Process* button to create the statement. Review the statement on the Preview screen and check for accuracy. Note the patient's name at the top of the statement and the statement information. Check the bottom of each statement and note the dunning message. Check your work with Figure WB9-4.

4. Next, print the statement for your records, or check if they are to be turned in to your instructor.

Douglasville Medicine Associates
5076 Brand Blvd., Suite 401
Douglasville, NY 01234
Ph: (123) 456-7890
Fax: (123) 456-7891
Email: admin@dfma.com
Website: www.dfma.com

REMAINDER STATEMENT

ISABEL DURAND
15721 Spring Way
Douglasville, NY 01234

Date:
Account No: DUR001
Student No: Student1

Date	Patient	Procedure	Total Charges	Patient Co-Pay	Insurance Payment	Adjust-ments	Deduct-ibles	Current Balance
13-Nov-09	Isabel Durand	99307	$68.00	$0.00	$28.50	$32.38	$0	$14.24
		Totals:	$68.00	$0.00	$28.50	$32.38	$0	$14.24

Please make checks payable to:
Douglasville Medicine Associates

BALANCE DUE $14.24

Important Note:

Figure WB9-4 *(Delmar/Cengage Learning)*

Critical Thinking: Patient Accounts Hartsfeld and Herbert

Instructions: Create one patient statement for each patient, Deanna Hartsfeld and Nancy Herbert, and include the dunning messages previously prepared. When finished, check your work with Figures WB9-5 and WB9-6. Print the statements for your records, or check if they are to be turned in to your instructor.

Douglasville Medicine Associates
5076 Brand Blvd., Suite 401
Douglasville, NY 01234
Ph: (123) 456-7890
Fax: (123) 456-7891
Email: admin@dfma.com
Website: www.dfma.com

REMAINDER STATEMENT

DEANNA HARTSFELD
8821 Golden Ave
Douglasville, NY 01235

Date:
Account No: HAR001
Student No: Student1

Date	Patient	Procedure	Total Charges	Patient Co-Pay	Insurance Payment	Adjust-ments	Deduct-ibles	Current Balance
22-Oct-09	Deanna Hartsfeld	99214	$180.00	$0.00	$23.57	$75.54	$75	$161.78
		Totals:	$180.00	$0.00	$23.57	$75.54	$75	$161.78

Please make checks payable to:
Douglasville Medicine Associates

BALANCE DUE	$161.78

Important Note:
Medicare has paid; your secondary insurance has been billed and is pending payment.

Figure WB9-5 *(Delmar/Cengage Learning)*

Douglasville Medicine Associates
5076 Brand Blvd., Suite 401
Douglasville, NY 01234
Ph: (123) 456-7890
Fax: (123) 456-7891
Email: admin@dfma.com
Website: www.dfma.com

REMAINDER STATEMENT

NANCY HERBERT

9768 Golden Ave

Douglasville, NY 01235

Date:

Account No: HER001

Student No: Student1

Date	Patient	Procedure	Total Charges	Patient Co-Pay	Insurance Payment	Adjust-ments	Deduct-ibles	Current Balance
22-Oct-09	Nancy Herbert	99215	$249.00	$0.00	$112.25	$108.69	$0	$56.12
		Totals:	$249.00	$0.00	$112.25	$108.69	$0	$56.12

Please make checks payable to:

Douglasville Medicine Associates

BALANCE DUE	$56.12

Important Note:

Medicare has paid; your secondary insurance has been billed and is pending payment.

Figure WB9-6 *(Delmar/Cengage Learning)*

BUILDING SKILLS 9-5: PREPARE PATIENT STATEMENTS FOR MEDICARE PATIENTS WHO OWE A REMAINDER BALANCE

Instructions: Using the Billing and Payments report from Building Skills 9-3 and data obtained from each of the Workbook patients, prepare patient statements with dunning messages. When completed, the statements are to be printed for mailing.

Patient Account: Sean McKay

1. From the Main Menu in MOSS, click on the *Patient Billing* button on the Main Menu. This opens the Patient Billing window, ready to input settings.

2. As previously done, create a Remainder Statement for Patient McKay, using an appropriate dunning message. Check your Patient Billing screen with Figure WB9-7 before proceeding.

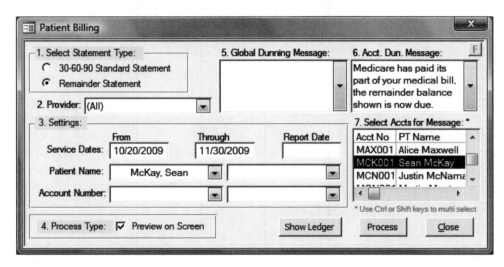

Figure WB9-7 *(Delmar/Cengage Learning)*

3. Process the statement, review it for accuracy, and check your work with Figure WB9-8. When finished, print the statement for your records or check with your instructor for further directions for turning in your work.

Douglasville Medicine Associates
5076 Brand Blvd., Suite 401
Douglasville, NY 01234
Ph: (123) 456-7890
Fax: (123) 456-7891
Email: admin@dfma.com
Website: www.dfma.com

REMAINDER STATEMENT

SEAN MCKAY
521 East Marble Way
Douglasville, NY 01235

Date:
Account No: MCK001
Student No: Student1

Date	Patient	Procedure	Total Charges	Patient Co-Pay	Insurance Payment	Adjust-ments	Deduct-ibles	Current Balance
20-Nov-09	Sean McKay	99221	$145.00	$0.00	$73.86	$52.67	$0	$18.47
		Totals:	$145.00	$0.00	$73.86	$52.67	$0	$18.47

Please make checks payable to:
Douglasville Medicine Associates

BALANCE DUE	$18.47

Important Note:

Medicare has paid its part of your medical bill, the remainder balance shown is now due.

Figure WB9-8 *(Delmar/Cengage Learning)*

Critical Thinking: Patient Account Joel Royzin

Instructions: Create one patient statement for Patient Royzin and include the dunning message previously prepared. When finished, check your work with Figure WB9-9. Print the statement for your records, or check with your instructor for further directions for turning in your work.

Douglasville Medicine Associates
5076 Brand Blvd., Suite 401
Douglasville, NY 01234
Ph: (123) 456-7890
Fax: (123) 456-7891
Email: admin@dfma.com

REMAINDER STATEMENT
Website: www.dfma.com

JOEL ROYZIN
14321 Wilson Drive
Douglasville, NY 01234

Date:
Account No: ROY001
Student No: Student1

Date	Patient	Procedure	Total Charges	Patient Co-Pay	Insurance Payment	Adjust-ments	Deduct-ibles	Current Balance
13-Nov-09	Joel Royzin	99308	$113.00	$0.00	$47.25	$53.94	$0	$11.81
		Totals:	$113.00	$0.00	$47.25	$53.94	$0	$11.81

Please make checks payable to:
Douglasville Medicine Associates

BALANCE DUE $11.81

Important Note:
Medicare has paid its part of your medical bill, the remainder balance shown is now due.

Figure WB9-9 *(Delmar/Cengage Learning)*

BUILDING SKILLS 9-6: PREPARE STATEMENTS FOR PATIENTS WHO OWE A REMAINDER BALANCE AFTER PRIVATE INSURANCE HAS PAID AND THERE IS NO SECONDARY PLAN

Instructions: Using the Billing and Payments report from Building Skills 9-3 and data obtained from each of the Workbook patients, prepare patient statements with dunning messages. When completed, the statements are to be printed for mailing.

Patient Account: Harold Engleman

1. From the Main Menu in MOSS, click on the *Patient Billing* button on the Main Menu. This opens the Patient Billing window, ready to input settings.

2. As previously done, create a Remainder Statement for Patient Engleman, using an appropriate dunning message. Check your Patient Billing screen with Figure WB9-10 before proceeding.

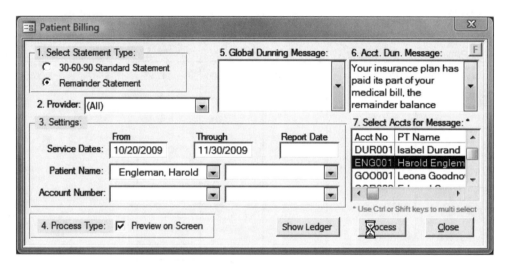

Figure WB9-10 *(Delmar/Cengage Learning)*

3. Process the statement, review it for accuracy, and check your work with Figure WB9-11. When finished, print the statement for your records or check with your instructor for further directions for turning in your work.

Douglasville Medicine Associates
5076 Brand Blvd., Suite 401
Douglasville, NY 01234
Ph: (123) 456-7890
Fax: (123) 456-7891
Email: admin@dfma.com
Website: www.dfma.com

REMAINDER STATEMENT

HAROLD ENGLEMAN
58682 Pebble Trail
Douglasville, NY 01234

Date:
Account No: ENG001
Student No: Student1

Date	Patient	Procedure	Total Charges	Patient Co-Pay	Insurance Payment	Adjust-ments	Deduct-ibles	Current Balance
22-Oct-09	Harold Engleman	99205	$358.00	$0.00	$260.80	$0.00	$0	$97.20
		Totals:	$358.00	$0.00	$260.80	$0.00	$0	$97.20

Please make checks payable to:
Douglasville Medicine Associates

BALANCE DUE	$97.20

Important Note:
Your insurance plan has paid its part of your medical bill, the remainder balance shown is now due.

Figure WB9-11 *(Delmar/Cengage Learning)*

Critical Thinking: Patient Accounts Hedensten and Jouharian

Instructions: Create one patient statement for each patient, Mark Hedensten and Siran Jouharian, and include the dunning messages previously prepared. When finished, check your work with Figures WB9-12 and WB9-13. Print the statements for your records, or check if they are to be turned in to your instructor.

Douglasville Medicine Associates
5076 Brand Blvd., Suite 401
Douglasville, NY 01234
Ph: (123) 456-7890
Fax: (123) 456-7891
Email: admin@dfma.com
Website: www.dfma.com

REMAINDER STATEMENT

MARK HEDENSTEN
12341 Slate Court
Douglasville, NY 01235

Date:
Account No: HED001
Student No: Student1

Date	Patient	Procedure	Total Charges	Patient Co-Pay	Insurance Payment	Adjust-ments	Deduct-ibles	Current Balance
22-Nov-09	Mark Hedensten	99221	$145.00	$0.00	$116.00	$0.00	$0	$29.00
		Totals:	$145.00	$0.00	$116.00	$0.00	$0	$29.00

Please make checks payable to:
Douglasville Medicine Associates

BALANCE DUE	$29.00

Important Note:

Your insurance plan has paid its part of your medical bill, the remainder balance shown is now due.

Figure WB9-12 *(Delmar/Cengage Learning)*

REMAINDER STATEMENT

<u>Douglasville Medicine Associates</u>
5076 Brand Blvd., Suite 401
Douglasville, NY 01234
Ph: (123) 456-7890
Fax: (123) 456-7891
Email: admin@dfma.com
Website: www.dfma.com

SIRAN JOUHARIAN
11234 Long Point
Douglasville, NY 01234

Date:
Account No: JOU001
Student No: Student1

Date	Patient	Procedure	Total Charges	Patient Co-Pay	Insurance Payment	Adjust-ments	Deduct-ibles	Current Balance
12-Nov-09	Siran Jouharian	99282	$147.00	$0.00	$108.00	$12.00	$0	$27.00
		Totals:	$147.00	$0.00	$108.00	$12.00	$0	$27.00

Please make checks payable to:
Douglasville Medicine Associates

BALANCE DUE $27.00

Important Note:

Your insurance plan has paid its part of your medical bill, the remainder balance shown is now due.

Figure WB9-13 *(Delmar/Cengage Learning)*

BUILDING SKILLS 9-7: PREPARE STATEMENTS FOR PATIENTS WHO OWE AN AMOUNT THAT WAS APPLIED TO THE ANNUAL DEDUCTIBLE FOR THEIR INSURANCE PLAN

Instructions: Using the Billing and Payments report from Building Skills 9-3 and data obtained from each of the Workbook patients, prepare patient statements with dunning messages. When completed, the statements are to be printed for mailing.

Patient Account: Dennis Johnsen

1. From the Main Menu in MOSS, click on the *Patient Billing* button on the Main Menu. This opens the Patient Billing window, ready to input settings.

2. As previously done, create a Remainder Statement for Patient Johnsen, using an appropriate dunning message. Check your Patient Billing screen with Figure WB9-14 before proceeding.

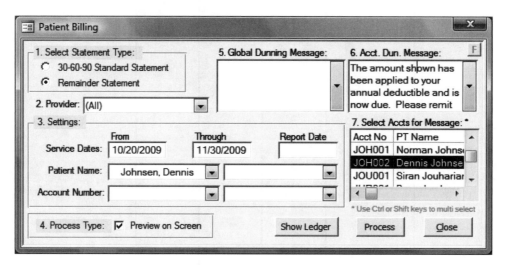

Figure WB9-14 *(Delmar/Cengage Learning)*

3. Process the statement, review it for accuracy, and check your work with Figure WB9-15. When finished, print the statement for your records or check with your instructor for further directions for turning in your work.

Douglasville Medicine Associates
5076 Brand Blvd., Suite 401
Douglasville, NY 01234
Ph: (123) 456-7890
Fax: (123) 456-7891
Email: admin@dfma.com
Website: www.dfma.com

REMAINDER STATEMENT

DENNIS JOHNSEN
8965 Pebble Way
Douglasville, NY 01235

Date:
Account No: JOH002
Student No: Student1

Date	Patient	Procedure	Total Charges	Patient Co-Pay	Insurance Payment	Adjust-ments	Deduct-ibles	Current Balance
09-Nov-09	Dennis Johnsen	99282	$147.00	$0.00	$0.00	$12.00	$135	$135.00
		Totals:	$147.00	$0.00	$0.00	$12.00	$135	$135.00

Please make checks payable to:
Douglasville Medicine Associates

BALANCE DUE	$135.00

Important Note:

The amount shown has been applied to your annual deductible and is now due. Please remit payment today.

Figure WB9-15 *(Delmar/Cengage Learning)*

Critical Thinking: Patient Account Karen Ross

Instructions: Create one patient statement for patient Karen Ross and include the dunning message previously prepared. When finished, check your work with Figure WB9-16. Print the statement for your records, or check if it is to be turned in to your instructor.

Douglasville Medicine Associates
5076 Brand Blvd., Suite 401
Douglasville, NY 01234
Ph: (123) 456-7890
Fax: (123) 456-7891
Email: admin@dfma.com
Website: www.dfma.com

REMAINDER STATEMENT

KAREN ROSS
5831 Pebble Way
Douglasville, NY 01235

Date:
Account No: ROS001
Student No: Student1

Date	Patient	Procedure	Total Charges	Patient Co-Pay	Insurance Payment	Adjust-ments	Deduct-ibles	Current Balance
17-Nov-09	Karen Ross	99221	$145.00	$0.00	$0.00	$11.40	$134	$133.60
		Totals:	$145.00	$0.00	$0.00	$11.40	$134	$133.60

Please make checks payable to:
Douglasville Medicine Associates

BALANCE DUE $133.60

Important Note:
The amount shown has been applied to your annual deductible and is now due. Please remit payment today.

Figure WB9-16 *(Delmar/Cengage Learning)*

BUILDING SKILLS 9-8: PREPARE STATEMENTS FOR PATIENTS COVERED BY AN HRA PLAN WHO OWE A BALANCE

Instructions: Using the Billing and Payments report from Building Skills 9-3 and data obtained from each of the Workbook patients, prepare patient statements with dunning messages. When completed, the statements are to be printed for mailing.

Patient Account: Tina Rizzo

1. From the Main Menu in MOSS, click on the *Patient Billing* button on the Main Menu. This opens the Patient Billing window, ready to input settings.

2. As previously done, create a Remainder Statement for Patient Rizzo, using an appropriate dunning message. Check your Patient Billing screen with Figure WB9-17 before proceeding.

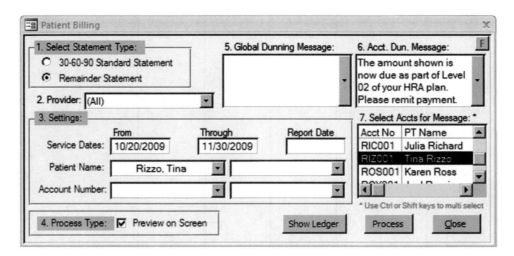

Figure WB9-17 *(Delmar/Cengage Learning)*

3. Process the statement, review it for accuracy, and check your work with Figure WB9-18. When finished, print the statement for your records or check with your instructor for further directions for turning in your work.

Douglasville Medicine Associates
5076 Brand Blvd., Suite 401
Douglasville, NY 01234
Ph: (123) 456-7890
Fax: (123) 456-7891
Email: admin@dfma.com
Website: www.dfma.com

REMAINDER STATEMENT

TINA RIZZO
4936 Columbine Street
Douglasville, NY 01234

Date:
Account No: RIZ001
Student No: Student1

Date	Patient	Procedure	Total Charges	Patient Co-Pay	Insurance Payment	Adjust-ments	Deduct-ibles	Current Balance
22-Oct-09	Tina Rizzo	36415	$18.00	$0.00	$0.00	$13.00	$0	$5.00
22-Oct-09	Tina Rizzo	85031	$11.00	$0.00	$0.00	$2.00	$0	$9.00
22-Oct-09	Tina Rizzo	99214	$180.00	$0.00	$0.00	$11.30	$0	$168.70
		Totals:	$209.00	$0.00	$0.00	$26.30	$0	$182.70

Please make checks payable to:
Douglasville Medicine Associates

BALANCE DUE	$182.70

Important Note:

The amount shown is now due as part of Level 02 of your HRA plan. Please remit payment.

Figure WB9-18 *(Delmar/Cengage Learning)*

Critical Thinking: Patient Account Wynona Sheridan

Instructions: Create one patient statement for patient Wynona Sheridan and include the dunning message previously prepared. When finished, check your work with Figure WB9-19. Print the statement for your records, or check if it is to be turned in to your instructor.

Douglasville Medicine Associates
5076 Brand Blvd., Suite 401
Douglasville, NY 01234
Ph: (123) 456-7890
Fax: (123) 456-7891
Email: admin@dfma.com
Website: www.dfma.com

REMAINDER STATEMENT

WYNONA SHERIDAN
12390 Marble Way
Douglasville, NY 01234

Date:
Account No: SHE002
Student No: Student1

Date	Patient	Procedure	Total Charges	Patient Co-Pay	Insurance Payment	Adjust-ments	Deduct-ibles	Current Balance
27-Oct-09	Wynona Sheridan	99203	$200.00	$0.00	$0.00	$4.00	$0	$196.00
		Totals:	$200.00	$0.00	$0.00	$4.00	$0	$196.00

Please make checks payable to:
Douglasville Medicine Associates

BALANCE DUE	$196.00

Important Note:

The amount shown is now due as part of Level 02 of your HRA plan. Please remit payment.

Figure WB9-19 *(Delmar/Cengage Learning)*

BUILDING SKILLS 9-9: PATIENT PAYMENTS BY PERSONAL CHECK REVIEW

1. When receiving a personal check as a payment from a patient, there are a number of items that should be checked before posting the payment to the patient's account. Describe at least five of these items.

   A. _____
      _____
      _____
      _____

   B. _____
      _____
      _____
      _____

   C. _____
      _____
      _____
      _____

   D. _____
      _____
      _____
      _____

   E. _____
      _____
      _____
      _____

2. Describe where a restrictive endorsement is placed on a personal check, and the purpose of the endorsement.

_____

_____

_____

_____

_____

3. Why is it a good business practice to promptly cash personal checks from patients?

_____

_____

_____

_____

_____

4. Is a bank obligated to honor a post-dated check and not release payment until that time? Explain why or why not.

_____

_____

_____

_____

_____

BUILDING SKILLS 9-10: POSTING PERSONAL CHECK PAYMENTS TO PATIENT ACCOUNTS

Instructions: On Monday, 12/21/2009, the mail is brought to the office from the mailboxes located in the lobby of the medical building. Included in the mail are some personal checks sent by patients who recently received the statements that were sent out to them a couple of weeks ago. Post the payments to each patient's account as indicated below.

Patient Sean McKay

1. From the Main Menu in MOSS, click on the *Posting Payments* button. Select Sean McKay from the list and click on the *Apply Payment* button.

2. Select the line item so that the $18.47 balance due appears in Field 13. Enter a posting date of 12/21/2009. Check your work with Figure WB9-20.

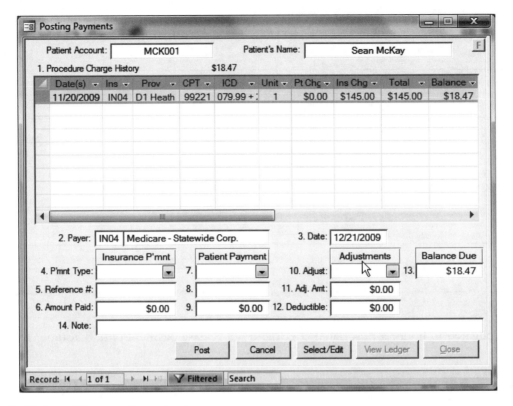

Figure WB9-20 *(Delmar/Cengage Learning)*

3. Next, refer to the personal check from Patient McKay shown on Source Document WB9-1 in the back of the workbook. Enter the payment details on the Posting Payments screen and then check your work with Figure WB9-21 before posting.

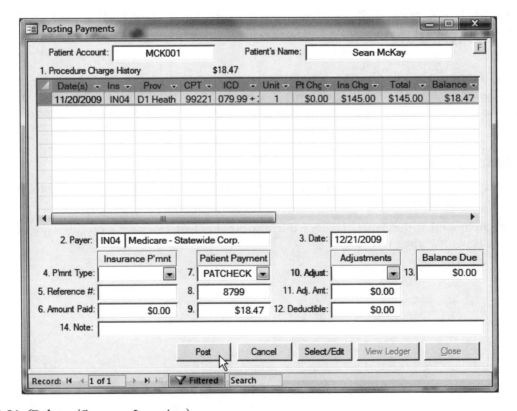

Figure WB9-21 *(Delmar/Cengage Learning)*

4. Click on the *Post* button to apply the payment. View the Patient Ledger and check your work with Figure WB9-22.

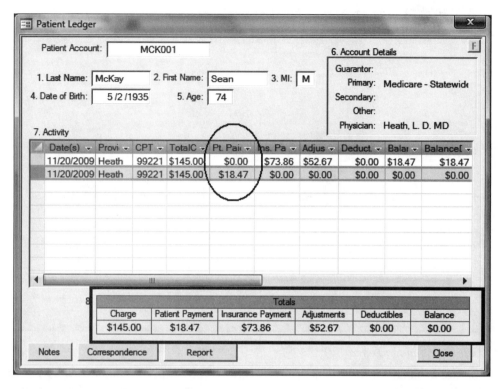

Figure WB9-22 *(Delmar/Cengage Learning)*

5. Close all open windows and return to the Patient Selection list for Posting Payments.

Patient Joel Royzin

1. From the Main Menu in MOSS, click on the *Posting Payments* button. Select Joel Royzin from the list and click on the *Apply Payment* button.

2. Select the line item so that the $11.81 balance due appears in Field 13. Enter a posting date of 12/21/2009. Check your work with Figure WB9-23.

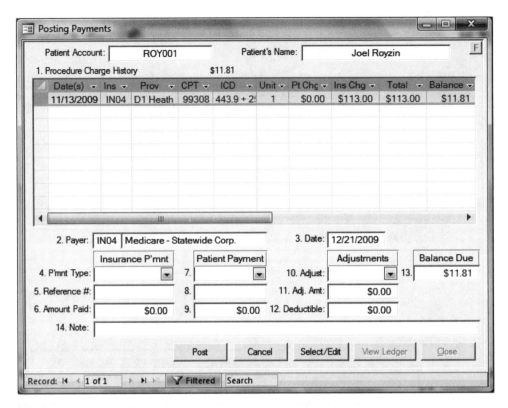

Figure WB9-23 *(Delmar/Cengage Learning)*

3. Next, refer to the personal check from Patient Royzin shown on Source Document WB9-2 in the back of the workbook. Enter the payment details on the Posting Payments screen and then check your work with Figure WB9-24 before posting.

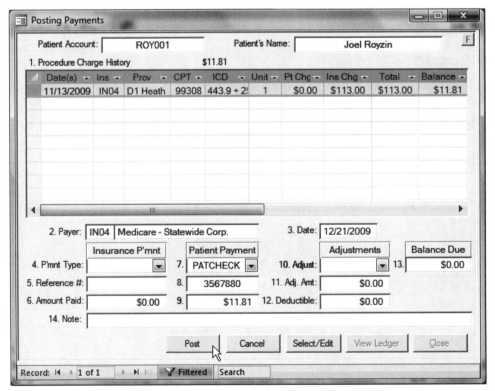

Figure WB9-24 *(Delmar/Cengage Learning)*

4. Click on the *Post* button to apply the payment. View the Patient Ledger and check your work with Figure WB9-25.

5. Close all open windows and return to the Patient Selection list for Posting Payments.

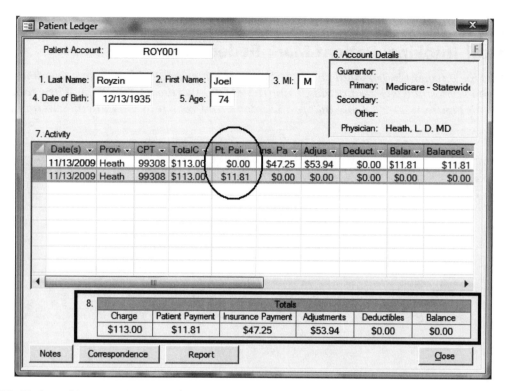

Figure WB9-25 *(Delmar/Cengage Learning)*

Critical Thinking: Patient Siran Jouharian

Instructions: Post the payment by personal check for Patient Jouharian. Refer to Source Document WB9-3 in the back of the workbook. Post the payment details, using 12/21/2009 as the posting date. When finished, check the Patient Ledger with Figure WB9-26. Close all open windows and return to the Patient Selection list for Posting Payments.

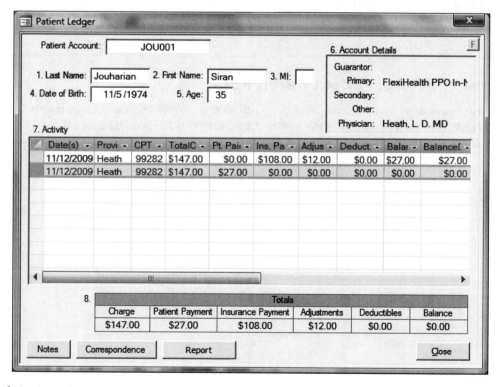

Figure WB9-26 *(Delmar/Cengage Learning)*

Critical Thinking: Patient Mark Hedensten

Instructions: Post the payment by personal check for Patient Hedensten. Refer to Source Document WB9-4 in the back of the workbook. Post the payment details, using 12/21/2009 as the posting date. When finished, check the Patient Ledger with Figure WB9-27. Close all open windows and return to the Patient Selection list for Posting Payments.

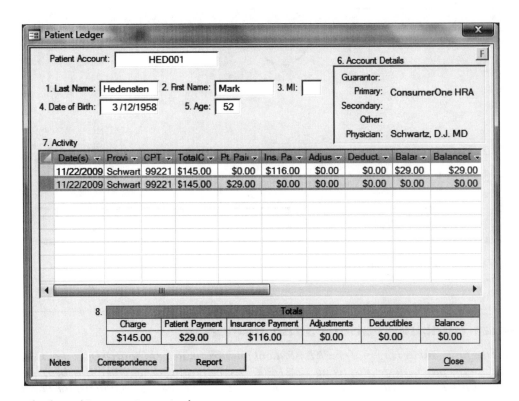

Figure WB9-27 *(Delmar/Cengage Learning)*

Critical Thinking: Patient Karen Ross

Instructions: Post the payment by personal check for Patient Ross. Refer to Source Document WB9-5 in the back of the workbook. Post the payment details, using 12/21/2009 as the posting date. When finished, check the Patient Ledger with Figure WB9-28. Close all open windows and return to the Patient Selection list for Posting Payments.

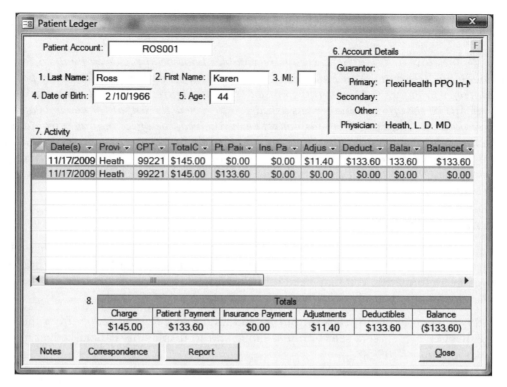

Figure WB9-28 *(Delmar/Cengage Learning)*

 ## Critical Thinking: Patient Tina Rizzo

Instructions: Post the payment by personal check for Patient Rizzo. Refer to Source Document WB9-6 in the back of the workbook. Post the payment details, using 12/21/2009 as the posting date. (HINT: When posting one check that applies to multiple line items, post that part of the payment that applies to each individual service.) When finished, check the Patient Ledger with Figure WB9-29. Close all open windows and return to the Patient Selection list for Posting Payments.

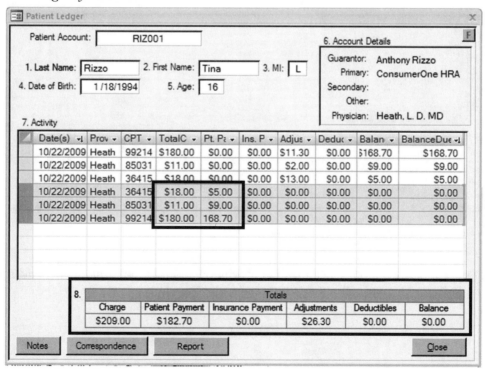

Figure WB9-29 *(Delmar/Cengage Learning)*

BUILDING SKILLS 9-11: WRITING COLLECTION LETTERS

Instructions: On Wednesday, 01/06/2010, accounts receivables have been reviewed by the office manager at Douglasville Medicine Associates. You have been given three statements for the following patients: Harold Engleman (refer to Figure 9-13), Dennis Johnsen (refer to Figure 9-15), and Wynona Sheridan (refer to Figure 9-19). Using MOSS, the office manager has asked you to review the unpaid statements against the patient ledgers for all three patients. Since payment has not yet been received, the office manager would like you to write a reminder collection letter to each of the patients on behalf of the respective doctor. Include details on how much is due, why the balance is due, and offer alternatives for payment, including credit card or payment plan, and give a two-week time line to pay. If payment is not received in two weeks, telephone calls will be initiated. The letter will be signed by each patient's doctor.

Patient Harold Engleman

1. On a piece of paper, or using a word processor, prepare a draft of the collection letter that will be sent to Patient Engleman. Refer to MOSS as needed to review details on the Patient Ledger, registration form, and other areas to gather information you may need to include. When you are ready to write the letter on the practice letterhead, continue with the steps below.

2. From the pull-down menu in MOSS, click on *Billing* and then select *Patient Ledger* from the drop-down list. From the Patient Ledger screen, select *Patient Engleman* to display his Patient Ledger and transaction details, as shown in Figure WB9-30.

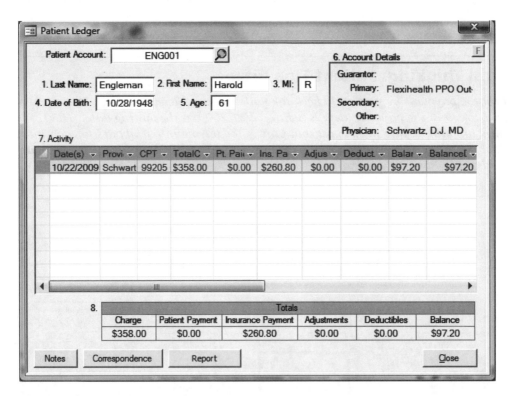

Figure WB9-30 *(Delmar/Cengage Learning)*

3. Click on the *Correspondence* button. When the Output window opens, type a unique filename for the collection letter. An example is: "engleman_collection letter_your name," as shown in Figure WB9-31.

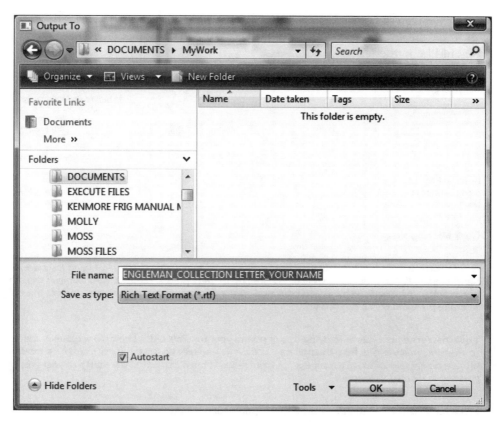

Figure WB9-31 *(Delmar/Cengage Learning)*

4. Select a location for the collection letter to be saved on the hard drive of your computer, or to a flash drive, CD, or other location as directed by your instructor. Remember the location and name of your file. Next, click on *OK* to continue.

5. A letterhead document will open in your word processor, as shown on Figure WB9-32. You may now *delete* the place that reads "Type message here," and begin writing the final collection letter onto the letterhead. Be

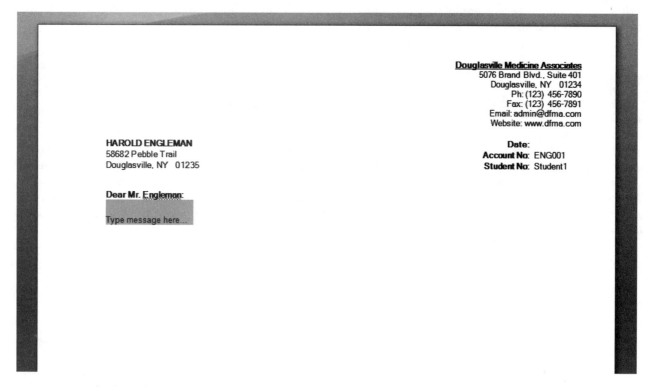

Figure WB9-32 *(Delmar/Cengage Learning)*

sure to periodically save your document as you work, and again when completed. The body of your letter may differ from the example shown on Figure WB9-33; however, the main points you were asked to include by the office manager should be in the letter.

Douglasville Medicine Associates
5076 Brand Blvd., Suite 401
Douglasville, NY 01234
Ph: (123) 456-7890
Fax: (123) 456-7891
Email: admin@dfma.com
Website: www.dfma.com

HAROLD ENGLEMAN
58682 Pebble Trail
Douglasville, NY 01235

Date:
Account No: ENG001
Student No: Student1

Dear Mr. Engleman:

Our Office Manager has brought your past due account to my attention.   Have you forgotten to send payment?   In order to keep your account up to date, please remit $97.20 within in the next two weeks.   An envelope has been enclosed for your convenience, or you may contact the office to make payment with a credit card.

Your insurance plan has already paid their part of your medical bill.   The balance due is the remainder, which is due from the patient.   If there is any reason full payment cannot be made, please contact my office to arrange a payment plan.   I have instructed my staff to assist you in any needed to resolve this matter.

I look forward to your timely response to this payment reminder.

Sincerely,

D.J. Schwartz, MD

Figure WB9-33 *(Delmar/Cengage Learning)*

6. When the letter has been completed, print it for your records, and follow the directions of your instructor for turning in your work.

Critical Thinking: Patient Dennis Johnsen

Instructions: Prepare a collection letter for Patient Johnsen. First, write a draft, and then type it on the practice letterhead, using MOSS. Review the details of this patient on his statement and Patient Ledger as needed, and include the main points as directed by the office manager. Name the file and save it to a location on your computer or removable media. When the letter has been completed, print it for your records, and follow the directions of your instructor for turning in your work. Compare your letter to the example shown on Figure WB9-34. The body of your letter may differ from the example shown; however, the main points you were asked to include should be in the letter.

Douglasville Medicine Associates
5076 Brand Blvd., Suite 401
Douglasville, NY 01234
Ph: (123) 456-7890
Fax: (123) 456-7891
Email: admin@dfma.com
Website: www.dfma.com

DENNIS JOHNSEN
9865 Pebble Way
Douglasville, NY 01235

Date:
Account No: JOH002
Student No: Student1

Dear Mr. Johnsen:

Our Office Manager has brought your past due balance to my attention. This letter is a reminder that the balance due on your account is a portion of your medical bill that was applied to your annual deductible. As you know, deductibles are payable by the patient out-of-pocket each year. Please remit payment within the next two weeks so that your account will be up date. An envelope has been enclosed for your convenience, or you may call the office to pay with a credit card if this is more convenient.

If there is any reason that a full payment cannot be made, a payment plan can be arranged with the billing department. I have instructed my staff to assist you in any way possible. I look forward to your prompt attention to this matter. Thank you.

Sincerely,

L.D. Heath, MD

Figure WB9-34 *(Delmar/Cengage Learning)*

Critical Thinking: Patient Wynona Sheridan

Instructions: Prepare a collection letter for Patient Sheridan. First, write a draft, and then type it on the practice letterhead, using MOSS. Review the details of this patient on her statement and Patient Ledger as needed, and include the main points as directed by the office manager. Name the file and save it to a location on your computer or removable media. When the letter has been completed, print it for your records, and follow the directions of your instructor for turning in your work. Compare your letter to the example shown on Figure WB9-35. The body of your letter may differ from the example shown; however, the main points you were asked to include should be in the letter.

```
                                              Douglasville Medicine Associates
                                                  5076 Brand Blvd., Suite 401
                                                    Douglasville, NY  01234
                                                       Ph: (123) 456-7890
                                                       Fax: (123) 456-7891
                                                    Email: admin@dfma.com
                                                    Website: www.dfma.com

   WYNONA SHERIDAN                                         Date:
   12390 Marble Way                              Account No: SHE002
   Douglasville, NY  01234                       Student No: Student1

   Dear Ms. Sheridan:

   Our Office Manager has brought your past due balance to my attention.  This letter is a reminder that the balance
   due on your account is part of the level two portion of your ConsumerONE HRA plan.  As you know, whenever
   medical expenses fall into level two, the patient is responsible for 100% of the network fee schedule out-of-pocket,
   up to your plan's limit.  Please remit payment within the next two weeks so that your account will be up date.  An
   envelope has been enclosed for your convenience, or you may call the office to pay with a credit card if this is
   more convenient.

   If there is any reason that a full payment cannot be made, a payment plan can be arranged with the billing
   department. I have instructed my staff to assist you in any way possible.  I look forward to your prompt attention
   to this matter. Thank you.

   Sincerely,


   L.D. Heath, MD
```

Figure WB9-35 *(Delmar/Cengage Learning)*

BUILDING SKILLS 9-12: TELEPHONE COLLECTIONS REVIEW

Instructions: There are several guidelines that can be followed when placing telephone calls for the purpose of collections in a medical office. Some of the more common guidelines that adhere to most state and federal regulations were discussed in the book. Answer the follow questions as a review.

1. At what times of the day should collections calls be placed and limited to?

_____

_____

_____

_____

_____

2. Why are collections calls that are placed at other times, such as early morning or late at night, or made three or four times in one day for the same collections attempt, not permitted under the general guidelines?

_____

_____

_____

_____

_____

3. A collection call is made to a debtor's place of work. The debtor's boss informs you that personal calls cannot be made at the workplace, and that the debtor cannot accept the call. Is the collector permitted to call back under the general guidelines? What is the minimum the collector should do in this case?

_____

_____

_____

_____

_____

4. Describe examples of misrepresentations by a collector that are not permitted when making collections calls.

_____

_____

_____

_____

_____

5. Whenever discussing any personal matter from a medical office with a patient, whether sensitive medical information or a collections call for a debt, be certain you are speaking to the appropriate person. Explain why disclosing information to a third party is not permitted under the general guidelines. Suggest how you might identify the person you are speaking with.

_____

_____

_____

_____

_____

6. Referring to a debtor as a delinquent, freeloader, deadbeat, bum, or other descriptive names are not permitted under the general guidelines of collections calls. If such tactics are used, what are the consequences?

_____

_____

_____

_____

_____

BUILDING SKILLS 9-13: ROLE-PLAY PRACTICE: TELEPHONE COLLECTIONS CALLS

Instructions: Practice the dialogue below for each case study with a classmate or study partner.

Case Study 1: Harold Engleman

On 01/26/2010, the office manager has reviewed accounts receivables and asks you to place a collection call to Mr. Engleman. Refer to Figure WB9-33, which is the reminder letter sent on 01/06/2010. It is helpful to review the EOB from FlexiHealth, Source Document WB8-4 in the back of the workbook. Mr. Engleman has not responded to the letter or sent payment, and a call will be made to attempt to collect the remainder balance of $97.20.

Collector: Hello, this is (your name) from Douglasville Medicine Associates. Am I speaking with Mr. Harold Engleman?

Patient: Yes, this is Harold, who is this?

Collector: Good (morning, afternoon), Mr. Engleman. My name is (your name) from Douglasville Medicine Associates. Dr. Schwartz has asked me to call you today regarding your past due account. Your insurance plan has paid its portion of your medical bill. We have mailed a statement and a reminder letter for the remaining balance, but have not received payment from you.

Patient: Yes, I've been getting those.

Collector: Mr. Engleman, we would like to bring your account up to date. Can you pay your balance of $97.20 with a credit card on the phone today?

Patient: Well, I'm not really sure why I owe this much money to the doctor. I have good insurance, and it should be taken care of by FlexiHealth. Don't these doctors just take what the insurance pays?

Collector: I'm sorry if there has been a misunderstanding, Mr. Engleman. Our office bills for services according to the benefits offered by your plan. You received services from Dr. Schwartz, who is an out-of-network doctor with your plan. The $97.20 is the 20% remainder, plus the noncovered amount.

Patient: I don't understand. I thought your office participated with my insurance. Dr. Schwartz was highly recommended by my urologist; that's why I saw him.

Collector: At Douglasville Medicine, only Dr. Heath participates as an in-network doctor with FlexiHealth PPO plans. Since Dr. Schwartz does not participate with FlexiHealth, your benefits are paid as an out-of-network provider.

Patient: Well, I didn't know that when I made my appointment. I thought I was just going to pay my $20.00 copayment, and the rest would be taken care of.

Collector: Mr. Engleman, I would be happy to have you speak with Dr. Schwartz about your situation and possibly changing doctors so that you may continue your care using your in-network benefits at our office. In the meantime, payment for the services provided by Dr. Schwartz will need to be made.

Patient: Well, I really liked Dr. Schwartz, and he did help with my problem. I'm not sure I want to see someone else now that I saw him. I'll pay this now and talk to him at my follow-up appointment.

Collector: Very well, Mr. Engleman. Would you like to pay by credit card on the phone?

Patient: No, I'll send a check out today. You should have it soon in the mail.

Collector: Thank you. I will document on your record that you will be sending a payment of $97.20 in the mail today, and will inform Dr. Schwartz.

Patient: Thank you. Good-bye.

Collector: Good-bye. Have a good day.

Next, document the pertinent details of the telephone call. Record the agreement that was made in the notes section of Patient Engleman's account as follows:

1. Click on the *Billing* drop-down menu in MOSS and select *Patient Ledger*, as shown in Figure WB9-36. Select the account for *Harold Engleman* to open his ledger for viewing.

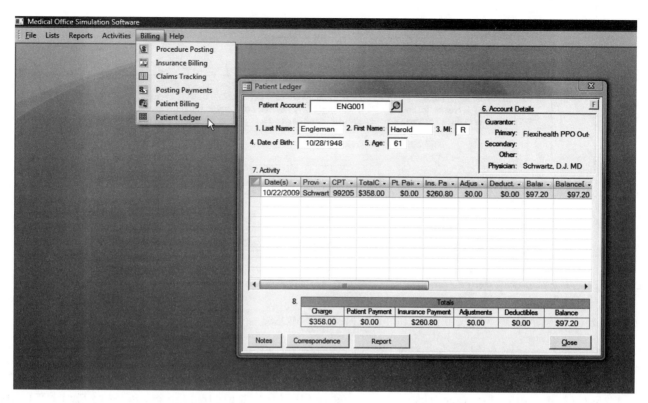

Figure WB9-36 *(Delmar/Cengage Learning)*

2. Click on the *Notes* button located at the bottom left of the Ledger screen, as shown in Figure WB9-37. When the Notes window opens, click on the *Add* button in order to add a new note to the record.

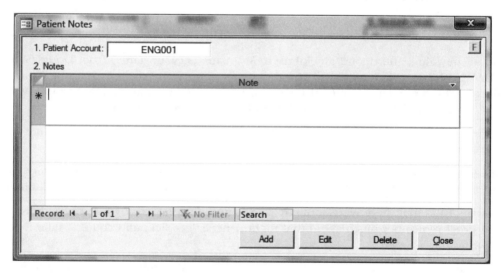

Figure WB9-37 *(Delmar/Cengage Learning)*

3. Click inside the *Note box* and type the following: "01/26/2010 – Spoke to patient on the telephone; patient agreed to send $97.20 by check in mail today. Discussed reason for balance. Patient thought Dr. Schwartz participated with FlexiHealth PPO. Will talk to doctor at next follow-up visit about this and make decision to change doctor or not." (Type your last name at the end of the note.) Compare your note to the example in Figure WB9-38.

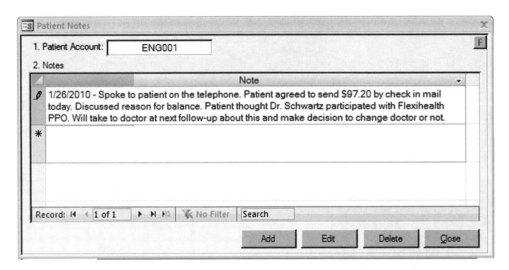

Figure WB9-38 *(Delmar/Cengage Learning)*

4. Close all open windows and return to the Main Menu of MOSS.

Case Study 2: Dennis Johnsen

On 01/26/2010, the office manager asks you to place a collection call to Mr. Johnsen. Refer to Figure WB9-34, which is the reminder letter sent on 01/06/2010. It is helpful to review the EOB from FlexiHealth, Source Document WB8-3, and the Emergency Care and Treatment form, Source Document WB5-8 in the back of the workbook. Mr. Johnsen has not responded to the letter or sent payment, and a call will be made to attempt to collect the balance of $135.00 that was applied to the annual deductible.

Collector: Hello, this is (your name) from Douglasville Medicine Associates. Am I speaking with Mr. Dennis Johnsen?

Patient: Yes, this is Dennis.

Collector: Good (morning, afternoon), Mr. Johnsen. My name is (your name) from Douglasville Medicine Associates. Dr. Heath has asked me to call you today regarding your past due account. Your insurance plan has been billed and has applied $135.00 of your charges towards your annual deductible. We have mailed a statement and a reminder letter for this balance, but have not received payment from you.

Patient: I haven't made a payment on this because I don't know who Dr. Heath is. I'm not going to pay someone I don't even know.

Collector: Mr. Johnsen, Dr. Heath was the attending doctor who treated you at Community Hospital Emergency Room on November 9, 2009. Did you visit the emergency room on that date at Community Hospital?

Patient: Well, yes I did, but there were so many nurses and doctors I saw while I was there. I was in a lot of pain, and I don't remember much about that night. I never get sick, and couldn't take it anymore, and just went down to the hospital.

Collector: I can understand there being a lot going on when you're in pain and visiting the emergency room. It is not unusual for patients to not remember the doctors who saw them in a hospital. However, Dr. Heath did treat your condition at the hospital, and requested that you follow up with him in one week at our office. I do not have a record that you returned in follow-up. How is your leg doing now?

Patient: My leg is much better, thanks. I went back to see another doctor who is closer to my office and easier to drive to for appointments. When I started getting all these bills, I didn't remember who anybody was.

Collector: Your insurance plan applied the allowed charges to your annual deductible. Can we have you pay the balance of $135.00 on a credit card on the phone today?

Patient: My cards are just about maxed out. Can I send half by check in the mail now, and pay the other half on March 1?

Collector: Mr. Johnsen, I would be happy to accept a check by mail now, and have you commit to paying off the other half later. Can I have you pay the second half sooner, by February 15, so that we can bring your account up to date?

Patient: Yes, I'll do that. Can you give me the address where I send the payments to?

Collector: Certainly. Please make your checks out to Douglasville Medicine Associates. The mailing address is: 5076 Brand Blvd., Suite 401, Douglasville, NY 01234. I will also send a letter to your address at 9865 Pebble Way in Douglasville to confirm the agreement. I'll enclose a mailing envelope for your convenience.

Patient: Thank you.

Collector: Mr. Johnsen, I have documented on your record that you will be sending a payment of $67.50 in the mail today, and I will inform Dr. Heath that you will send the second payment of $67.50 no later than February 15, 2010. Is there any other way I can assist you today?

Patient: No, thank you. Good-bye.

Collector: Good-bye. Have a good day.

Next, document the pertinent details of the telephone call. Record the agreement that was made in the Notes section of the Patient Johnsen's account. Check you work with Figure WB9-39. Your actual note may vary from the one in the Figure.

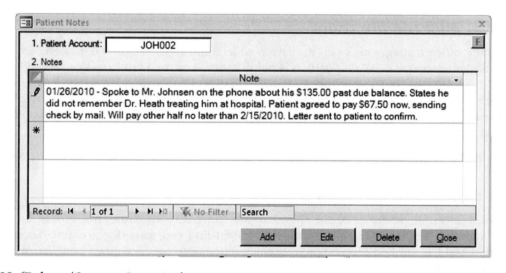

Figure WB9-39 *(Delmar/Cengage Learning)*

Last, using the *Correspondence* button of the Patient Ledger screen for Patient Johnsen, prepare the confirmation letter, dated 01/26/2010, that will be sent to the patient outlining the details of the payment agreement he has made. Check your letter with the example on Figure WB9-40. The body of your letter may vary, but should contain the main points of the discussion.

Douglasville Medicine Associates
5076 Brand Blvd., Suite 401
Douglasville, NY 01234
Ph: (123) 456-7890
Fax: (123) 456-7891
Email: admin@dfma.com
Website: www.dfma.com

DENNIS JOHNSEN
9865 Pebby Way
Douglasville, NY 01235

Date: 01/26/2010
Account No: JOH002
Student No: Student1

Dear Mr. Johnsen:

As per our conversation on the phone today regarding your past due balance of $135.00, this letter confirms that you have committed to making a payment by mail today in the amount of $67.50 by personal check. You have agreed to send the second payment no later than February 15, 2010, also in the amount of $67.50, to bring your account up to date. I have enclosed a mailing envelope for your convenience.

Thank you for your attention to this matter. If I can assist you in any way, please do not hesitate contacting me.

Sincerely,

Your name
Administrative Medical Assistant

Figure WB9-40 *(Delmar/Cengage Learning)*

Case Study 3: Wynona Sheridan

On 01/26/2010, the office manager asks you to place a collection call to Ms. Sheridan. Refer to Figure WB9-35, which is the reminder letter sent on 01/06/2010. It is helpful to review the EOB from ConsumerONE HRA, Source Document WB8-1, in the back of the workbook. Ms. Sheridan has not responded to the letter or sent payment, and a call will be made to attempt to collect the balance of $196.00. Recall that once the employer-provided funds (EPA) are exhausted at level one of the HRA plan, the patient pays up to $500.00 in level two out-of-pocket for medical expenses.

Collector: Hello, this is (your name) from Douglasville Medicine Associates. Am I speaking with Ms. Wynona Sheridan?

Patient: Yes, this is Wynona. Can I help you?

Collector: Good (morning, afternoon), Ms. Sheridan. My name is (your name) from Douglasville Medicine Associates. Dr. Heath has asked me to call you today regarding your past due account. Your insurance plan has been billed and has applied $196.00 of your charges towards your level-two benefits. We have mailed a statement and a reminder letter for this balance, but have not received payment from you.

Patient: Oh, yes, I know, I've just forgotten all about that. I've been so busy and have had some personal family problems; I really haven't had money to send in towards that.

Collector: Ms. Sheridan, I would be happy to assist you in either taking a payment with a credit card over the phone today, or setting up a payment plan so that you can take care of your balance as soon as possible. Will you be making a payment with a credit card today?

Patient: No, I don't like to give my credit card number to anyone over the telephone. What is this about a payment plan? I could probably use that.

Collector: I understand. If you would like to set up a payment plan, we could split up your balance into smaller, monthly installments until it is paid in full. On your balance of $196.00, we could accept $65.00 each month for three months. Are you able to agree to that payment plan?

Patient: Oh, no, $65.00 a month is entirely more than I can afford! I'm having my hours cut at work and can just barely hang on to my job so I can have these medical benefits.

Collector: Ms. Sheridan, is there an amount that you are comfortable with that you can send each month to pay down your balance?

Patient: Well, I think I can send about $25.00 a month. But that's about all. Can I do that?

Collector: If you can commit to $25.00 at the first of each month until your balance is paid, I would be happy to set up a payment plan for you today. We can set up a seven-month payment plan of $25.00, due on the first of each month. At month eight, your last payment would be $21.00. May I set up this payment plan for you now?

Patient: Well, what happens if I need to see the doctor again? I still have to pay up to $500.00 out of my own pocket.

Collector: I understand your concern. So long as you continue to keep current on your payments, we can adjust the amount due and add in future services if you need to put them on this payment plan.

Patient: Is there interest I have to pay on this plan?

Collector: No, Ms. Sheridan. As long as you stay current, Douglasville Medicine Associates will not charge any interest on the balance due.

Patient: That's great. Yes, please set up a payment plan for me.

Collector: Very well. I have documented on your record that you will be sending a payment of $25.00 now, for your February 1 payment. Thereafter, $25.00 is due at the first of each month until your balance is paid. On month eight, the final payment will be $21.00, unless we need to adjust this agreement for future medical services. Are you in agreement with this payment plan?

Patient: Yes, thank you very much. I feel so much better now!

Collector: I'm glad, Ms. Sheridan. Please send your first payment today of $25.00. I will mail you a letter confirming our conversation and agreement today. Thank you. Is there anything else I can assist you with?

Patient: No, thank you. Good-bye.

Collector: Good-bye. Have a good day.

Next, document the pertinent details of the telephone call. Record the agreement that was made in the Notes section of Patient Sheridan's ledger. Check you work with Figure WB9-41. Your actual note may vary from the one in the Figure.

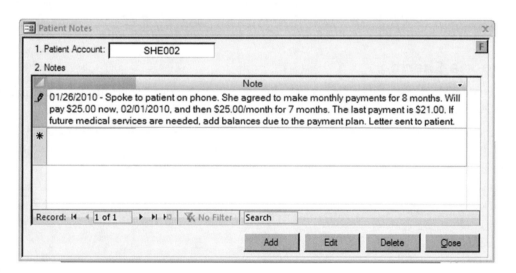

Figure WB9-41 *(Delmar/Cengage Learning)*

Last, using the *Correspondence* button of the Patient Ledger screen for Patient Sheridan, prepare the confirmation letter, dated 01/26/2010, that will be sent to the patient outlining the details of the payment agreement she has made. Be sure to include when the first payment is expected, and for how much, the number of months, and the final payment amount. Check your letter with the example on Figure WB9-42. The body of your letter may vary, but should contain the main points of the discussion.

WYNONA SHERIDAN
12390 Marble Way
Douglasville, NY 01234

Date: 01/26/10
Account No: SHE002
Student No: Student1

Dear Ms. Sheridan:

As per our conversation on the phone today regarding your past due balance of $196.00, this letter confirms that you have committed to a payment plan.   You have agreed to pay on the following schedule:

Due
02/01/2010	$25.00
03/01/2010	$25.00
04/01/2010	$25.00
05/01/2010	$25.00
06/01/2010	$25.00
07/01/2010	$25.00
08/01/2010	$25.00
09/01/2010	$21.00

I have enclosed some envelopes for your convenience.   Thank you for your attention to this matter.   If I can assist you in any way, please do not hesitate contacting me.

Sincerely,

Your name
Administrative Medical Assistant

Figure WB9-42 *(Delmar/Cengage Learning)*

BUILDING SKILLS 9-14: POSTING PERSONAL CHECK PAYMENTS RECEIVED AFTER COLLECTIONS ACTIVITY

Instructions: The mail was brought to the office from the mailboxes on 02/04/2010. Personal checks were received from patients Sheridan, Johnsen, and Engelman. These patients recently were contacted by reminder letters and collections calls to pay on past due balances on their respective accounts. Refer to Source Documents WB9-7, WB9-8, and WB9-9 in the back of the workbook and post the payments as indicated below.

Patient Wynona Sheridan

1. From the Main Menu in MOSS, select *Posting Payments*. Select *Wynona Sheridan* from the patient list, and then click on *Apply Payment*.

2. Select the line item for services rendered on 10/27/2009 for $196.00. Using Source Document WB9-7, post the personal check payment to the account. Use the Note area in Field 14 to document that this is payment #1 of the payment plan set up with the patient. Check your work with Figure WB9-43.

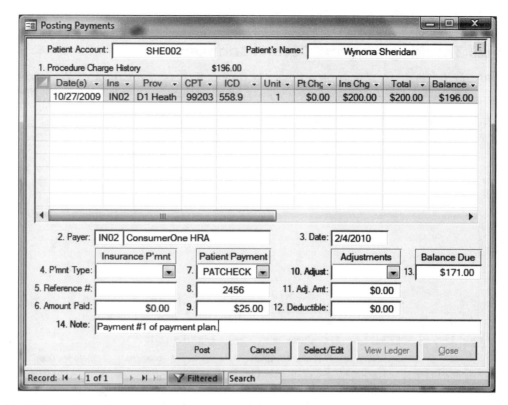

Figure WB9-43 *(Delmar/Cengage Learning)*

3. Post the payment, and then check your work with the Patient Ledger, as shown in Figure WB9-44.

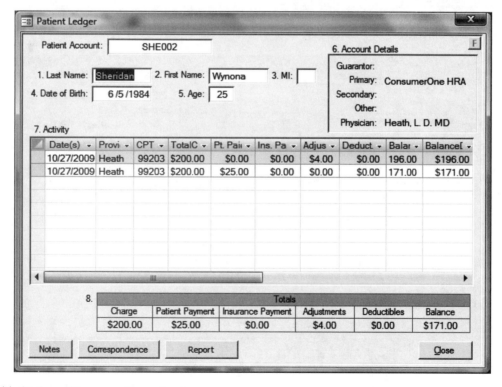

Figure WB9-44 *(Delmar/Cengage Learning)*

4. Close all open windows and return to the Main Menu.

Critical Thinking: Patient Dennis Johnsen

Instructions: Apply the payment as shown on Source Document WB9-8 in the back of the workbook to Patient Johnsen's account. Be sure to include a note. Check your work with Figures WB9-45 and WB9-46.

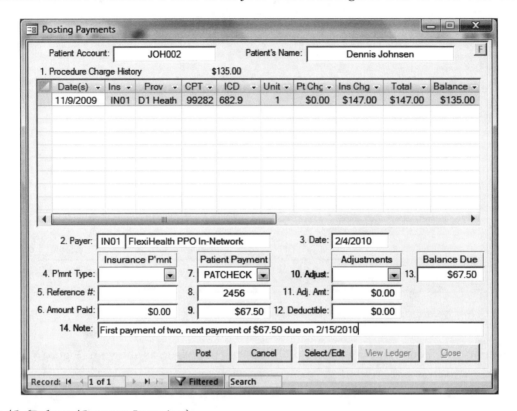

Figure WB9-45 *(Delmar/Cengage Learning)*

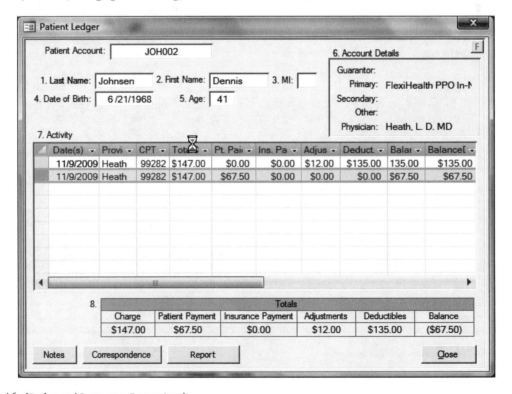

Figure WB9-46 *(Delmar/Cengage Learning)*

Critical Thinking: Patient Harold Engleman

Instructions: Apply the payment as shown on Source Document WB9-9 in the back of the workbook to Patient Engleman's account. Check your work with Figures WB9-47 and WB9-48.

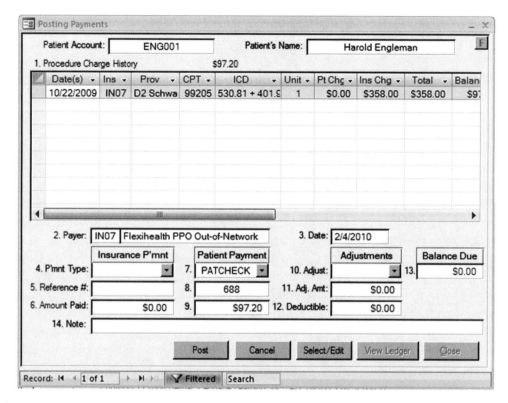

Figure WB9-47 *(Delmar/Cengage Learning)*

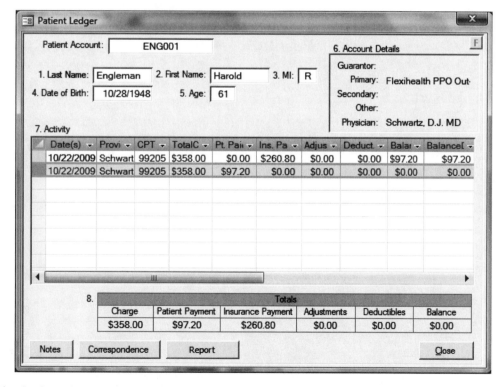

Figure WB9-48 *(Delmar/Cengage Learning)*

U N I T **1 0**

Posting Secondary Insurance Payments and Electronic RA Payments

BUILDING SKILLS 10-1: POSTING PAYMENTS FROM SECONDARY INSURANCE PLANS: CENTURY SENIORGAP

Instructions: Post the payments from the secondary insurance plan, Century SeniorGap, for each of the patients below. Refer to Source Documents WB10-1, WB10-2, and WB10-3 in the back of the workbook.

Note: Building Skills 10-1 and 10-2 includes using the *Primary Billing Ledger Adjustment* feature in MOSS as a bonus skill. The adjustment of balances in MOSS after secondary insurance payments have been completed can be included or excluded, in both this Workbook and the student book at the instructor's discretion.

Patient Deanna Hartsfeld

1. At the Main Menu of MOSS, click on *Posting Payments*. Select *Patient Hartsfeld* from the patient list and click *Apply Payment* to open the Posting Payments windows.

2. Refer to Source Document WB10-1. Read the EOB from Century SeniorGap and answer the following questions regarding Patient Hartsfeld's services.

Cover the answers using the tear-off bookmark from the cover of your textbook. Check your work before entering data into MOSS to be sure you have correctly interpreted the source documents.

A.	How much did the SeniorGap plan pay?	$80.89
B.	Did SeniorGap pay the patient's deductible?	Yes, the $80.89 does include the $75.00 deductible.
C.	Did SeniorGap pay the patient's co-insurance?	Yes, the $80.89 does include the $5.89 Medicare co-insurance.

3. Since this is a payment made by the secondary insurance, select the *Secondary Plan* with the locator bar on the bottom left of the screen. Click so that Record 2 is shown on the screen, indicated by Field 2 displaying Century SeniorGap. Check your screen with Figure WB10-1 before proceeding.

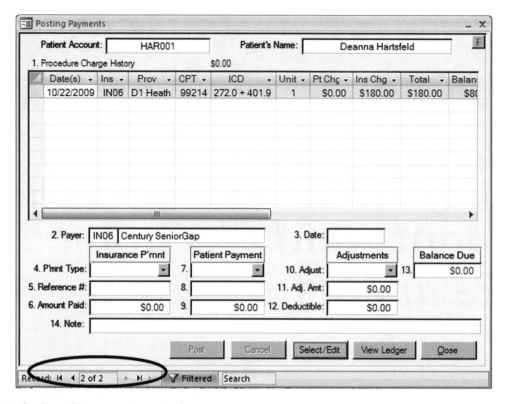

Figure WB10-1 *(Delmar/Cengage Learning)*

4. Post the payment, using 01/04/2010 as the posting date and SeniorGap Claim Number as the reference number. Before clicking Post, check your work with Figure WB10-2.

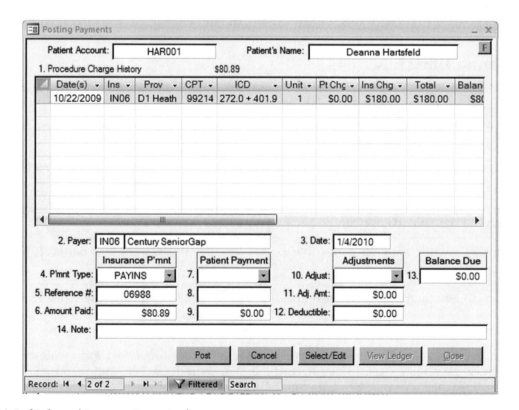

Figure WB10-2 *(Delmar/Cengage Learning)*

5. View the Patient Ledger for Patient Hartsfeld and check your screen with Figure WB10-3.

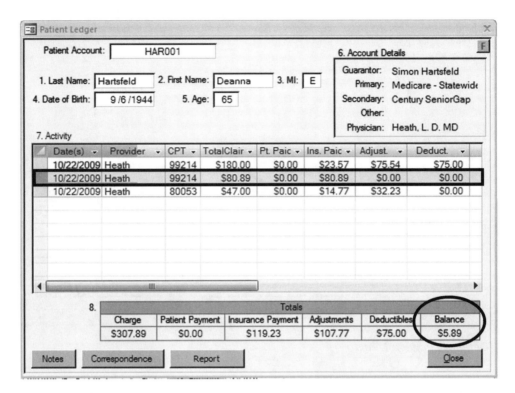

Figure WB10-3 *(Delmar/Cengage Learning)*

6. Note that $5.89 is showing as due. Since this portion was already paid by the secondary insurance, a Primary Billing Ledger Adjustment will be made to the primary insurance balance to zero out the account balance. Close the Patient Ledger to return to the Posting Payments screen.

7. Use the *locator bar* on the bottom left of the screen to return to Record 1 of 2, the Primary Insurance, Medicare—Statewide Corp.

8. Now, select the *99214 line item* for the 10/22/2009 service. Use 01/04/2010 as the posting date. Next, select *Primary Billing Ledger Adjustment* from the list in Field 10. Enter $5.89 in Field 11, and check your work with Figure WB10-4. Note that the Balance Due field reads $75.00; this represents the patient's deductible.

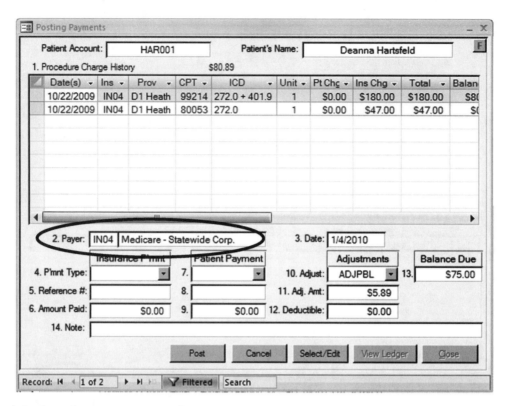

Figure WB10-4 *(Delmar/Cengage Learning)*

9. Click on *Post* and then view the Patient Ledger. Check your work with Figure WB10-5.

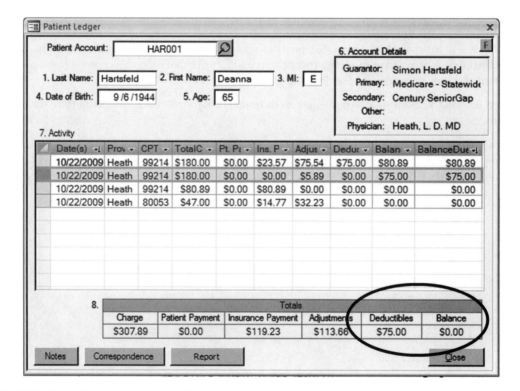

Figure WB10-5 *(Delmar/Cengage Learning)*

10. When finished, close all open windows and return to the Main Menu in MOSS.

Patient Nancy Herbert

1. At the Main Menu of MOSS, click on *Posting Payments*. Select *Patient Herbert* from the patient list to open the Posting Payments windows.

2. Refer to Source Document WB10-2. Read the EOB from Century SeniorGap and answer the following question regarding Patient Herbert's services.

A.	How much did the SeniorGap plan pay?	$28.06

3. Click the *locator bar* to display Record 2 on the screen, indicated by Field 2 displaying Century SeniorGap.

4. Post the payment, using 01/04/2010 as the posting date and SeniorGap Claim Number as the reference number. Check your work with Figure WB10-6.

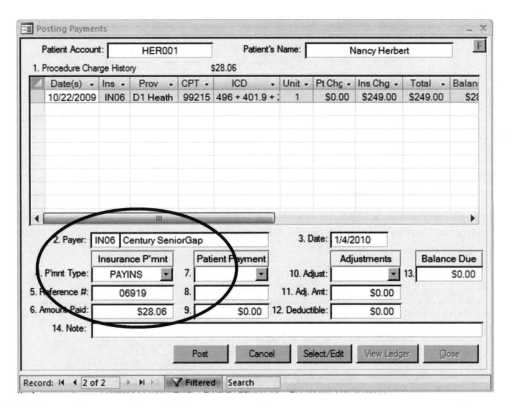

Figure WB10-6 *(Delmar/Cengage Learning)*

5. View the Patient Ledger for *Patient Herbert* and check your screen with Figure WB10-7. Note that $28.06 is showing as due. Since this portion was already paid by the secondary insurance, a Primary Billing Ledger Adjustment will be made to zero out the account balance.

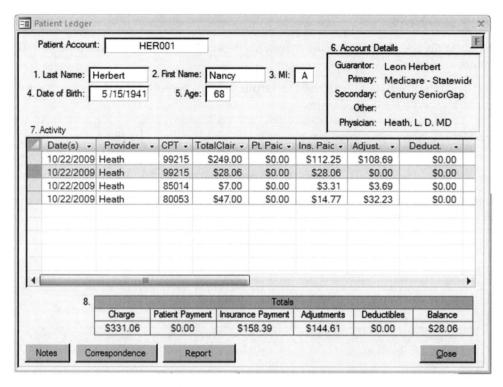

Figure WB10-7 *(Delmar/Cengage Learning)*

6. Close the Patient Ledger to return to the Posting Payments screen. Use the *locator bar* on the bottom left of the screen to return to the primary insurance, Medicare—Statewide Corp.

7. Select the *line item* for the 10/22/2009 service. Use 01/04/2010 as the posting date. Next, select *Primary Billing Ledger Adjustment* from the list in Field 10. Enter $28.06 in Field 11, and check your work with Figure WB10-8.

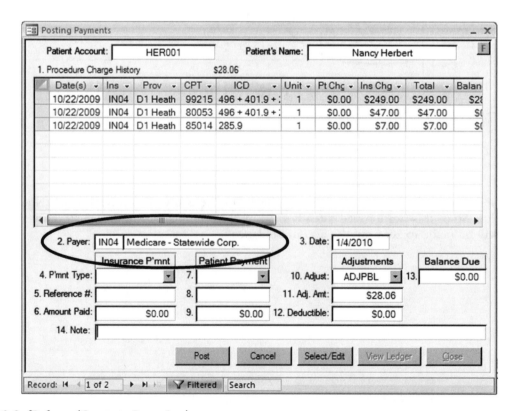

Figure WB10-8 *(Delmar/Cengage Learning)*

8. Click on *Post*, and then view the Patient Ledger. Check your work with Figure WB10-9. The balance on the account should now read zero.

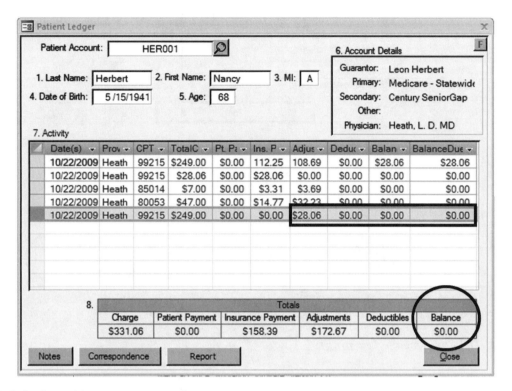

Figure WB10-9 *(Delmar/Cengage Learning)*

9. When finished, close all open windows and return to the Main Menu in MOSS.

Critical Thinking: Patient William Bernardo

Instructions: Refer to Source Document WB10-3 in the back of the workbook. Post the secondary insurance payment as shown on the EOB from Century SeniorGap for services done on 11/9/2009. Use the Primary Billing Ledger Adjustment to zero out the account when posting is complete. Check your work with Figures WB10-10 and WB10-11.

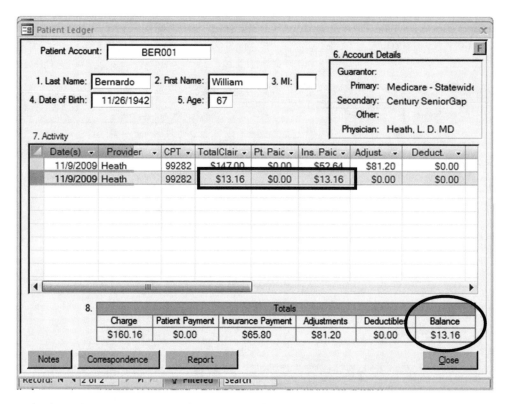

Figure WB10-10 *(Delmar/Cengage Learning)*

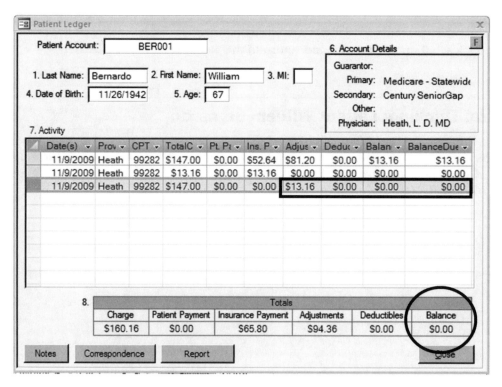

Figure WB10-11 *(Delmar/Cengage Learning)*

BUILDING SKILLS 10-2: POSTING PAYMENTS FROM SECONDARY INSURANCE PLANS: MEDICAID

Instructions: Post the payments from the secondary insurance plan Medicaid for Patient Isabel Durand. Refer to Source Documents WB10-4 in the back of the workbook.

Patient Isabel Durand

1. At the Main Menu of MOSS, click on *Posting Payments*. Select *Patient Durand* from the patient list to open the Posting Payments windows.

2. Refer to Source Document WB10-4. Read the Remittance Advice from Medicaid and answer the following question regarding Patient Durand's services.

A.	How much did Medicaid pay?	$7.12

3. Click the *locator bar* to display Record 2 on the screen, indicated by Field 2 displaying Medicaid.

4. Post the payment, using 01/05/2010 as the posting date and the RA Number as the reference number. Check your work with Figure WB10-12.

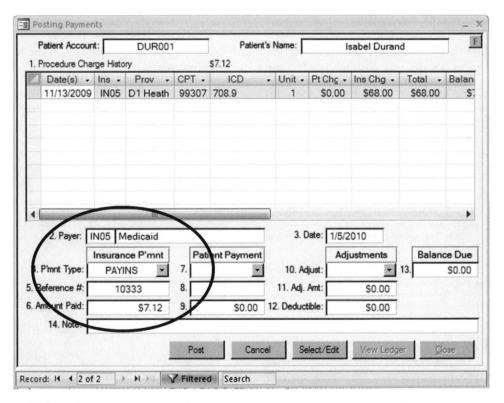

Figure WB10-12 *(Delmar/Cengage Learning)*

5. View the Patient Ledger for *Patient Durand* and check your screen with Figure WB10-13. Note that $7.12 is showing as due. Since this portion was already paid by the secondary insurance, a Primary Billing Ledger Adjustment will be made to zero out the account balance.

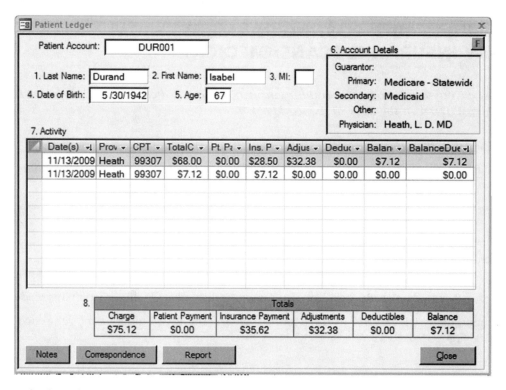

Figure WB10-13 *(Delmar/Cengage Learning)*

6. Close the Patient Ledger to return to the Posting Payments screen. Use the *locator bar* on the bottom left of the screen to return to the primary insurance, Medicare—Statewide Corp.

7. At the Posting Payment screen for Patient Durand, select the *line item* for the 11/13/2009 service. Use 01/04/2010 as the posting date. Next, select *Primary Billing Ledger Adjustment* from the list in Field 10. Enter $7.12 in Field 11, and check your work with Figure WB10-14.

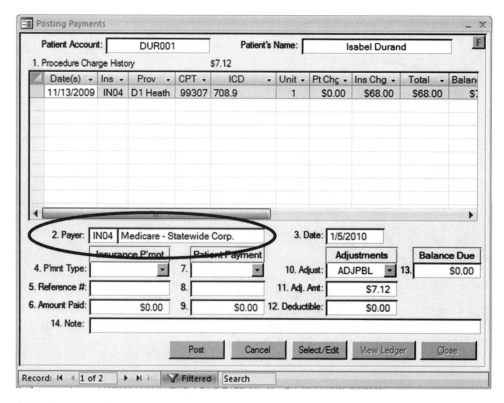

Figure WB10-14 *(Delmar/Cengage Learning)*

8. Click on *Post*, and then view the Patient Ledger. Check your work with Figure WB10-15. The balance due on the account should now read zero.

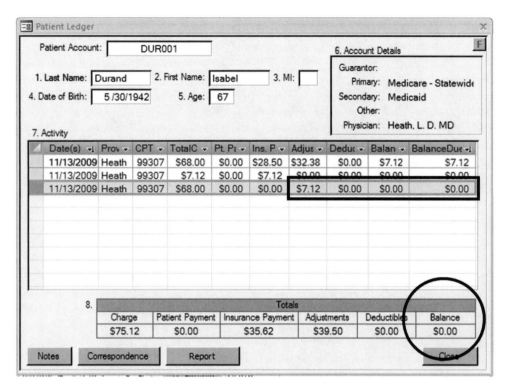

Figure WB10-15 *(Delmar/Cengage Learning)*

9. When finished, close all open windows and return to the Main Menu in MOSS.

U N I T **11**

Insurance Claims Follow-up and Dispute Resolution

BUILDING SKILLS 11-1: TRACKING AND FOLLOW-UP OF OUTSTANDING INSURANCE CLAIMS REVIEW

Instructions: Tell whether the following statements are true or false. In the lines below, explain your answer.

1. True or False? Patients with dual insurance coverage will typically have a longer wait time before all payments return for medical services.

   _____

   _____

   _____

   _____

2. True or False? Tracking and follow-up of claims should be done promptly, as many insurance companies have time limits for submitting an appeal or review.

   _____

   _____

   _____

   _____

3. True or False? It is best to gather and accumulate a number of problem claims that require follow-up and pursue the claims all at once.

   _____

   _____

   _____

   _____

Instructions: Select the correct answer for each of the following.

4. A claim that may require more information from the provider, or is being reviewed by medical professionals who represent the insurance company, is called a

   a. lost claim.

   b. suspended/pending claim.

   c. denied claim.

   d. None of the above

5. A claim that has not been paid, and the insurance company has given a reason, is referred to as a

   a. denied claim.

   b. suspended/pending claim.

   c. lost claim.

   d. None of the above

6. Claims that have not been paid due to omissions made by the medical office, or because incorrectly submitted information was provided on the claim, will most likely be a

   a. suspended/pending claim.

   b. denied claim.

   c. lost claim.

   d. None of the above

7. An insurance company has requested medical documentation, such as a surgical report, before considering a claim for payment. A notice is sent to the office requesting that this documentation be forwarded. This claim is most likely a

   a. denied claim.

   b. lost claim.

   c. suspended/pending claim.

   d. None of the above

8. Coding errors involving the CPT and/or ICD codes submitted with a claim are most likely to result in a

   a. denied claim.

   b. suspended/pending claim.

   c. lost claim.

   d. None of the above

BUILDING SKILLS 11-2: CLAIMS REVIEW AND APPEALS REVIEW

1. Explain what a review and appeal of a claim is.

   _____

   _____

   _____

   _____

   _____

   _____

2. When a medical office experiences claims that are denied payment, or for which the payment has been reduced, describe some solutions for isolating and addressing these problems.

_____

_____

_____

_____

_____

_____

3. If a claim needs to be reviewed, provide some suggestions as to where instructions for requesting a review might be found for a particular insurance company.

_____

_____

_____

_____

_____

_____

4. Describe information that can be included in a written request for review of a claim that might be helpful to the insurance company considering a review.

_____

_____

_____

_____

_____

_____

BUILDING SKILLS 11-3: THE MEDICARE APPEALS PROCESS REVIEW

1. Describe the function of the Medicare Recovery Audit Contractor (RAC) program.

_____

_____

_____

2. Arrange the following steps in the Medicare Appeals Process Review in the order they need to be done by writing "1st step", "2nd step", "3rd step", and "4th step" in the blanks provided:

a. ALJ Hearing   _____

b. Redetermination   _____

c. MAC review   _____

d. Reconsideration   _____

3. Match the appropriate CMS form that must be used for each of the following Medicare appeal steps:

   _ Redetermination   A. CMS20034

   _ Reconsideration   B. CMS20027

   _ ALJ Hearing   C. CMS20033

BUILDING SKILLS 11-4: COLLECTIONS TACTICS FOR PRIVATE THIRD-PARTY PAYERS REVIEW

1. Whenever placing telephone calls to insurance companies to make inquiries about denied or problem claims, or for any matter, describe some of the information a medical assistant should document during the conversation to help with future communications.

2. How can the intervention of the patient, or insured, be helpful when attempting to resolve problem claims or other issues that need further attention?

3. List important information that should be included in all letters requesting a review of denied or suspended claims that are sent to private third-party payers.

BUILDING SKILLS 11-5: PREPARE A MEDICARE REDETERMINATION REQUEST FORM

Instructions: Using the information in each case study below, prepare a Medicare CMS-20027 form requesting a review as indicated for each.

Case Study 1: Patient Joan Mandeville

On 01/07/2010, a Medicare RA was received with a payment for services rendered on 12/17/2009, as shown on Source Document WB11-1 in the back of the workbook. While posting the payment, the medical assistant noticed that procedure 99214 was allowed at a lower amount than what is customary. As such, the payment from Medicare was lower for the service.

1. Can you find another instance on a Medicare RA used with this book where CPT 99214 was allowed at a higher rate?

2. Using the CMS20027 form shown in Source Document WB11-2 in the back of the workbook, fill out a redetermination request so that the service will be considered for the correct allowed amount.

3. The form will be prepared on behalf of Dr. Heath as the requester, using the date of 1/7/2010.

4. Attach a copy of the Medicare RA with the error, and also include a copy of an RA from a correctly paid claim found on another Medicare RA as evidence. Check your form with Figure WB11-1.

5. Follow the directions of your instructor for turning in your work.

Case Study 2: Patient Franklin Ritter

On 01/07/2010, a Medicare RA was received with a payment for services rendered on 12/21/2009, as shown on Source Document WB11-3 in the back of the workbook. While posting the payment, the medical assistant noticed that procedure 99215 was allowed at a lower amount than what is customary. As such, the payment from Medicare was lower for the service.

1. Can you find another instance on a Medicare RA used with this book where CPT 99215 was allowed at a higher rate?

2. Using the CMS20027 form shown in Source Document W11-4 in the back of the workbook, fill out a redetermination request so that the service will be considered for the correct allowed amount.

3. The form will be prepared on behalf of Dr. Heath as the requester, using the date of 1/7/2010.

4. Attach a copy of the Medicare RA with the error, and also include a copy of an RA from a correctly paid claim found on another Medicare RA as evidence. Check your form with Figure WB11-2.

5. Follow the directions of your instructor for turning in your work.

DEPARTMENT OF HEALTH AND HUMAN SERVICES
CENTERS FOR MEDICARE & MEDICAID SERVICES

MEDICARE REDETERMINATION REQUEST FORM

1. Beneficiary's Name: *JOAN MANDEVILLE*

2. Medicare Number: *999613122 B*

3. Description of Item or Service in Question: *CPT 99214*

4. Date the Service or Item was Received: *12/17/2009*

5. I do not agree with the determination of my claim. MY REASONS ARE:

AMOUNT ALLOWED IS NOT THE USUAL & CUSTOMARY

ALLOWED AMOUNT, 99214 IS USUALLY ALLOWED AT $104.46

6. Date of the initial determination notice _*01/07/2010*_
(If you received your initial determination notice more than 120 days ago, include your reason for not making this request earlier.)

7. Additional Information Medicare Should Consider: *OUR OFFICE HAS PREVIOUSLY BEEN ALLOWED $104.46*

FOR CPT 99214

8. Requester's Name: *LD HEATH, MD*

9. Requester's Relationship to the Beneficiary: *PHYSICIAN*

10. Requester's Address: *5076 BRAND BLVD SUITE 401*

DOUGLASVILLE, NY 01234

11. Requester's Telephone Number: *(123) 456 – 7890*

12. Requester's Signature: _____

13. Date Signed: _____

14. ☒ I have evidence to submit. (Attach such evidence to this form.)
☐ I do not have evidence to submit.

NOTICE: Anyone who misrepresents or falsifies essential information requested by this form may upon conviction be subject to fine or imprisonment under Federal Law.

Form CMS-20027 (05/05) EF 05/2005

Figure WB11-1 *(Courtesy of the Centers for Medicare & Medicaid Services.)*

DEPARTMENT OF HEALTH AND HUMAN SERVICES
CENTERS FOR MEDICARE & MEDICAID SERVICES

MEDICARE REDETERMINATION REQUEST FORM

1. Beneficiary's Name: _FRANKLIN RITTER_

2. Medicare Number: _999231125 A_

3. Description of Item or Service in Question: _CPT 99215_

4. Date the Service or Item was Received: _12/21/2009_

5. I do not agree with the determination of my claim. MY REASONS ARE:

AMOUNT ALLOWED IS NOT THE USUAL & CUSTOMARY

ALLOWED AMOUNT, 99215 IS USUALLY ALLOWED AT $140.31

6. Date of the initial determination notice _01/07/2010_

(If you received your initial determination notice more than 120 days ago, include your reason for not making this request earlier.)

7. Additional Information Medicare Should Consider: _OUR OFFICE HAS PREVIOUSLY BEEN ALLOWED $140.31_

FOR CPT 99215

8. Requester's Name: _LD HEATH, MD_

9. Requester's Relationship to the Beneficiary: _PHYSICIAN_

10. Requester's Address: _5076 BRAND BLVD SUITE 401_

DOUGLASVILLE, NY 01234

11. Requester's Telephone Number: _(123) 456 – 7890_

12. Requester's Signature: _____

13. Date Signed: _____

14. ☒ I have evidence to submit. (Attach such evidence to this form.)
   ❏ I do not have evidence to submit.

NOTICE: Anyone who misrepresents or falsifies essential information requested by this form may upon conviction be subject to fine or imprisonment under Federal Law.

Form CMS-20027 (05/05) EF 05/2005

Figure WB11-2 *(Courtesy of the Centers for Medicare & Medicaid Services.)*

Comprehensive Final Examination

The Comprehensive Final Examination will evaluate your understanding of how to perform common medical-office tasks using practice management software. Carefully read the instructions for each section below and complete the medical-office tasks using Medical Office Simulation Software (MOSS). Follow the directions of your instructor for turning in your work.

EVALUATION 1 – NEW PATIENT REGISTRATION

Patient Sharon Riley

Instructions: Refer to the registration form and copy of insurance card in Figures WBE 1-1 and WBE 1-2. Using Monday, April 5, 2010, as the date, enter the new patient information using MOSS and document that the office privacy notice was given to the patient and signed.

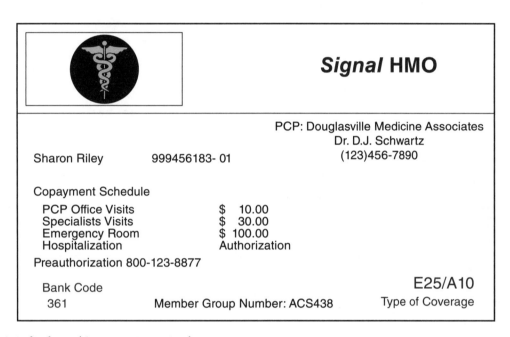

Figure WBE 1-1 *(Delmar/Cengage Learning)*

Welcome To Our Office
PLEASE PRINT

NEW PATIENT INFORMATION

DATE _____

LAST NAME	FIRST NAME	MI	SSN		GENDER	MARITAL STATUS	DATE OF BIRTH
Riley	Sharon	A.	999-45-6183		Female	Single	12/04/1982

ADDRESS	APT/UNIT	CITY	STATE	ZIP	HOME PH (123)	WORK PH (123) EXT:
438 State Court	302	Douglasville	NY	01235	457-3310	457-1000

EMPLOYER/SCHOOL	EMPLOYER ADDRESS	CITY	STATE	ZIP
ACE Corner Stores, Inc	123 Industry Way	Douglasville	NY	01234

REFERRING PHYSICIAN (LAST NAME, FIRST NAME)	ADDRESS	CITY	STATE	ZIP	PHONE

GUARANTOR - Person responsible for payment: ☒ self ☐ spouse/other ☐ parent ☐ legal guardian If not "self", please complete the following:

LAST NAME	FIRST NAME	MI	SSN		GENDER	DATE OF BIRTH

ADDRESS (IF DIFFERENT FROM PATIENT)	CITY	STATE	ZIP	HOME PH ( )	ALT. PHONE

EMPLOYER NAME	EMPLOYER ADDRESS	CITY	STATE	ZIP	WORK PHONE EXT

OTHER RESPONSIBLE PARTY:

LAST NAME	FIRST NAME	MI	SSN	GENDER	DATE OF BIRTH

ADDRESS (IF DIFFERENT FROM PATIENT)	CITY	STATE	ZIP	HOME PH ( )	ALT. PHONE

EMPLOYER NAME	EMPLOYER ADDRESS	CITY STATE	ZIP	WORK PHONE EXT

INSURANCE - PRIMARY

PLAN NAME	PATIENT RELATIONSHIP TO INSURED:
Signal HMO	☒ self ☐ spouse ☐ child ☐ other

POLICYHOLDER INFORMATION

LAST NAME	FIRST NAME	MI	DATE OF BIRTH	ID#	POLICY #	GROUP #
Riley	Sharon	A.	12/04/1982	999456183-01		ACS438

EMPLOYER NAME	PCP NAME, IF APPLICABLE:
ACE Corner Stores	DJ Schwartz

INSURANCE - SECONDARY

PLAN NAME	PATIENT RELATIONSHIP TO INSURED: ☐ self ☐ spouse ☐ child ☐ other
None	

POLICYHOLDER INFORMATION

LAST NAME	FIRST NAME	MI	DATE OF BIRTH	ID#	POLICY #	GROUP #

EMPLOYER NAME	PCP NAME, IF APPLICABLE:

ACCIDENT? ☐ YES ☒ NO IF YES, DATE OF INJURY	OCCUR AT WORK? ☐ YES ☒ NO	AUTO INVOLVED: ☐ YES ☒ NO	STATE

NAME OF ATTORNEY	PHONE NUMBER EXT.		

INSURANCE AUTHORIZATION AND ASSIGNMENT

Name of Policy Holder _____ HIC Number _____

I request that payment of authorized Medicare/Other Insurance company benefits be made either to me or on my behalf to ___Dr. Schwartz___
For any services furnished me by that party who accepts assignment/physician. Regulations pertaining to Medicare assignment of benefits apply.
I authorize the release of protected health information to the Social Security Administration and Centers for Medicare and Medicaid Services or its intermediaries or carriers any information needed for this or a related Medicare claim/other Insurance Company claim...(Section 11288 f the Social Security Act and if 31 U.S.C. Sections 3801-3812 provides penalties for withholding this information).

Signature ____*Sharon Riley*____ Date_____

Figure WBE 1-2 (Used with permission. InHealth Record Systems, Inc. 5076 Winters Chapel Road, Atlanta, GA 30360, 800-477-7374. http://www.inhealthrecords.com)

Patient George Manfred

Instructions: Refer to the registration form and copy of insurance cards in Figures WBE 1-3A, WBE 1-3B, and WBE1–4. Using Monday, April 5, 2010, as the date, enter the new patient information using MOSS and document that the office privacy notice was given to the patient and signed.

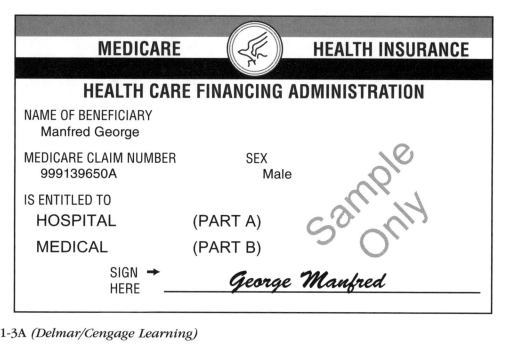

Figure WBE 1-3A *(Delmar/Cengage Learning)*

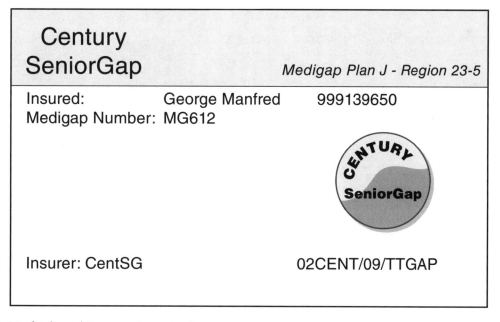

Figure WBE 1-3B *(Delmar/Cengage Learning)*

Welcome To Our Office   **NEW PATIENT INFORMATION**   DATE _____

PLEASE PRINT

LAST NAME	FIRST NAME	MI	SSN	GENDER	MARITAL STATUS	DATE OF BIRTH
Manfred	George	L.	999-13-9650	Male	Married	01/28/1925

ADDRESS	APT/UNIT	CITY	STATE	ZIP	HOME PH (123)	WORK PH ( ) EXT:
4012 Marble Way		Douglasville	NY	01234	457-1161	

EMPLOYER/SCHOOL	EMPLOYER ADDRESS	CITY	STATE	ZIP
Retired				

REFERRING PHYSICIAN (LAST NAME, FIRST NAME)	ADDRESS	CITY	STATE	ZIP	PHONE

GUARANTOR - Person responsible for payment: ☒ self ☐ spouse/other ☐ parent ☐ legal guardian If not "self", please complete the following:

LAST NAME	FIRST NAME	MI	SSN	GENDER	DATE OF BIRTH

ADDRESS (IF DIFFERENT FROM PATIENT)	CITY	STATE	ZIP	HOME PH ( )	ALT. PHONE

EMPLOYER NAME	EMPLOYER ADDRESS	CITY	STATE	ZIP	WORK PHONE	EXT

OTHER RESPONSIBLE PARTY:

LAST NAME	FIRST NAME	MI	SSN	GENDER	DATE OF BIRTH	
Manfred	Louis	A.		Female	09/18/1943	

ADDRESS (IF DIFFERENT FROM PATIENT)	CITY	STATE	ZIP	HOME PH (123)	ALT. PHONE
Same				457-1161	

EMPLOYER NAME	EMPLOYER ADDRESS	CITY STATE	ZIP	WORK PHONE	EXT
Retired					

INSURANCE - PRIMARY

PLAN NAME	PATIENT RELATIONSHIP TO INSURED:
Medicare Statewide	☒ self ☐ spouse ☐ child ☐ other

POLICYHOLDER INFORMATION

LAST NAME	FIRST NAME	MI	DATE OF BIRTH	ID#	POLICY #	GROUP #
Manfred	George		01/28/1925	999139650A		

EMPLOYER NAME	PCP NAME, IF APPLICABLE:
	LD Heath

INSURANCE - SECONDARY

PLAN NAME	PATIENT RELATIONSHIP TO INSURED:
Century Senior GAP	☒ self ☐ spouse ☐ child ☐ other

POLICYHOLDER INFORMATION

LAST NAME	FIRST NAME	MI	DATE OF BIRTH	ID#	POLICY #	GROUP #
Manfred	George			999139650		MG612

EMPLOYER NAME	PCP NAME, IF APPLICABLE:

ACCIDENT? ☐ YES ☒ NO IF YES, DATE OF INJURY	OCCUR AT WORK? ☐ YES ☐ NO	AUTO INVOLVED: ☐ YES ☒ NO	STATE

NAME OF ATTORNEY	PHONE NUMBER EXT.

INSURANCE AUTHORIZATION AND ASSIGNMENT

Name of Policy Holder ___George Manfred_____   HIC Number __999139650A____

I request that payment of authorized Medicare/Other Insurance company benefits be made either to me or on my behalf to ___Dr. Heath___
For any services furnished me by that party who accepts assignment/physician. Regulations pertaining to Medicare assignment of benefits apply.
I authorize the release of protected health information to the Social Security Administration and Centers for Medicare and Medicaid Services or its intermediaries or carriers any information needed for this or a related Medicare claim/other Insurance Company claim...(Section 11288 f the Social Security Act and if 31 U.S.C. Sections 3801-3812 provides penalties for withholding this information).

Signature ___*George Manfred*_____   Date_____

Figure WBE 1-4 *(Used with permission. InHealth Record Systems, Inc. 5076 Winters Chapel Road, Atlanta, GA 30360, 800-477-7374. http://www.inhealthrecords.com)*

Patient Emma Lansford

Instructions: Refer to the registration form and copy of insurance card in Figures WBE 1-5 and WBE 1-6. Using Monday, April 5, 2010, as the date, enter the new patient information using MOSS and document that the office privacy notice was given to the patient and signed.

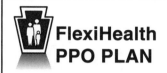

		Insurer 81564
FlexiHealth **PPO PLAN**		*Your Health First* ᴿᴹ

Insured: Lansford, Emma 999119315-01
Employer: Vander Solutions, LLC Network 45A-2
Group: VS2210

Individual Group Benefits
In-network - YES

Physician Co-pay: $20.00
Hospital Services: $400.00
Surgery & Hospitalization: Requires preauthorization 800-123-3654

Figure WBE 1-5 *(Delmar/Cengage Learning)*

Welcome To Our Office   **NEW PATIENT INFORMATION**   *DATE* _____

PLEASE PRINT

LAST NAME Lansford	FIRST NAME Emma	MI S.	SSN 999-11-9315	GENDER Female	MARITAL STATUS Single	DATE OF BIRTH 12/23/1985

ADDRESS 5220 Gravel Street	APT/UNIT	CITY Douglasville	STATE NY	ZIP 01234	HOME PH (123) 457-0188	WORK PH (123) EXT: 457-1200 x31

EMPLOYER/SCHOOL Vander Solutions, LLC	EMPLOYER ADDRESS PO Box 3521	CITY Douglasville	STATE NY	ZIP 01235

REFERRING PHYSICIAN (LAST NAME, FIRST NAME)	ADDRESS	CITY	STATE	ZIP	PHONE

GUARANTOR - Person responsible for payment: ☒ self ☐ spouse/other ☐ parent ☐ legal guardian <u>If not "self", please complete the following:</u>

LAST NAME	FIRST NAME	MI	SSN	GENDER	DATE OF BIRTH

ADDRESS (IF DIFFERENT FROM PATIENT)	CITY	STATE	ZIP	HOME PH ( )	ALT. PHONE

EMPLOYER NAME	EMPLOYER ADDRESS	CITY	STATE	ZIP	WORK PHONE	EXT

OTHER RESPONSIBLE PARTY:

LAST NAME	FIRST NAME	MI	SSN	GENDER	DATE OF BIRTH

ADDRESS (IF DIFFERENT FROM PATIENT)	CITY	STATE	ZIP	HOME PH ( )	ALT. PHONE

EMPLOYER NAME	EMPLOYER ADDRESS	CITY STATE	ZIP	WORK PHONE	EXT

INSURANCE - PRIMARY

PLAN NAME Flexi Health PPO	PATIENT RELATIONSHIP TO INSURED: ☒ self ☐ spouse ☐ child ☐ other

POLICYHOLDER INFORMATION

LAST NAME Lansford	FIRST NAME Emma	MI S.	DATE OF BIRTH 12/23/1985	ID# 999119315-01	POLICY #	GROUP # VS2210

EMPLOYER NAME Vander Solutions, LLC	PCP NAME, IF APPLICABLE: LD Heath

INSURANCE - SECONDARY

PLAN NAME None	PATIENT RELATIONSHIP TO INSURED: ☐ self ☐ spouse ☐ child ☐ other

POLICYHOLDER INFORMATION

LAST NAME	FIRST NAME	MI	DATE OF BIRTH	ID#	POLICY #	GROUP #

EMPLOYER NAME	PCP NAME, IF APPLICABLE:

ACCIDENT? ☐ YES ☒ NO IF YES, DATE OF INJURY	OCCUR AT WORK? ☐ YES ☒ NO	AUTO INVOLVED: ☐ YES ☒ NO	STATE

NAME OF ATTORNEY	PHONE NUMBER EXT.		

INSURANCE AUTHORIZATION AND ASSIGNMENT

Name of Policy Holder _____ HIC Number _____

I request that payment of authorized Medicare/Other Insurance company benefits be made either to me or on my behalf to _____**Dr. Heath**_____

For any services furnished me by that party who accepts assignment/physician. Regulations pertaining to Medicare assignment of benefits apply.

I authorize the release of protected health information to the Social Security Administration and Centers for Medicare and Medicaid Services or its intermediaries or carriers any information needed for this or a related Medicare claim/other Insurance Company claim...(Section 11288 f the Social Security Act and if 31 U.S.C. Sections 3801-3812 provides penalties for withholding this information).

Signature _____*Emma Lansford*_____ Date_____

Figure WBE 1-6 *(Used with permission. InHealth Record Systems, Inc. 5076 Winters Chapel Road, Atlanta, GA 30360, 800-477-7374. http://www.inhealthrecords.com)*

Patient Timothy Meade

Instructions: Refer to the registration form and copy of insurance card in Figures WBE 1-7 and WBE 1-8. Using Monday, April 5, 2010, as the date, enter the new patient information using MOSS and document that the office privacy notice was given to the patient and signed.

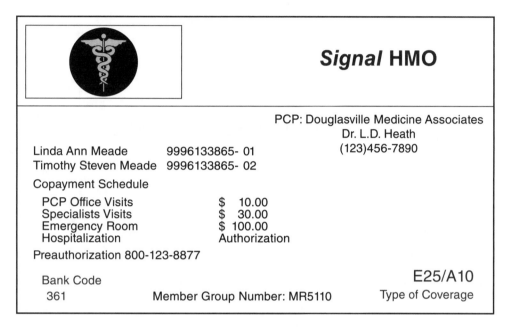

Figure WBE 1-7 *(Delmar/Cengage Learning)*

Welcome To Our Office
PLEASE PRINT

NEW PATIENT INFORMATION   DATE _____

LAST NAME	FIRST NAME	MI	SSN		GENDER	MARITAL STATUS	DATE OF BIRTH
Meade	Timothy	S.	999-61-3386		Male	Married	07/04/1978

ADDRESS	APT/UNIT	CITY	STATE	ZIP	HOME PH (123)	WORK PH ( ) EXT:
913 Pebble Road	101	Douglasville	NY	01235	457-1361	

EMPLOYER/SCHOOL	EMPLOYER ADDRESS	CITY	STATE	ZIP
Unemployed				

REFERRING PHYSICIAN (LAST NAME, FIRST NAME)	ADDRESS	CITY	STATE	ZIP	PHONE

GUARANTOR - Person responsible for payment: ☐ self   ☒ spouse/other   ☐ parent   ☐ legal guardian *If not "self", please complete the following:*

LAST NAME	FIRST NAME	MI	SSN		GENDER	DATE OF BIRTH
Meade	Linda	A.	999312611		Female	11/24/1972

ADDRESS (IF DIFFERENT FROM PATIENT)	CITY	STATE	ZIP	HOME PH ( )	ALT. PHONE
Same					

EMPLOYER NAME	EMPLOYER ADDRESS	CITY STATE	ZIP	WORK PHONE 123 EXT
Midway Radiology, P.C.	11610 Midway Boulevard	Douglasville, NY	01234	457-3300 x2

OTHER RESPONSIBLE PARTY:

LAST NAME	FIRST NAME	MI	SSN	GENDER	DATE OF BIRTH

ADDRESS (IF DIFFERENT FROM PATIENT)	CITY	STATE	ZIP	HOME PH ( )	ALT. PHONE

EMPLOYER NAME	EMPLOYER ADDRESS	CITY STATE	ZIP	WORK PHONE EXT

INSURANCE - PRIMARY

PLAN NAME	PATIENT RELATIONSHIP TO INSURED:
Signal HMO	☐ self ☒ spouse ☐ child ☐ other

POLICYHOLDER INFORMATION

LAST NAME	FIRST NAME	MI	DATE OF BIRTH	ID#	POLICY #	GROUP #
Meade	Linda		11/24/1972	9996133865-02		MR5110

EMPLOYER NAME	PCP NAME, IF APPLICABLE:
Midway Radiology, PC	LD Heath

INSURANCE - SECONDARY

PLAN NAME	PATIENT RELATIONSHIP TO INSURED: ☒ self ☐ spouse ☐ child ☐ other
None	

POLICYHOLDER INFORMATION

LAST NAME	FIRST NAME	MI	DATE OF BIRTH	ID#	POLICY #	GROUP #

EMPLOYER NAME	PCP NAME, IF APPLICABLE:

ACCIDENT? ☐ YES ☒ NO IF YES, DATE OF INJURY	OCCUR AT WORK? ☐ YES ☒ NO	AUTO INVOLVED: ☐ YES ☒ NO	STATE

NAME OF ATTORNEY	PHONE NUMBER EXT.

INSURANCE AUTHORIZATION AND ASSIGNMENT

Name of Policy Holder _____   HIC Number _____

I request that payment of authorized Medicare/Other Insurance company benefits be made either to me or on my behalf to _____ **Dr. Heath** _____

For any services furnished me by that party who accepts assignment/physician. Regulations pertaining to Medicare assignment of benefits apply.

I authorize the release of protected health information to the Social Security Administration and Centers for Medicare and Medicaid Services or its intermediaries or carriers any information needed for this or a related Medicare claim/other Insurance Company claim...(Section 11288 f the Social Security Act and if 31 U.S.C. Sections 3801-3812 provides penalties for withholding this information).

Signature _____ *Timothy Meade* _____   Date_____

Figure WBE 1-8 *(Used with permission. InHealth Record Systems, Inc. 5076 Winters Chapel Road, Atlanta, GA 30360, 800-477-7374. http://www.inhealthrecords.com)*

EVALUATION 2 – VERIFY PATIENT BENEFITS USING ONLINE ELIGIBILITY

Instructions: For new patients Riley, Manfred, Lansford, and Meade, verify the insurance benefits using the online eligibility tool in MOSS. Print and/or save the report for each patient.

EVALUATION 3 – PATIENT CHECK-OUT: POSTING PROCEDURES, PAYMENTS, AND APPOINTMENT SCHEDULING

Patient Sharon Riley

Instructions: Complete the following tasks on 4/5/2010:

a. Refer to the superbill in Figure WBE 1-9 and enter the procedure(s) for Patient Riley using MOSS.

b. Refer to the personal check in Figure WBE 1-10 and post the payment made by the patient.

c. Schedule a follow-up appointment as requested by the physician for 15 minutes.

PLEASE RETURN THIS FORM TO RECEPTIONIST

NAME _Sharon Riley_

Ref # E001

PLACE OF SERVICE:
(X) OFFICE
( ) NEW YORK COUNTY HOSPITAL
( ) COMMUNITY GENERAL HOSPITAL
( ) RETIREMENT INN NURSING HOME
( ) _____

DATE OF SERVICE _04/05/2010_

A. OFFICE VISITS - New Patient

	Code	History	Exam	Dec.	Time	
	99201	Prob. Foc.	Prob. Foc.	Straight	10 min.	
	99202	Ex. Prob. Foc.	Ex. Prob. Foc.	Straight	20 min.	
X	99203	Detail	Detail	Low	30 min.	1, 2
	99204	Comp.	Comp.	Mod.	45 min.	
	99205	Comp.	Comp.	High	60 min.	

B. OFFICE VISIT - Established Patient

Code	History	Exam	Dec.	Time	
99211	Minimal	Minimal	Minimal	5 min.	
99212	Prob. Foc.	Prob. Foc.	Straight	10min.	
99213	Ex. Prob. Foc.	Ex. Prob. Foc.	Low	15 min.	
99214	Detail	Detail	Mod.	25 min.	
99215	Comp.	Comp.	High	40 min.	

C. HOSPITAL CARE

		Dx	Units	
1.	Initial Hospital Care (30 min)		99221	
2.	Subsequent Care		99231	
3.	Critical Care (30-74 min)		99291	
4.	each additional 30 min.		99292	
5.	Discharge Services		99238	
6.	Emergency Room		99282	

D. NURSING HOME CARE

		Dx	Units	
	Initial Care - New Pt.			
1.	Expanded		99322	
2.	Detailed		99323	
	Subsequent Care - Estab. Pt.			
3.	Problem Focused		99307	
4.	Expanded		99308	
5.	Detailed		99309	
5.	Comprehensive		99310	

E. PROCEDURES

1.	Arthrocentesis, Small Jt.		20600
2.	Colonoscopy		45378
3.	EKG w/interpretation		93000
4.	X-Ray Chest, PA/LAT		71020

F. LAB

1.	Blood Sugar		82947	
2.	CBC w/differential	1	85031	X
3.	Cholesterol		82465	
4.	Comprehensive Metabolic Panel		80053	
5.	ESR		85651	
6.	Hematocrit		85014	
7.	Mono Screen		86308	
8.	Pap Smear		88150	
9.	Potassium		84132	
10.	Preg. Test, Quantitative		84702	
11.	Routine Venipuncture		36415	

F. Cont'd

			Dx	Units	
12.	Strep Screen			87081	
13.	UA, Routine w/Micro			81000	
14.	UA, Routine w/o Micro	1		81002	X
15.	Uric Acid			84550	
16.	VDRL			86592	
17.	Wet Prep			82710	
18.	_____				

G. INJECTIONS

1.	Influenza Virus Vaccine		90658
2.	Pneumoccocal Vaccine		90772
3.	Tetanus Toxoids		90703
4.	Therapeutic Subcut/IM		90732
5.	Vaccine Administration		90471
6.	Vaccine - each additional		90472

H. MISCELLANEOUS
1. _____
2. _____

AMOUNT PAID $ _10.00_

Mark diagnosis with (1=Primary, 2=Secondary, 3=Tertiary)

DIAGNOSIS NOT LISTED BELOW _____

DIAGNOSIS	ICD-9-CM 1, 2, 3	DIAGNOSIS	ICD-9-CM 1, 2, 3	DIAGNOSIS	ICD-9-CM 1, 2, 3
Abdominal Pain	789.0	Dehydration	276.51	Otitis Media, Acute NOS	382.9
Allergic Rhinitis, Unspec.	477.9	Depression, NOS	311	Peptic Ulcer Disease	536.9
Angina Pectoris, Unspec.	413.9	Diabetes Mellitus, Type II Controlled	250.00	Peripheral Vascular Disease NOS	443.9
Anemia, Iron Deficiency, Unspec.	280.9	Diabetes Mellitus, Type II Controlled	250.02	Pharyngitis, Acute	462
Anemia, NOS	285.9	Drug Reaction, NOS	995.29	Pneumonia, Organism Unspec.	486
Anemia, Pernicious	281.0	Dysuria	788.1 2	Prostatitis, NOS	601.9
Asthma w/ Exacerbation	493.92	Eczema, NOS	692.2	PVC	427.69
Asthmatic Bronchitis, Unspec.	493.90	Edema	782.3	Rash, Non Specific	782.1
Atrial Fibrillation	427.31	Fever, Unknown Origin	780.6	Seizure Disorder NOS	780.39
Atypical Chest Pain, Unspec.	786.59	Gastritis, Acute w/o Hemorrhage	535.00	Serous Otitis Media, Chronic, Unspec.	381.10
Bronchiolitis, due to RSV	466.11	Gastroenteritis, NOS	558.9	Sinusitis, Acute NOS	461.9
Bronchitis, Acute	466.0	Gastroesophageal Reflux	530.81	Tonsillitis, Acute	463.
Bronchitis, NOS	490	Hepatitis A, Infectious	070.1	Upper Respiratory Infection, Acute NOS	465.9
Cardiac Arrest	427.5	Hypercholesterolemia, Pure	272.0	Urinary Tract Infection, Unspec.	599.0 1
Cardiopulmonary Disease, Chronic, Unspec.	416.9	Hypertension, Unspec.	401.9	Urticaria, Unspec.	708.9
Cellulitis, NOS	682.9	Hypoglycemia NOS	251.2	Vertigo, NOS	780.4
Congestive Heart Failure, Unspec.	428.0	Hypokalemia	276.8	Viral Infection NOS	079.99
Contact Dermatitis NOS	692.9	Impetigo	684	Weakness, Generalized	780.79
COPD NOS	496	Lymphadenitis, Unspec.	289.3	Weight Loss, Abnormal	783.21
CVA, Acute, NOS	434.91	Mononucleosis	075		
CVA, Old or Healed	438.9	Myocardial Infarction, Acute, NOS	410.9		
Degenerative Arthritis (Specify Site)	715.9	Organic Brain Syndrome	310.9		
		Otitis Externa, Acute NOS	380.10		

ABN: I UNDERSTAND THAT MEDICARE PROBABLY WILL NOT COVER THE SERVICES LISTED BELOW

A. _____ B. _____ C. _____

Patient

Date _____ Signature _____

Doctor's Signature _D.J. Schwartz MD_

RETURN: _____ Days _2_ Weeks _____ Months

REF# 122949 SB (05.07.09) TO REORDER CALL INHEALTH RECORD SYSTEMS 800-477-7374

DOUGLASVILLE MEDICINE ASSOCIATES
5076 BRAND BLVD., SUITE 401
DOUGLASVILLE, NY 01234
PHONE No. (123) 456-7890
□ L.D. HEATH, M.D.   ☒ D.J. SCHWARTZ, M.D.
NPI# 9995010111   NPI# 9995020212
EIN# 00-1234560

Figure WBE 1-9 *(Used with permission. InHealth Record Systems, Inc. 5076 Winters Chapel Road, Atlanta, GA 30360, 800-477-7374. http://www.inhealthrecords.com)*

Figure WBE 1-10 *(Delmar/Cengage Learning)*

Patient George Manfred

Instructions: Complete the following tasks on 4/5/2010:

a. Refer to the superbill in Figure WBE 1-11 and enter the procedure(s) for Patient Manfred using MOSS.

b. Schedule a follow-up appointment as requested by the physician for 15 minutes.

PLEASE RETURN THIS FORM TO RECEPTIONIST

NAME *George Manfred*

Ref # E002

PLACE OF SERVICE:
(X) OFFICE
( ) NEW YORK COUNTY HOSPITAL
( ) COMMUNITY GENERAL HOSPITAL
( ) RETIREMENT INN NURSING HOME
( ) _____

DATE OF SERVICE *04/05/2010*

A. OFFICE VISITS - New Patient

Code	History	Exam	Dec.	Time	
____ 99201	Prob. Foc.	Prob. Foc.	Straight	10 min.	_____
____ 99202	Ex. Prob. Foc.	Ex. Prob. Foc.	Straight	20 min.	_____
____ 99203	Detail	Detail	Low	30 min.	_____
X 99204	Comp.	Comp.	Mod.	45 min.	1, 2, 3
____ 99205	Comp.	Comp.	High	60 min.	_____

B. OFFICE VISIT - Established Patient

Code	History	Exam	Dec.	Time	
____ 99211	Minimal	Minimal	Minimal	5 min.	_____
____ 99212	Prob. Foc.	Prob. Foc.	Straight	10min.	_____
____ 99213	Ex. Prob. Foc.	Ex. Prob. Foc.	Low	15 min.	_____
____ 99214	Detail	Detail	Mod.	25 min.	_____
____ 99215	Comp.	Comp.	High	40 min.	_____

C. HOSPITAL CARE

		Dx	Units	
1. Initial Hospital Care (30 min)	____	____	99221	_____
2. Subsequent Care	____	____	99231	_____
3. Critical Care (30-74 min)	____	____	99291	_____
4. each additional 30 min.	____	____	99292	_____
5. Discharge Services	____	____	99238	_____
6. Emergency Room	____	____	99282	_____

D. NURSING HOME CARE

	Dx	Units	
Initial Care - New Pt.			
1. Expanded	____	____	99322
2. Detailed	____	____	99323
Subsequent Care - Estab. Pt.			
3. Problem Focused	____	____	99307
4. Expanded	____	____	99308
5. Detailed	____	____	99309
5. Comprehensive	____	____	99310

E. PROCEDURES

1. Arthrocentesis, Small Jt.	____	20600	
2. Colonoscopy	____	45378	
3. EKG w/interpretation	____	93000	
4. X-Ray Chest, PA/LAT	____	71020	

F. LAB

1. Blood Sugar	____	82947		
2. CBC w/differential	____	85031		
3. Cholesterol	3	82465	X	
4. Comprehensive Metabolic Panel	1, 2	80053	X	
5. ESR	____	85651		
6. Hematocrit	1, 2	85014	X	
7. Mono Screen	____	86308		
8. Pap Smear	____	88150		
9. Potassium	____	84132		
10. Preg. Test, Quantitative	____	84702		
11. Routine Venipuncture	____	36415		

F. Cont'd

		Dx	Units	
12. Strep Screen		____	87081	_____
13. UA, Routine w/Micro		____	81000	_____
14. UA, Routine w/o Micro		____	81002	_____
15. Uric Acid		____	84550	_____
16. VDRL		____	86592	_____
17. Wet Prep		____	82710	_____
18. _____		____	_____	_____

G. INJECTIONS

1. Influenza Virus Vaccine	____	90658	_____
2. Pneumococcal Vaccine	____	90772	_____
3. Tetanus Toxoids	____	90703	_____
4. Therapeutic Subcut/IM	____	90732	_____
5. Vaccine Administration	____	90471	_____
6. Vaccine - each additional	____	90472	_____

H. MISCELLANEOUS

1. _____	_____	_____
2. _____	_____	_____

AMOUNT PAID $ ___ 0 ___

Mark diagnosis with
(1=Primary, 2=Secondary, 3=Tertiary)

DIAGNOSIS NOT LISTED BELOW _____

DIAGNOSIS	ICD-9-CM	1, 2, 3	DIAGNOSIS	ICD-9-CM	1, 2, 3	DIAGNOSIS	ICD-9-CM	1, 2, 3
Abdominal Pain	789.0_		Dehydration	276.51		Otitis Media, Acute NOS	382.9	
Allergic Rhinitis, Unspec.	477.9		Depression, NOS	311		Peptic Ulcer Disease	536.9	
Angina Pectoris, Unspec.	413.9		Diabetes Mellitus, Type II Controlled	250.00		Peripheral Vascular Disease NOS	443.9	
Anemia, Iron Deficiency, Unspec.	280.9		Diabetes Mellitus, Type II Controlled	250.02		Pharyngitis, Acute	462	
Anemia, NOS	285.9	2	Drug Reaction, NOS	995.29		Pneumonia, Organism Unspec.	486	
Anemia, Pernicious	281.0		Dysuria	788.1		Prostatitis, NOS	601.9	
Asthma w/ Exacerbation	493.92		Eczema, NOS	692.2		PVC	427.69	
Asthmatic Bronchitis, Unspec.	493.90		Edema	782.3		Rash, Non Specific	782.1	
Atrial Fibrillation	427.31		Fever, Unknown Origin	780.6		Seizure Disorder NOS	780.39	
Atypical Chest Pain, Unspec.	786.59		Gastritis, Acute w/o Hemorrhage	535.00		Serous Otitis Media, Chronic, Unspec.	381.10	
Bronchiolitis, due to RSV	466.11		Gastroenteritis, NOS	558.9		Sinusitis, Acute NOS	461.9	
Bronchitis, Acute	466.0		Gastroesophageal Reflux	530.81		Tonsillitis, Acute	463.	
Bronchitis, NOS	490		Hepatitis A, Infectious	070.1		Upper Respiratory Infection, Acute NOS	465.9	
Cardiac Arrest	427.5		Hypercholesterolemia, Pure	272.0	3	Urinary Tract Infection, Unspec.	599.0	
Cardiopulmonary Disease, Chronic, Unspec.	416.9		Hypertension, Unspec.	401.9		Urticaria, Unspec.	708.9	
Cellulitis, NOS	682.9		Hypoglycemia NOS	251.2		Vertigo, NOS	780.4	
Congestive Heart Failure, Unspec.	428.0	1	Hypokalemia	276.8		Viral Infection NOS	079.99	
Contact Dermatitis NOS	692.9		Impetigo	684		Weakness, Generalized	780.79	
COPD NOS	496		Lymphadenitis, Unspec.	289.3		Weight Loss, Abnormal	783.21	
CVA, Acute, NOS	434.91		Mononucleosis	075				
CVA, Old or Healed	438.9		Myocardial Infarction, Acute, NOS	410.9				
Degenerative Arthritis			Organic Brain Syndrome	310.9				
(Specify Site) _____	715.9		Otitis Externa, Acute NOS	380.10				

ABN: I UNDERSTAND THAT MEDICARE PROBABLY WILL NOT COVER THE SERVICES LISTED BELOW

A. _____ B. _____ C. _____

Patient

Date _____ Signature _____

Doctor's Signature *LD Heath*

RETURN: _____ Days _____ Weeks ___ 1 ___ Months

REF# 122949 SB (05.07.09) TO REORDER CALL INHEALTH RECORD SYSTEMS 800-477-7374

DOUGLASVILLE MEDICINE ASSOCIATES
5076 BRAND BLVD., SUITE 401
DOUGLASVILLE, NY 01234
PHONE No. (123) 456-7890
☒ L.D. HEATH, M.D. ☐ D.J. SCHWARTZ, M.D.
NPI# 9995010111   NPI# 9995020212
EIN# 00-1234560

Figure WBE 1-11 *(Used with permission. InHealth Record Systems, Inc. 5076 Winters Chapel Road, Atlanta, GA 30360, 800-477-7374. http://www.inhealthrecords.com)*

Patient Emma Lansford

Instructions: Complete the following tasks on 4/5/2010:

a. Refer to the superbill in Figure WBE 1-12 and enter the procedure(s) for Patient Lansford using MOSS.

PLEASE RETURN THIS FORM TO RECEPTIONIST

NAME Emma Lansford

Ref # E003

PLACE OF SERVICE:
(X) OFFICE
( ) NEW YORK COUNTY HOSPITAL
( ) COMMUNITY GENERAL HOSPITAL
( ) RETIREMENT INN NURSING HOME
( ) _____

DATE OF SERVICE 04/05/2010

A. OFFICE VISITS - New Patient

Code	History	Exam	Dec.	Time	
99201	Prob. Foc.	Prob. Foc.	Straight	10 min.	
X 99202	Ex. Prob. Foc.	Ex. Prob. Foc.	Straight	20 min.	1
99203	Detail	Detail	Low	30 min.	
99204	Comp.	Comp.	Mod.	45 min.	
99205	Comp.	Comp.	High	60 min.	

B. OFFICE VISIT - Established Patient

Code	History	Exam	Dec.	Time	
99211	Minimal	Minimal	Minimal	5 min.	
99212	Prob. Foc.	Prob. Foc.	Straight	10min.	
99213	Ex. Prob. Foc.	Ex. Prob. Foc.	Low	15 min.	
99214	Detail	Detail	Mod.	25 min.	
99215	Comp.	Comp.	High	40 min.	

C. HOSPITAL CARE

		Dx	Units	
1. Initial Hospital Care (30 min)		____	____ 99221	____
2. Subsequent Care		____	____ 99231	____
3. Critical Care (30-74 min)		____	____ 99291	____
4. each additional 30 min.		____	____ 99292	____
5. Discharge Services		____	____ 99238	____
6. Emergency Room		____	____ 99282	____

D. NURSING HOME CARE

	Dx	Units	
Initial Care - New Pt.			
1. Expanded	____	____ 99322	____
2. Detailed	____	____ 99323	____
Subsequent Care - Estab. Pt.			
3. Problem Focused	____	____ 99307	____
4. Expanded	____	____ 99308	____
5. Detailed	____	____ 99309	____
5. Comprehensive	____	____ 99310	____

E. PROCEDURES

	Dx		
1. Arthrocentesis, Small Jt.	____	20600	
2. Colonoscopy	____	45378	
3. EKG w/interpretation	____	93000	
4. X-Ray Chest, PA/LAT	____	71020	

F. LAB

1. Blood Sugar	____	82947	____
2. CBC w/differential	____	85031	____
3. Cholesterol	____	82465	____
4. Comprehensive Metabolic Panel	____	80053	____
5. ESR	____	85651	____
6. Hematocrit	____	85014	____
7. Mono Screen	____	86308	____
8. Pap Smear	____	88150	____
9. Potassium	____	84132	____
10. Preg. Test, Quantitative	____	84702	____
11. Routine Venipuncture	____	36415	____

F. Cont'd

	Dx	Units	
12. Strep Screen	____	87081	____
13. UA, Routine w/Micro	____	81000	____
14. UA, Routine w/o Micro	____	81002	____
15. Uric Acid	____	84550	____
16. VDRL	____	86592	____
17. Wet Prep	____	82710	____
18. _____	____	____	____

G. INJECTIONS

1. Influenza Virus Vaccine	____	90658	
2. Pneumoccocal Vaccine	____	90772	
3. Tetanus Toxoids	____	90703	
4. Therapeutic Subcut/IM	____	90732	
5. Vaccine Administration	____	90471	
6. Vaccine - each additional	____	90472	

H. MISCELLANEOUS

1. _____ ____ _____
2. _____ ____ _____

AMOUNT PAID $ 20.00

Mark diagnosis with
(1=Primary, 2=Secondary, 3=Tertiary)

DIAGNOSIS NOT LISTED BELOW _____

DIAGNOSIS	ICD-9-CM 1, 2, 3	DIAGNOSIS	ICD-9-CM 1, 2, 3	DIAGNOSIS	ICD-9-CM 1, 2, 3
Abdominal Pain	789.0	Dehydration	276.51	Otitis Media, Acute NOS	382.9
Allergic Rhinitis, Unspec.	477.9	Depression, NOS	311	Peptic Ulcer Disease	536.9
Angina Pectoris, Unspec.	413.9	Diabetes Mellitus, Type II Controlled	250.00	Peripheral Vascular Disease NOS	443.9
Anemia, Iron Deficiency, Unspec.	280.9	Diabetes Mellitus, Type II Controlled	250.02	Pharyngitis, Acute	462
Anemia, NOS	285.9	Drug Reaction, NOS	995.29	Pneumonia, Organism Unspec.	486
Anemia, Pernicious	281.0	Dysuria	788.1	Prostatitis, NOS	601.9
Asthma w/ Exacerbation	493.92	Eczema, NOS	692.2	PVC	427.69
Asthmatic Bronchitis, Unspec.	493.90	Edema	782.3	Rash, Non Specific	782.1
Atrial Fibrillation	427.31	Fever, Unknown Origin	780.6	Seizure Disorder NOS	780.39
Atypical Chest Pain, Unspec.	786.59	Gastritis, Acute w/o Hemorrhage	535.00	Serous Otitis Media, Chronic, Unspec.	381.10
Bronchiolitis, due to RSV	466.11	Gastroenteritis, NOS	558.9	Sinusitis, Acute NOS	461.9
Bronchitis, Acute	466.0	Gastroesophageal Reflux	530.81	Tonsillitis, Acute	463.
Bronchitis, NOS	490	Hepatitis A, Infectious	070.1	Upper Respiratory Infection, Acute NOS	465.9
Cardiac Arrest	427.5	Hypercholesterolemia, Pure	272.0	Urinary Tract Infection, Unspec.	599.0
Cardiopulmonary Disease, Chronic, Unspec.	416.9	Hypertension, Unspec.	401.9	Urticaria, Unspec.	708.9
Cellulitis, NOS	682.9	Hypoglycemia NOS	251.2	Vertigo, NOS	780.4
Congestive Heart Failure, Unspec.	428.0	Hypokalemia	276.8	Viral Infection NOS	079.99
Contact Dermatitis NOS	692.9	Impetigo	684 1	Weakness, Generalized	780.79
COPD NOS	496	Lymphadenitis, Unspec.	289.3	Weight Loss, Abnormal	783.21
CVA, Acute, NOS	434.91	Mononucleosis	075		
CVA, Old or Healed	438.9	Myocardial Infarction, Acute, NOS	410.9		
Degenerative Arthritis		Organic Brain Syndrome	310.9		
(Specify Site) _____	715.9	Otitis Externa, Acute NOS	380.10		

ABN: I UNDERSTAND THAT MEDICARE PROBABLY WILL NOT COVER THE SERVICES LISTED BELOW

A. _____ B. _____ C. _____
Patient

Date _____ Signature _____

Doctor's Signature *LD Heath*

RETURN: _____ Days 3 Weeks _____ Months _____

REF# 122949 SB (05.07.09)   TO REORDER CALL INHEALTH RECORD SYSTEMS 800-477-7374

DOUGLASVILLE MEDICINE ASSOCIATES
5076 BRAND BLVD., SUITE 401
DOUGLASVILLE, NY 01234
PHONE No. (123) 456-7890
☒ L.D. HEATH, M.D.   ☐ D.J. SCHWARTZ, M.D.
NPI# 9995010111   NPI# 9995020212
EIN# 00-1234560

Figure WBE 1-12 *(Used with permission. InHealth Record Systems, Inc. 5076 Winters Chapel Road, Atlanta, GA 30360, 800-477-7374. http://www.inhealthrecords.com)*

b. Refer to the personal check in Figure WBE 1-13 and post the payment made by the patient.

c. Schedule a follow-up appointment as requested by the physician for 15 minutes.

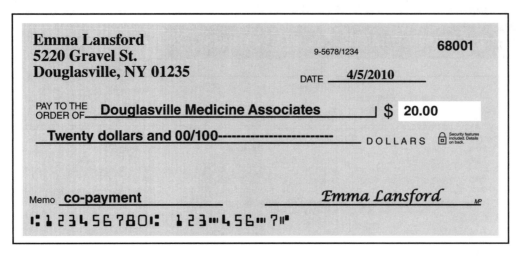

Figure WBE 1-13 *(Delmar/Cengage Learning)*

Patient Timothy Meade

Instructions: Complete the following tasks on 4/5/2010:

a. Refer to the superbill in Figure WBE 1-14 and enter the procedure(s) for Patient Meade using MOSS.

b. Refer to the personal check in Figure WBE 1-15 and post the payment made by the patient.

c. Schedule a follow-up appointment as requested by the physician for 15 minutes.

PLEASE RETURN THIS FORM TO RECEPTIONIST

NAME Timothy Meade

Ref # E004

PLACE OF SERVICE:
(X) OFFICE
( ) NEW YORK COUNTY HOSPITAL
( ) COMMUNITY GENERAL HOSPITAL
( ) RETIREMENT INN NURSING HOME
( ) _____

DATE OF SERVICE _____

A. OFFICE VISITS - New Patient

Code	History	Exam	Dec.	Time	
99201	Prob. Foc.	Prob. Foc.	Straight	10 min.	
99202	Ex. Prob. Foc.	Ex. Prob. Foc.	Straight	20 min.	
99203	Detail	Detail	Low	30 min.	
X 99204	Comp.	Comp.	Mod.	45 min.	1, 2
99205	Comp.	Comp.	High	60 min.	

B. OFFICE VISIT - Established Patient

Code	History	Exam	Dec.	Time	
99211	Minimal	Minimal		5 min.	
99212	Prob. Foc.	Prob. Foc.	Straight	10min.	
99213	Ex. Prob. Foc.	Ex. Prob. Foc.	Low	15 min.	
99214	Detail	Detail	Mod.	25 min.	
99215	Comp.	Comp.	High	40 min.	

C. HOSPITAL CARE

		Dx	Units	
1.	Initial Hospital Care (30 min)		99221	
2.	Subsequent Care		99231	
3.	Critical Care (30-74 min)		99291	
4.	each additional 30 min.		99292	
5.	Discharge Services		99238	
6.	Emergency Room		99282	

D. NURSING HOME CARE

		Dx	Units	
Initial Care - New Pt.				
1.	Expanded		99322	
2.	Detailed		99323	
Subsequent Care - Estab. Pt.				
3.	Problem Focused		99307	
4.	Expanded		99308	
5.	Detailed		99309	
5.	Comprehensive		99310	

E. PROCEDURES

1.	Arthrocentesis, Small Jt.		20600	
2.	Colonoscopy		45378	
3.	EKG w/interpretation		93000	
4.	X-Ray Chest, PA/LAT	1, 2	71020	X

F. LAB

1.	Blood Sugar		82947	
2.	CBC w/differential		85031	
3.	Cholesterol		82465	
4.	Comprehensive Metabolic Panel		80053	
5.	ESR		85651	
6.	Hematocrit		85014	
7.	Mono Screen		86308	
8.	Pap Smear		88150	
9.	Potassium		84132	
10.	Preg. Test, Quantitative		84702	
11.	Routine Venipuncture		36415	

F. Cont'd

		Dx	Units	
12.	Strep Screen		87081	
13.	UA, Routine w/Micro		81000	
14.	UA, Routine w/o Micro		81002	
15.	Uric Acid		84550	
16.	VDRL		86592	
17.	Wet Prep		82710	
18.	_____			

G. INJECTIONS

1.	Influenza Virus Vaccine		90658	
2.	Pneumoccocal Vaccine		90772	
3.	Tetanus Toxoids		90703	
4.	Therapeutic Subcut/IM		90732	
5.	Vaccine Administration		90471	
6.	Vaccine - each additional		90472	

H. MISCELLANEOUS

1. _____ ____
2. _____ ____

AMOUNT PAID $ 10.00

Mark diagnosis with (1=Primary, 2=Secondary, 3=Tertiary)

DIAGNOSIS NOT LISTED BELOW _____

DIAGNOSIS	ICD-9-CM	1,2,3	DIAGNOSIS	ICD-9-CM	1,2,3	DIAGNOSIS	ICD-9-CM	1,2,3
Abdominal Pain	789.0		Dehydration	276.51		Otitis Media, Acute NOS	382.9	
Allergic Rhinitis, Unspec.	477.9		Depression, NOS	311		Peptic Ulcer Disease	536.9	
Angina Pectoris, Unspec.	413.9		Diabetes Mellitus, Type II Controlled	250.00		Peripheral Vascular Disease NOS	443.9	
Anemia, Iron Deficiency, Unspec.	280.9		Diabetes Mellitus, Type II Controlled	250.02		Pharyngitis, Acute	462	
Anemia, NOS	285.9		Drug Reaction, NOS	995.29		Pneumonia, Organism Unspec.	486	
Anemia, Pernicious	281.0		Dysuria	788.1		Prostatitis, NOS	601.9	
Asthma w/ Exacerbation	493.92	1	Eczema, NOS	692.2		PVC	427.69	
Asthmatic Bronchitis, Unspec.	493.90		Edema	782.3		Rash, Non Specific	782.1	
Atrial Fibrillation	427.31		Fever, Unknown Origin	780.6		Seizure Disorder NOS	780.39	
Atypical Chest Pain, Unspec.	786.59		Gastritis, Acute w/o Hemorrhage	535.00		Serous Otitis Media, Chronic, Unspec.	381.10	
Bronchiolitis, due to RSV	466.11		Gastroenteritis, NOS	558.9		Sinusitis, Acute NOS	461.9	
Bronchitis, Acute	466.0		Gastroesophageal Reflux	530.81		Tonsillitis, Acute	463.	
Bronchitis, NOS	490		Hepatitis A, Infectious	070.1		Upper Respiratory Infection, Acute NOS	465.9	2
Cardiac Arrest	427.5		Hypercholesterolemia, Pure	272.0		Urinary Tract Infection, Unspec.	599.0	
Cardiopulmonary Disease, Chronic, Unspec.	416.9		Hypertension, Unspec.	401.9		Urticaria, Unspec.	708.9	
Cellulitis, NOS	682.9		Hypoglycemia NOS	251.2		Vertigo, NOS	780.4	
Congestive Heart Failure, Unspec.	428.0		Hypokalemia	276.8		Viral Infection NOS	079.99	
Contact Dermatitis NOS	692.9		Impetigo	684		Weakness, Generalized	780.79	
COPD NOS	496		Lymphadenitis, Unspec.	289.3		Weight Loss, Abnormal	783.21	
CVA, Acute, NOS	434.91		Mononucleosis	075				
CVA, Old or Healed	438.9		Myocardial Infarction, Acute, NOS	410.9				
Degenerative Arthritis (Specify Site)	715.9		Organic Brain Syndrome	310.9				
			Otitis Externa, Acute NOS	380.10				

ABN: I UNDERSTAND THAT MEDICARE PROBABLY WILL NOT COVER THE SERVICES LISTED BELOW

A. _____ B. _____ C. _____

Patient

Date _____ Signature _____

Doctor's Signature *LD Heath*

RETURN: 10 Days _____ Weeks _____ Months _____

DOUGLASVILLE MEDICINE ASSOCIATES
5076 BRAND BLVD., SUITE 401
DOUGLASVILLE, NY 01234
PHONE No. (123) 456-7890
☒ L.D. HEATH, M.D. ☐ D.J. SCHWARTZ, M.D.
NPI# 9995010111 NPI# 9995020212
EIN# 00-1234560

REF# 122949 SB (05.07.09) TO REORDER CALL INHEALTH RECORD SYSTEMS 800-477-7374

Figure WBE 1-14 *(Used with permission. InHealth Record Systems, Inc. 5076 Winters Chapel Road, Atlanta, GA 30360, 800-477-7374. http://www.inhealthrecords.com)*

Figure WBE 1-15 *(Delmar/Cengage Learning)*

EVALUATION 4 – REPORT GENERATION – DAILY TRANSACTIONS

Instructions: Generate a report showing daily transactions by running a Billing and Payment Report for the date of April 5, 2010. Print the report or follow the directions from your instructor.

EVALUATION 5 – BILL PRIMARY INSURANCE PLANS FOR SERVICES ON 4/5/2010

Instructions: Prepare the insurance billing for primary insurance plans for services provided to patients Riley, Manfred, Lansford, and Meade on April 5, 2010.

a. Print a Prebilling Worksheet using MOSS.

b. Submit the claims electronically or on paper, as directed by your instructor.

c. Print reports as directed by your instructor.

EVALUATION 6 – POST INSURANCE PAYMENTS TO PATIENT ACCOUNTS FROM A PAPER EOB AND RA

Instructions: Refer to the Explanation of Benefits from FlexiHeath PPO and the Medicare Remittance Advice shown in Figures WBE 1-16 and WBE 1-17. Post the payments as indicated, using "Eval 6" as the reference number in Field 5 for each posting and 5/15/2010 as the date of posting.

Explanation of Medical Benefits – EVALUATION 6   **FlexiHealth PPO Plan**

Service Date	Type of Service	Charge(s) Submitted	Not Covered or Discount	Amount Covered	Patient Co-payment Co-insurance Deductible	Covered Balance	Plan Liability	See Note
Insured Name **LANSFORD, EMMA**		Insured/Patient ID **999119315-01**			Patient Name **LANSFORD, EMMA**			
Provider Name: L.D. Heath, MD – In-Network Provider Reference Number: EVAL 6								
04/05/10	99202 Office Service	$147.00	$ 15.00	$132.00	$20.00 co-pay	$112.00	$112.00	A
						Total Paid:	$112.00	

Notes on Benefit Determination:
A – Preferred provider discount. Patient is not required to pay this amount.
B – Patient is responsible for non-covered amounts for Out-of-Network providers

Figure WBE 1-16 *(Delmar/Cengage Learning)*

```
Medicare Remittance Advice (MOSS Sample)
-------------------------------------------------------------------------
05-15-2010 MEDICARE CLAIMS SUBMITTED FOR L.D. Heath, MD 999501
-------------------------------------------------------------------------

MANFRED, GEORGE
  HIC      999139650A       BILLED  ALLOWED DEDUCT  COINS PROV-PD MC-ADJUSTMENT
  ACNT     MAN003           ASG Y   ICN     97333671

0405       040510 11 99204  283.00  160.15  0        32.03 128.12  122.85

0405       040510 11 80053   47.00   14.77  0         0.00  14.77   32.83

0405       040510 11 82465   14.00    6.08  0         0.00   6.08    7.92

0405       040510 11 85014    7.00    3.31  0         0.00   3.31    3.69

           CLAIM TOTALS: 351.00  184.31  0        32.03 152.28  166.69

TOTAL PAID TO PROVIDER: $152.28
```

Figure WBE 1-17 *(Delmar/Cengage Learning)*

EVALUATION 7 – POST INSURANCE PAYMENTS TO PATIENT ACCOUNTS FROM AN ELECTRONIC RA

Instructions: Using the Claims Tracking feature in MOSS, obtain the electronic RA for services on 04/05/2010 paid by Signal HMO. Print the RA and refer to it to post the payments as indicated. Use "Eval 7" as the reference number in Field 5 for each posting and 5/15/2010 as the date of posting. If required, refer to the electronic RA in Figure WBE 1-18 to complete your work. Post the payments as indicated.

PROVIDER PAYMENT ADVICE
Signal HMO
Student1

Patient Name Timothy Meade (MEA001)

Claim ID	DOS	Procedure	Charges	Allowed Amount	Patient Responsibility	Rejected Amount	Paid to Provider	Remarks
1000445	4/5/2010	71020	$53.00	$46.91	$0.00	$0.00	$46.91	A
1000444	4/5/2010	99204	$283.00	$250.46	$10.00	$0.00	$240.46	A
Patient Totals			$336.00	$297.37	$10.00	$0.00	$287.37	

Patient Name Sharon Riley (RIL001)

Claim ID	DOS	Procedure	Charges	Allowed Amount	Patient Responsibility	Rejected Amount	Paid to Provider	Remarks
1000438	4/5/2010	81002	$9.00	$7.97	$0.00	$0.00	$7.97	A
1000437	4/5/2010	85031	$11.00	$9.74	$0.00	$0.00	$9.74	A
1000436	4/5/2010	99203	$200.00	$177.00	$10.00	$0.00	$167.00	A
Patient Totals			$220.00	$194.71	$10.00	$0.00	$184.71	

Figure WBE 1-18 *(Delmar/Cengage Learning)*

EVALUATION 8 – PREPARE AND PRINT A STATEMENT FOR PATIENT BILLING

Instructions: Prepare a remainder statement for Patient George Manfred. Since his secondary insurance will be billed and is expected to pay the balance, include a dunning message that advises the patient that the office is waiting for payment from the secondary insurance. Print the statement to be mailed to the patient.

EVALUATION 9 – REPORT GENERATION – ALL EXAMINATION TRANSACTIONS

Instructions: Generate a final report showing all transactions for this examination by running a Billing and Payment Report for the date of April 5, 2010. Print the report or follow the directions from your instructor for turning in your work, including your flash or other storage media drive, or additional materials or test papers that were provided, as requested for grading.

Source Documents

SOURCE DOCUMENT WB5-1

Welcome To Our Office	NEW PATIENT INFORMATION	DATE __10/22/2009__

PLEASE PRINT

LAST NAME	FIRST NAME	MI	SSN		GENDER	MARITAL STATUS	DATE OF BIRTH
Trimble	Devon	L.	999-21-1655		Male	Single	08/25/1972

ADDRESS	APT/UNIT	CITY	STATE	ZIP	HOME PH (123)	WORK PH (123) EXT:
774 Marble Way	206	Douglasville	NY	01234	970-4578	537-2210

EMPLOYER/SCHOOL	EMPLOYER ADDRESS	CITY	STATE	ZIP
Morgan Associates	5811 Main Street	Douglasville	NY	01235

REFERRING PHYSICIAN (LAST NAME, FIRST NAME)	ADDRESS	CITY	STATE	ZIP	PHONE

GUARANTOR - Person responsible for payment: ☒ self   ☐ spouse/other   ☐ parent   ☐ legal guardian If not "self", please complete the following:

LAST NAME	FIRST NAME	MI	SSN	GENDER	DATE OF BIRTH

ADDRESS (IF DIFFERENT FROM PATIENT)	CITY	STATE	ZIP	HOME PH ( )	ALT. PHONE

EMPLOYER NAME	EMPLOYER ADDRESS	CITY	STATE	ZIP	WORK PHONE EXT

OTHER RESPONSIBLE PARTY:

LAST NAME	FIRST NAME	MI	SSN	GENDER	DATE OF BIRTH	

ADDRESS (IF DIFFERENT FROM PATIENT)	CITY	STATE	ZIP	HOME PH ( )	ALT. PHONE

EMPLOYER NAME	EMPLOYER ADDRESS	CITY STATE	ZIP	WORK PHONE EXT

INSURANCE - PRIMARY

PLAN NAME	PATIENT RELATIONSHIP TO INSURED:
Signal HMO	☒ self ☐ spouse ☐ child ☐ other

POLICYHOLDER INFORMATION

LAST NAME	FIRST NAME	MI	DATE OF BIRTH	ID#	POLICY #	GROUP #
Trimble	Devon		08/25/1972	999211655		MA8991

EMPLOYER NAME	PCP NAME, IF APPLICABLE:
Morgan Associates	

INSURANCE - SECONDARY

PLAN NAME	PATIENT RELATIONSHIP TO INSURED: ☐ self ☐ spouse ☐ child ☐ other

POLICYHOLDER INFORMATION

LAST NAME	FIRST NAME	MI	DATE OF BIRTH	ID#	POLICY #	GROUP #

EMPLOYER NAME	PCP NAME, IF APPLICABLE:

ACCIDENT? ☐ YES ☒ NO IF YES, DATE OF INJURY	OCCUR AT WORK? ☐ YES ☐ NO	AUTO INVOLVED: ☐ YES ☐ NO	STATE

NAME OF ATTORNEY	PHONE NUMBER EXT.

INSURANCE AUTHORIZATION AND ASSIGNMENT

Name of Policy Holder _____**Devon Trimble**_____   HIC Number _____

I request that payment of authorized Medicare/Other Insurance company benefits be made either to me or on my behalf to _____**Dr. Heath**_____

For any services furnished me by that party who accepts assignment/physician. Regulations pertaining to Medicare assignment of benefits apply.

I authorize the release of protected health information to the Social Security Administration and Centers for Medicare and Medicaid Services or its intermediaries or carriers any information needed for this or a related Medicare claim/other Insurance Company claim...(Section 11288 f the Social Security Act and if 31 U.S.C. Sections 3801-3812 provides penalties for withholding this information).

Signature ____*Devon Trimble*_____   Date ____10/20/2009_____

(Used with permission. InHealth Record Systems, Inc. 5076 Winters Chapel Road, Atlanta, GA 30360, 800-477-7374. http://www.inhealthrecords.com)

SOURCE DOCUMENT WB5-2

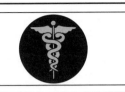

Signal HMO

PCP: Douglasville Medicine Associates
Dr. L.D. Heath
(123)456-7890

Devon Trimble   999211655   01

Copayment Schedule

PCP Office Visits $ 10.00
Specialists Visits $ 30.00
Emergency Room $ 100.00
Hospitalization   Authorization
Preauthorization 800-123-8877

Bank Code
361   Member Group Number: MA8991

E25/A10
Type of Coverage

(Delmar/Cengage Learning)

SOURCE DOCUMENT WB5-3

Welcome To Our Office
PLEASE PRINT

NEW PATIENT INFORMATION

DATE 10/27/2009

LAST NAME	FIRST NAME	MI	SSN		GENDER	MARITAL STATUS	DATE OF BIRTH
Sheridan	Wynona		999-32-0169		Female	Single	06/05/1984

ADDRESS	APT/UNIT	CITY	STATE	ZIP	HOME PH (123)	WORK PH (123) EXT:
12390 Marble Way	333	Douglasville	NY	01234	970-6123	537-0211 6

EMPLOYER/SCHOOL	EMPLOYER ADDRESS	CITY	STATE	ZIP
Midway Investments	301 Main Street	Douglasville	NY	01234

REFERRING PHYSICIAN (LAST NAME, FIRST NAME)	ADDRESS	CITY	STATE	ZIP	PHONE

GUARANTOR - Person responsible for payment: ☒ self   ☐ spouse/other   ☐ parent   ☐ legal guardian If not "self", please complete the following:

LAST NAME	FIRST NAME	MI	SSN		GENDER	DATE OF BIRTH

ADDRESS (IF DIFFERENT FROM PATIENT)	CITY	STATE	ZIP	HOME PH ( )	ALT. PHONE

EMPLOYER NAME	EMPLOYER ADDRESS	CITY	STATE	ZIP	WORK PHONE	EXT

OTHER RESPONSIBLE PARTY:

LAST NAME	FIRST NAME	MI	SSN	GENDER	DATE OF BIRTH

ADDRESS (IF DIFFERENT FROM PATIENT)	CITY	STATE	ZIP	HOME PH ( )	ALT. PHONE

EMPLOYER NAME	EMPLOYER ADDRESS	CITY STATE	ZIP	WORK PHONE	EXT

INSURANCE - PRIMARY

PLAN NAME	PATIENT RELATIONSHIP TO INSURED:
Consumer One HRA	☒ self ☐ spouse ☐ child ☐ other

POLICYHOLDER INFORMATION

LAST NAME	FIRST NAME	MI	DATE OF BIRTH	ID#	POLICY #	GROUP #
Sheridan	Wynona		06/05/1984	999320169		MI5015

EMPLOYER NAME	PCP NAME, IF APPLICABLE:			
Midway Investments				

INSURANCE - SECONDARY

PLAN NAME	PATIENT RELATIONSHIP TO INSURED: ☐ self ☐ spouse ☐ child ☐ other

POLICYHOLDER INFORMATION

LAST NAME	FIRST NAME	MI	DATE OF BIRTH	ID#	POLICY #	GROUP #

EMPLOYER NAME	PCP NAME, IF APPLICABLE:			

ACCIDENT? ☐ YES ☐ NO IF YES, DATE OF INJURY	OCCUR AT WORK? ☐ YES ☐ NO	AUTO INVOLVED: ☐ YES ☐ NO	STATE

NAME OF ATTORNEY	PHONE NUMBER EXT.		

INSURANCE AUTHORIZATION AND ASSIGNMENT

Name of Policy Holder _____ Wynona Sheridan _____   HIC Number _____

I request that payment of authorized Medicare/Other Insurance company benefits be made either to me or on my behalf to _____ Dr. Heath _____
For any services furnished me by that party who accepts assignment/physician. Regulations pertaining to Medicare assignment of benefits apply.
I authorize the release of protected health information to the Social Security Administration and Centers for Medicare and Medicaid Services or its intermediaries or carriers any information needed for this or a related Medicare claim/other Insurance Company claim...(Section 11288 f the Social Security Act and if 31 U.S.C. Sections 3801-3812 provides penalties for withholding this information).

Signature _____ *Wynona Sheridan* _____   Date _____ 10/27/2009 _____

(Used with permission. InHealth Record Systems, Inc. 5076 Winters Chapel Road, Atlanta, GA 30360, 800-477-7374. http://www.inhealthrecords.com)

SOURCE DOCUMENT WB5-4

ConsumerONE

Health Reimbursement Arrangement

Participant: Sheridan, Wynona
ID Number: 999320169
Employer Group: MI5015

Preventative Care: 100%
EPA – Call 800-123-8253
Level 3 - 80/20

In-Network Preferred

Plan Code GP123123

(Delmar/Cengage Learning)

SOURCE DOCUMENT WB5-5

Welcome To Our Office   **NEW PATIENT INFORMATION**   DATE _____

PLEASE PRINT

LAST NAME	FIRST NAME	MI	SSN		GENDER	MARITAL STATUS	DATE OF BIRTH
Engleman	Harold	R.	999-81-1169		Male	Married	10/28/1948

ADDRESS	APT/UNIT	CITY	STATE	ZIP	HOME PH (123)	WORK PH (123) EXT:
58682 Pebble Trail		Douglasville	NY	01234	537-8823	970-5000

EMPLOYER/SCHOOL	EMPLOYER ADDRESS	CITY	STATE	ZIP
Eastern Auto Sales	505 Midway Boulevard	Douglasville	NY	01235

REFERRING PHYSICIAN (LAST NAME, FIRST NAME)	ADDRESS	CITY	STATE	ZIP	PHONE

GUARANTOR - Person responsible for payment: ☒ self   ☐ spouse/other   ☐ parent   ☐ legal guardian If not "self", please complete the following:

LAST NAME	FIRST NAME	MI	SSN		GENDER	DATE OF BIRTH

ADDRESS (IF DIFFERENT FROM PATIENT)	CITY	STATE	ZIP	HOME PH ( )	ALT. PHONE

EMPLOYER NAME	EMPLOYER ADDRESS	CITY	STATE	ZIP	WORK PHONE	EXT

OTHER RESPONSIBLE PARTY:

LAST NAME	FIRST NAME	MI	SSN		GENDER	DATE OF BIRTH

ADDRESS (IF DIFFERENT FROM PATIENT)	CITY	STATE	ZIP	HOME PH ( )	ALT. PHONE

EMPLOYER NAME	EMPLOYER ADDRESS	CITY STATE	ZIP	WORK PHONE	EXT

INSURANCE - PRIMARY

PLAN NAME	PATIENT RELATIONSHIP TO INSURED:
FlexiHealth PPO Out of Network	☒ self ☐ spouse ☐ child ☐ other

POLICYHOLDER INFORMATION

LAST NAME	FIRST NAME	MI	DATE OF BIRTH	ID#	POLICY #	GROUP #
Engleman	Harold		10/28/1948	999811169-01		EA51322

EMPLOYER NAME	PCP NAME, IF APPLICABLE:
Eastern Auto Sales	

INSURANCE - SECONDARY

PLAN NAME	PATIENT RELATIONSHIP TO INSURED: ☐ self ☐ spouse ☐ child ☐ other

POLICYHOLDER INFORMATION

LAST NAME	FIRST NAME	MI	DATE OF BIRTH	ID#	POLICY #	GROUP #

EMPLOYER NAME	PCP NAME, IF APPLICABLE:

ACCIDENT? ☐ YES ☐ NO IF YES, DATE OF INJURY	OCCUR AT WORK? ☐ YES ☐ NO	AUTO INVOLVED: ☐ YES ☐ NO	STATE

NAME OF ATTORNEY	PHONE NUMBER EXT.		

INSURANCE AUTHORIZATION AND ASSIGNMENT

Name of Policy Holder _____ **Harold Engleman** _____   HIC Number _____

I request that payment of authorized Medicare/Other Insurance company benefits be made either to me or on my behalf to _____ **Dr. Schwartz** _____
For any services furnished me by that party who accepts assignment/physician. Regulations pertaining to Medicare assignment of benefits apply.
I authorize the release of protected health information to the Social Security Administration and Centers for Medicare and Medicaid Services or its intermediaries or carriers any information needed for this or a related Medicare claim/other Insurance Company claim...(Section 11288 f the Social Security Act and if 31 U.S.C. Sections 3801-3812 provides penalties for withholding this information).

Signature _____ *Harold Englemen* _____   Date _____ 10/22/2009 _____

(Used with permission. InHealth Record Systems, Inc. 5076 Winters Chapel Road, Atlanta, GA 30360, 800-477-7374. http://www.inhealthrecords.com)

SOURCE DOCUMENT WB5-6

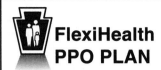

		Insurer 81564
FlexiHealth **PPO PLAN**		*Your Health First* SM

Insured: Engleman, Harold R.   999811169-01
Employer: Eastern Auto Sales   Network 45A-2
Group: EA51322

Individual Group Benefits

Out-of-Network: Co-insurance

Physician Co-pay: $ 20.00   In-network only
Hospital Services: $ 400.00
Surgery & Hospitalization: Requires preauthorization 800-123-3654

(Delmar/Cengage Learning)

SOURCE DOCUMENT WB5-7

Outside Services LOG
Drs. Heath and Schwartz

Ref. Number	Date(s) of Service	Patient Name	Facility Physician	Procedures Authorization #	Diagnosis (Primary/Secondary/Tertiary)
0018	11/12/2009	Jouharian, Siran	New York County Hospital Dr. Heath	99282 Emergency Room	Severe vertigo 780.4
0019	11/13/2009	Royzin, Joel	Retirement Inn Nursing Home Dr. Heath	99308 Est. Pt. Expanded	PVD and DM 443.9, 250.00
0020	11/13/2009	Durand, Isabel	Retirement Inn Nursing Home Dr. Heath	99307 Est. Pt. Problem focused	Urticaria 708.9

(Delmar/Cengage Learning)

SOURCE DOCUMENT WB5-8

(See Instructions on Back of this sheet)

EMERGENCY CARE AND TREATMENT *(Medical Record)*	TREATMENT FACILITY *(Stamp)* Community General Hospital	LOG NUMBER 12356

ARRIVAL	TRANSPORTATION TO HOSPITAL *(Attach care enroute sheet)*	CURRENT MEDS. *(tetanus immun- ization and other data)*	HISTORY OBTAINED FROM

DATE			TIME			
DAY 11	MONTH 09	YR. 09	10:35 PM	☒ PRIVATE VEHICLE ☐ AMBULANCE ☐ OTHER *(Specify)*	Aspirin	☒ PATIENT ☐ OTHER *(Specify)*

ALLERGIES: NKA

PATIENT?S HOME ADDRESS OR DUTY STATION *(City, State, and ZIP Code)*
8965 Pebble Way, Douglasville, NY 01235

HOME TELE. NO. *(Inc. area code)* (123) 456-3260

CHIEF COMPLAINT(S) *(Include symptom(s), duration)*
Pain Right Ankle and Calf

SEX: M AGE: 42

POSSIBLE THIRD PARTY PAYER? ☐ YES ☒ NO

VITAL SIGNS
TIME	10:40
BP	138/68
PULSE	101
RESP.	28
TEMP.	101.2
WT. *(Child)*	203

DESCRIBE (1) *Subjective data (Pertinent History)*; (2) *Objective data (Examination - include results of tests and x-rays)*; (3) *Assessment (Diagnosis)*; (4) *Plan (Treatment/Procedures - include medication given and follow-up)*

TIME SEEN BY PROVIDER: 11:15 PM

S — Patient c/o tenderness and pain right lower extremity + ankle. Got leg caught by metal screen door x 4 days ago, cut skin just below calf. States "excruiating", can't sleep.

O — Painful to touch, swelling + redness with mottled appearance. Closed laceration; good pedal pulses.

A — Probable cellulitis

P — 1. Start broad spectrum antibiotic
2. NSAIDS for pain management
3. Keep leg elevated
4. Culture affected Area

CATEGORY *(See reverse)*
EMERGENT	
URGENT	✓
NON-URGENT	

ORDERS	INITS.	TIME

ASSESSMENT/DIAGNOSIS
682.6

DISPOSITION *(Check all that apply)*
✓ HOME		FULL DUTY

QUARTERS
24 Hrs.	48 Hrs.	72 Hrs.

MODIFIED DUTY UNTIL:
DAY	MONTH	YEAR

REFERRED TO *(Indicate clinic)*

INSURANCE

EMERGENCY	TODAY
72 HOURS	ROUTINE

Primary FlexiHealth PPO in-network
SSN: 999529842 ID: 999529842-01

ADMIT. TO HOSP. UNIT/SERVICE

CONDITION UPON RELEASE
IMPROVED	✓ UNCHANGED
DETERIORATED	

Secondary None

TIME OF RELEASE:

PATIENT'S IDENTIFICATION *(Mechanical imprint)* FOR WRITTEN ENTRIES GIVE: *Name - last, first, middle; SSN; DOB, service status, name and relation of sponsor or next of kin.* *(IMPORTANT: LIST FACILITY HOLDING TREATMENT RECORD).*

Johnsen, Dennis
999-52-9842
DOB: 06/21/1968
MRN 000032136

SIGNATURE OF PROVIDER AND ID STAMP
L.D. Heath

INSTRUCTIONS TO PATIENT *(Include medications ordered, any limitations and follow-up plans)*
1. NSAIDS for pain, elevate leg
2. Rest for 4 days until relieved
3. Continue antibiotics
4. Follow-up to Dr. Heath in 1 week

EMERGENCY CARE AND TREATMENT
Medical Record Copy

(Delmar/Cengage Learning)

SOURCE DOCUMENT WB5-9

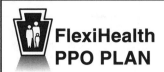

FlexiHealth **PPO PLAN**	Insurer 81564 *Your Health First* ^{SM}

Insured: Johnsen, Dennis   999529842-01
Employer: Cannon Networks, Inc.Network 45A-2
Group: EA51322

Individual Group Benefits

Physician Co-Pay: $ 20.00
Hospital Services: $ 400.00
Surgery & Hospitalization: Requires preauthorization 800-123-3654

(Delmar/Cengage Learning)

SOURCE DOCUMENT WB5-10

(See Instructions on Back of this sheet)

EMERGENCY CARE AND TREATMENT
(Medical Record)

TREATMENT FACILITY *(Stamp)* **Community General Hospital**	LOG NUMBER **12326**	

ARRIVAL

DATE			TIME
DAY	MONTH	YR.	**8:30 PM**
11	09	09	

TRANSPORTATION TO HOSPITAL
(Attach care enroute sheet)
- ☐ PRIVATE VEHICLE
- ☒ AMBULANCE
- ☐ OTHER *(Specify)*

CURRENT MEDS. *(tetanus immun-ization and other data)*
See below

HISTORY OBTAINED FROM *(Specify)*
- ☐ PATIENT ☒ OTHER **Daughter**

ALLERGIES
NKA

PATIENT?S HOME ADDRESS OR DUTY STATION *(City, State, and ZIP Code)*
13267 Gravel Way, Apt. 3, Douglasville, NY 01234

HOME TELE. NO. *(Inc. area code)*
(123) 456-1129

CHIEF COMPLAINT(S) *(Include symptom(s), duration)*
Palpitations, Shortness of Breath

SEX	AGE
M	68

POSSIBLE THIRD PARTY PAYER?
- ☐ YES ☒ NO

VITAL SIGNS

TIME	8:40	
BP	182/102	
PULSE	128	
RESP.	30	
TEMP.	97.4	
WT. *(Child)*	285	

TIME SEEN BY PROVIDER
8:50 PM

DESCRIBE (1) Subjective data *(Pertinent History)*; (2) Objective data *(Examination - include results of tests and x-rays)*; (3) Assessment *(Diagnosis)*; (4) Plan *(Treatment/Procedures - include medication given and follow-up)*

S — Carla Lacey, daughter, got call from patient with severe shortness of breath, chest pain, and palpitations. She called 911 for ambulance and met patient in E.R.

O — Patient in distress. Chest rales and crackles, B/P ↑, arrhythmia. Pulse rapid and weak. Difficult to control patient anxiety.

A — Exacerbation of COPD, congestive heart failure.

P — Continue current meds for blood pressure, start IV diuretic. Request cardiology consult. Admit tonight to CCU.

CATEGORY *(See reverse)*

✓	EMERGENT
	URGENT
	NON-URGENT

ORDERS	INITS.	TIME

ASSESSMENT/DIAGNOSIS
496, 428.0, 789.0

DISPOSITION *(Check all that apply)*

HOME		FULL DUTY	
QUARTERS			
24 Hrs.	48 Hrs.	72 Hrs.	

MODIFIED DUTY UNTIL:

DAY	MONTH	YEAR.

REFERRED TO *(Indicate clinic)*

EMERGENCY		TODAY
72 HOURS		ROUTINE

ADMIT. TO HOSP. UNIT/SERVICE
Cardiology

CONDITION UPON RELEASE

IMPROVED	✓	UNCHANGED
DETERIORATED		

TIME OF RELEASE:

INSURANCE

Primary   Medicare Statewide 999328652A

Secondary   MediGap - Century Senior GAP
                999328652   Policy: MG5133

PATIENT'S IDENTIFICATION *(Mechanical imprint)*
FOR WRITTEN ENTRIES GIVE: Name - last, first, middle; SSN; DOB, service status, name and relation of sponsor or next of kin.
(IMPORTANT: LIST FACILITY HOLDING TREATMENT RECORD).

Bernardo, William
999-32-8652
DOB: 11/26/1942
MRN: 000032269

SIGNATURE OF PROVIDER AND ID STAMP
Dr. L.D. Heath

INSTRUCTIONS TO PATIENT *(Include medications ordered, any limitations and follow-up plans)*
Admit to Hospital

EMERGENCY CARE AND TREATMENT
Medical Record Copy

(Delmar/Cengage Learning)

SOURCE DOCUMENT WB5-11

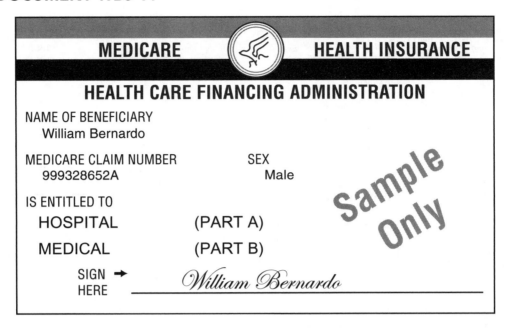

(Delmar/Cengage Learning)

SOURCE DOCUMENT WB5-12

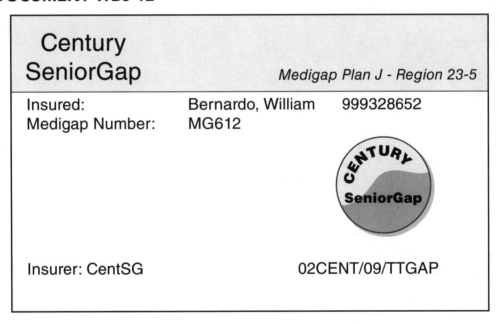

(Delmar/Cengage Learning)

SOURCE DOCUMENT WB5-13

(See Instructions on Back of this sheet)

EMERGENCY CARE AND TREATMENT *(Medical Record)*	TREATMENT FACILITY *(Stamp)*	LOG NUMBER 12388

ARRIVAL		TRANSPORTATION TO HOSPITAL *(Attach care enroute sheet)*	CURRENT MEDS. *(tetanus immun-ization and other data)*	HISTORY OBTAINED FROM

ARRIVAL

DATE			TIME	TRANSPORTATION TO HOSPITAL *(Attach care enroute sheet)*	CURRENT MEDS. *(tetanus immunization and other data)*	HISTORY OBTAINED FROM
DAY	MONTH	YR.	1:00 AM	☒ PRIVATE VEHICLE ☐ AMBULANCE ☐ OTHER *(Specify)*	None	☒ PATIENT ☐ OTHER *(Specify)*
11	10	09				ALLERGIES PCN

PATIENT?S HOME ADDRESS OR DUTY STATION *(City, State, and ZIP Code)*
1932 Slate Drive, Douglasville, NY 01234

HOME TELE. NO. *(Inc. area code)*
(123) 456-2432

CHIEF COMPLAINT(S) *(Include symptom(s), duration)* Vomit, diarrhea	SEX F	AGE 25	POSSIBLE THIRD PARTY PAYER? ☐ YES ☒ NO

TIME SEEN BY PROVIDER
2:10 AM

VITAL SIGNS

TIME	1:25	
BP	130/82	
PULSE	88	
RESP.	20	
TEMP.	99.2	
WT. *(Child)*	162	

DESCRIBE (1) *Subjective* data (Pertinent History); (2) *Objective* data (Examination - include results of tests and x-rays); (3) *Assessment* (Diagnosis); (4) *Plan* (Treatment/Procedures - include medication given and follow-up)

S — Presents with abdominal cramping, vomiting x 4 hrs and recent diarrhea. States was at seafood restuarant and may have had "bad shrimp" in heavy alfredo sauce.

O — Abdominal tenderness, vomit is clear bile now, no diarrhea relief with Pepto Bismol. No blood noted in stool or vomit material.

A — Gastroenteritis

P — Anti-emetic given to relieve nausea.
Increase clear ⬛uids; gradual to soft diet over 1–2 days.
Follow-up in one week, sooner if temp↑to 101°, chills start, and vomiting persists.

CATEGORY *(See reverse)*

EMERGENT	
URGENT	
✓ NON-URGENT	

ORDERS	INITS.	TIME

ASSESSMENT/DIAGNOSIS

558.9

DISPOSITION *(Check all that apply)*

✓ HOME	FULL DUTY

QUARTERS

24 Hrs.	48 Hrs.	72 Hrs.

MODIFIED DUTY UNTIL:

DAY	MONTH	YEAR.

REFERRED TO *(Indicate clinic)*

INSURANCE

EMERGENCY	TODAY
72 HOURS	ROUTINE

ADMIT. TO HOSP. UNIT/SERVICE

Primary   Signal HMO   999361238-02
Group: MISO15

CONDITION UPON RELEASE

IMPROVED	UNCHANGED
DETERIORATED	

Secondary   None

TIME OF RELEASE:

PATIENT'S IDENTIFICATION *(Mechanical imprint)*
FOR WRITTEN ENTRIES GIVE: Name - last, first, middle; SSN; DOB, service status, name and relation of sponsor or next of kin.
(IMPORTANT: LIST FACILITY HOLDING TREATMENT RECORD).

Souza, Janet
999-68-2118
DOB: 12/26/1985
MRN: 000032331

SIGNATURE OF PROVIDER AND ID STAMP
Dr. L.D. Heath

INSTRUCTIONS TO PATIENT   *(Include medications ordered, any limitations and follow-up plans)*

1. Push ⬛uids x 24°
2. Clear liquid to soft diet x 2 days
3. Follow-up in 1 week with Dr. Heath

EMERGENCY CARE AND TREATMENT
Medical Record Copy

(Delmar/Cengage Learning)

SOURCE DOCUMENT WB5-14

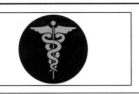

Signal HMO

PCP: Douglasville Medicine Associates
Dr. T.J. Pozzaro
(123)456-7890

Keven Souza 999361236 01
Janet Souza 999361238 02

Copayment Schedule

PCP Office Visits $ 10.00
Specialists Visits $ 30.00
Emergency Room $ 100.00
Hospitalization Authorization

Preauthorization 800-123-8877

Bank Code
361 Member Group Number: MIS015

E25/A10
Type of Coverage

(Delmar/Cengage Learning)

SOURCE DOCUMENT WB5-15

Community General Hospital						RECORD OF ADMISSION	

PATIENT NAME		ROOM NO.	HOSP. NO.	ADDRESS LINE - 1			ADDRESS LINE - 2
Karen Ross		401B		5831 Pebble Way			

AGE	BIRTHDATE	SEX	BIRTHPLACE	CITY	STATE	ZIP CODE	COUNTRY CODE
44	02/10/1966	F	Los Angeles, CA	Douglasville	NY	01235	

SSAN	NATIONALITY	CIVIL ST.	MILITARY	RELIGION	CHURCH		PATIENT TELEPHONE
999-61-2413				UNK			(123)465-2101

SPOUSE INFORMATION

NAME OF HUSBAND OR NAME OF WIFE		SPOUSE BIRTHPLACE		SPOUSE EMPLOYER NAME	
Thomas Ross				Extreme Electronics, Inc.	
Same	SPOUSE ADDRESS			SPOUSE EMPLOYER ADDRESS	

NAME OF FATHER	BIRTHPLACE	NAME OF MOTHER	BIRTHPLACE

NOTIFY IN CASE OF EMERGENCY

NAME	RELATIONSHIP	ADDRESS	TELEPHONE
Karen Muraski	Mother		(123)427-1160

PATIENT EMPLOYER NAME	EMPLOYER ADDRESS	EMPLOYER TELEPHONE	GUARANTOR OCCUPATION
Clearview Elementary	321 Industry Lane Douglasville, NY 01235	(123)423-8896	Sales

GUARANTOR NAME	GUARANTOR TELEPHONE	HOSPITALIZATION INSURANCE
Thomas Ross		FlexiHealth PPO In-Network

GUARANTOR ADDRESS - 1	CITY	ID Number: 999321611-02 Group: EXT213NY
Same		

GUARANTOR ADDRESS - 2	STATE	ZIP CODE	DATE	TIME	PLACE	EVENT	INJURY DUE TO ACCID.

ADMITTING PHYSICIAN	CONSULTING PHYSICIAN	ADMITTING SERVICE	SMOKER	ADMITTING DIAGNOSIS	
Heath		Medicine	No	Diabetes Mellitus	

ALLERGIES	DATE LAST ADM.	PREV. ADM. NO.	ADMISSION DATE	TIME OF ADMISSION	INITIALS	DISCHARGE DATE
NKA			11/17/2009	2:00 PM		

FINANCIAL CLASS	MEDICAL RECORDS NUMBER	ADMISSION CODE	HOME 1	SHORT TERM HOSPITAL 2	SKILLED NURSING FACILITY 3	INTERMEDIATE CARE FACILITY 4	OTHER 5	LEFT AMA 7	EXPIRED 20	TIME
	000213									

PRINCIPAL DIAGNOSIS:	ADVANCE DIRECTIVE =	CODE
DM 250.42		

SECONDARY DIAGNOSIS:		CPT
HTN 401.9	Preauthorization	
	obtained	99221
	FH002136	

PRINCIPAL OPERATION/DATE:

SECONDARY OPERATIONS:

Consultation With _____ *Marcie Pollanco, MD Endocrine Service Requested* _____

Results: ☐ Recovered ☒ Improved ☐ Not Improved ☐ Not Treated ☐ Diagnosis Only ☐ Died ☐ Released Against Advice

Cause of Death _____ Autopsy: ☐ Yes ☐ No

I have examined and approved this complete medical on _____ 20 ____

Signed _____ *L.D. Heath, MD* _____ Attending Physician

ADMISSION - SUMMARY SHEET

(Delmar/Cengage Learning)

SOURCE DOCUMENT WB5-16

| Community General Hospital | | | | | | | RECORD OF ADMISSION | |

PATIENT NAME	ROOM NO.	HOSP. NO.	ADDRESS LINE - 1	ADDRESS LINE - 2
Sean M. McKay	303C		521 East Marble Way	APT 3D

AGE	BIRTHDATE	SEX	BIRTHPLACE	CITY	STATE	ZIP CODE	COUNTRY CODE
75	05/02/1935	M		Douglasville	NY	01235	

SSAN	NATIONALITY	CIVIL ST.	MILITARY	RELIGION	CHURCH	PATIENT TELEPHONE
999-32-5576				Catholic		(123)466-3121

SPOUSE INFORMATION

NAME OF HUSBAND OR NAME OF WIFE	SPOUSE BIRTHPLACE	SPOUSE EMPLOYER NAME
None		
SPOUSE ADDRESS		SPOUSE EMPLOYER ADDRESS

NAME OF FATHER	BIRTHPLACE	NAME OF MOTHER	BIRTHPLACE

NOTIFY IN CASE OF EMERGENCY

NAME	RELATIONSHIP	ADDRESS	TELEPHONE
Patrick McKay	Son	518 East Marble Way	(123)466-3121

PATIENT EMPLOYER NAME	EMPLOYER ADDRESS	EMPLOYER TELEPHONE	GUARANTOR OCCUPATION
Retired			

GUARANTOR NAME	GUARANTOR TELEPHONE	HOSPITALIZATION INSURANCE
		Medicare-Statewide

GUARANTOR ADDRESS - 1	CITY	ID Number: 999325576 A

GUARANTOR ADDRESS - 2	STATE	ZIP CODE	DATE	TIME	PLACE	EVENT	INJURY DUE TO ACCID.

ADMITTING PHYSICIAN	CONSULTING PHYSICIAN	ADMITTING SERVICE	SMOKER	ADMITTING DIAGNOSIS				
Heath		Medicine		Viral Syndrome				

ALLERGIES	DATE LAST ADM.	PREV. ADM. NO.	ADMISSION DATE	TIME OF ADMISSION	INITIALS	DISCHARGE DATE
Sulfa			11/20/2009	9:00 AM		

FINANCIAL CLASS	MEDICAL RECORDS NUMBER	ADMISSION CODE	HOME 1	SHORT TERM HOSPITAL 2	SKILLED NURSING FACILITY 3	INTERMEDIATE CARE FACILITY 4	OTHER 5	LEFT AMA 7	EXPIRED 20	TIME
	000325									

PRINCIPAL DIAGNOSIS:
Viral Infection 079.99

ADVANCE DIRECTIVE =

CODE

CPT

SECONDARY DIAGNOSIS:
Dehydration 276.51

Preauthorization

obtained

99221

PRINCIPAL OPERATION/DATE:

SECONDARY OPERATIONS:

Consultation With _____

Results: ☐ Recovered   ☐ Improved   ☐ Not Improved   ☐ Not Treated   ☐ Diagnosis Only   ☐ Died   ☐ Released Against Advice

Cause of Death _____   Autopsy: ☐ Yes   ☐ No

I have examined and approved this complete medical on _____ 20 _____

Signed _____ *L.D. Heath, MD* _____   Attending Physician

ADMISSION - SUMMARY SHEET

(Delmar/Cengage Learning)

SOURCE DOCUMENT WB5-17

Community General Hospital				RECORD OF ADMISSION

PATIENT NAME	ROOM NO.	HOSP. NO.	ADDRESS LINE - 1		ADDRESS LINE - 2
Mark Hedensten	CCU		12341 Slate Court		

AGE	BIRTHDATE	SEX	BIRTHPLACE	CITY	STATE	ZIP CODE	COUNTRY CODE
52	03/12/1958	M	Buffalo, NY	Douglasville	NY	01235	

SSAN	NATIONALITY	CIVIL ST.	MILITARY	RELIGION	CHURCH	PATIENT TELEPHONE
999-54-1163			AR	Lutheran		(123)466-1120

SPOUSE INFORMATION

NAME OF HUSBAND OR NAME OF WIFE	SPOUSE BIRTHPLACE	SPOUSE EMPLOYER NAME
Tina Hedensten		
SPOUSE ADDRESS		SPOUSE EMPLOYER ADDRESS

NAME OF FATHER	BIRTHPLACE	NAME OF MOTHER	BIRTHPLACE

NOTIFY IN CASE OF EMERGENCY

NAME	RELATIONSHIP	ADDRESS	TELEPHONE
Tina Hedensten	Spouse	Same	

PATIENT EMPLOYER NAME	EMPLOYER ADDRESS	EMPLOYER TELEPHONE	GUARANTOR OCCUPATION
Concepts Media, LLC	110 Industry Lane, Douglasville, NY 01235	(123)467-1111	Manager

GUARANTOR NAME	GUARANTOR TELEPHONE	HOSPITALIZATION INSURANCE
Mark Hedensten		ConsumerONE HRA
GUARANTOR ADDRESS - 1	CITY	ID Number: 999541163 Group: CME89116

GUARANTOR ADDRESS - 2	STATE	ZIP CODE	DATE	TIME	PLACE	EVENT	INJURY DUE TO ACCID.

ADMITTING PHYSICIAN	CONSULTING PHYSICIAN	ADMITTING SERVICE	SMOKER	ADMITTING DIAGNOSIS
Schwartz		Medicine		Peptic Ulcer

ALLERGIES	DATE LAST ADM.	PREV. ADM. NO.	ADMISSION DATE	TIME OF ADMISSION	INITIALS	DISCHARGE DATE
Sulfa			11/22/2009	10:00 AM		

FINANCIAL CLASS	MEDICAL RECORDS NUMBER	ADMISSION CODE	HOME 1	SHORT TERM HOSPITAL 2	SKILLED NURSING FACILITY 3	INTERMEDIATE CARE FACILITY 4	OTHER 5	LEFT AMA 7	EXPIRED 20	TIME
	000398									

PRINCIPAL DIAGNOSIS:		
Angina 413.9	ADVANCE DIRECTIVE =	CODE
		CPT
SECONDARY DIAGNOSIS:		
PVC 427.69	Preauthorization	99221
	obtained	

PRINCIPAL OPERATION/DATE:

SECONDARY OPERATIONS:

Consultation With _*Cardiology: Service Requested for Consultation*_

Results: ☐ Recovered ☒ Improved ☐ Not Improved ☐ Not Treated ☐ Diagnosis Only ☐ Died ☐ Released Against Advice

Cause of Death _____ Autopsy: ☐ Yes ☐ No

I have examined and approved this complete medical on _____ 20 _____

Signed *D.J. Schwartz, MD* _____ Attending Physician

ADMISSION - SUMMARY SHEET

(Delmar/Cengage Learning)

SOURCE DOCUMENT WB6-1

PLEASE RETURN THIS FORM TO RECEPTIONIST	NAME Devon Trimble

Ref # WB001

PLACE OF SERVICE:
(X) OFFICE   ( ) RETIREMENT INN NURSING HOME
( ) NEW YORK COUNTY HOSPITAL
( ) COMMUNITY GENERAL HOSPITAL   ( ) _____

DATE OF SERVICE   10/20/2009

A. OFFICE VISITS - New Patient

Code	History	Exam	Dec.	Time	
__ 99201	Prob. Foc.	Prob. Foc.	Straight	10 min.	_____
__ 99202	Ex. Prob. Foc.	Ex. Prob. Foc.	Straight	20 min.	_____
__ 99203	Detail	Detail	Low	30 min.	_____
X 99204	Comp.	Comp.	Mod.	45 min.	1
__ 99205	Comp.	Comp.	High	60 min.	_____

B. OFFICE VISIT - Established Patient

Code	History	Exam	Dec.	Time	
__ 99211	Minimal	Minimal	Minimal	5 min.	_____
__ 99212	Prob. Foc.	Prob. Foc.	Straight	10 min.	_____
__ 99213	Ex. Prob. Foc.	Ex. Prob. Foc.	Low	15 min.	_____
__ 99214	Detail	Detail	Mod.	25 min.	_____
__ 99215	Comp.	Comp.	High	40 min.	_____

C. HOSPITAL CARE   Dx Units

1. Initial Hospital Care (30 min)	___ ___ 99221	_____
2. Subsequent Care	___ ___ 99231	_____
3. Critical Care (30-74 min)	___ ___ 99291	_____
4. each additional 30 min.	___ ___ 99292	_____
5. Discharge Services	___ ___ 99238	_____
6. Emergency Room	___ ___ 99282	_____

D. NURSING HOME CARE   Dx Units

Initial Care - New Pt.
1. Expanded	___ ___ 99322	_____
2. Detailed	___ ___ 99323	_____

Subsequent Care - Estab. Pt.
3. Problem Focused	___ ___ 99307	_____
4. Expanded	___ ___ 99308	_____
5. Detailed	___ ___ 99309	_____
5. Comprehensive	___ ___ 99310	_____

E. PROCEDURES
1. Arthrocentesis, Small Jt.	___	20600
2. Colonoscopy		45378
3. EKG w/interpretation	___	93000
4. X-Ray Chest, PA/LAT	___	71020

F. LAB
1. Blood Sugar	___	82947	_____
2. CBC w/differential	___	85031	_____
3. Cholesterol	___	82465	_____
4. Comprehensive Metabolic Panel	1	80053	X
5. ESR	___	85651	_____
6. Hematocrit	___	85014	_____
7. Mono Screen	___	86308	_____
8. Pap Smear	___	88150	_____
9. Potassium	___	84132	_____
10. Preg. Test, Quantitative	___	84702	_____
11. Routine Venipuncture	___	36415	_____

F. Cont'd   Dx Units
12. Strep Screen	___	87081	_____
13. UA, Routine w/Micro	___	81000	_____
14. UA, Routine w/o Micro	1	81002	X
15. Uric Acid	___	84550	_____
16. VDRL	___	86592	_____
17. Wet Prep	___	82710	_____
18. _____	___		_____

G. INJECTIONS
1. Influenza Virus Vaccine	___	90658	_____
2. Pneumococcal Vaccine	___	90772	_____
3. Tetanus Toxoids	___	90703	_____
4. Therapeutic Subcut/IM	___	90732	_____
5. Vaccine Administration	___	90471	_____
6. Vaccine - each additional	___	90472	_____

H. MISCELLANEOUS
1. _____   ____   ____
2. _____   ____   ____

AMOUNT PAID $ 10.00

Mark diagnosis with (1=Primary, 2=Secondary, 3=Tertiary)

DIAGNOSIS NOT LISTED BELOW _____

DIAGNOSIS	ICD-9-CM 1, 2, 3	DIAGNOSIS	ICD-9-CM 1, 2, 3	DIAGNOSIS	ICD-9-CM 1, 2, 3
Abdominal Pain	789.0_	Dehydration	276.51	Otitis Media, Acute NOS	382.9
Allergic Rhinitis, Unspec.	477.9	Depression, NOS	311	Peptic Ulcer Disease	536.9
Angina Pectoris, Unspec.	413.9	Diabetes Mellitus, Type II Controlled	250.00 1	Peripheral Vascular Disease NOS	443.9
Anemia, Iron Deficiency, Unspec.	280.9	Diabetes Mellitus, Type II Controlled	250.02	Pharyngitis, Acute	462
Anemia, NOS	285.9	Drug Reaction, NOS	995.29	Pneumonia, Organism Unspec.	486
Anemia, Pernicious	281.0	Dysuria	788.1	Prostatitis, NOS	601.9
Asthma w/ Exacerbation	493.92	Eczema, NOS	692.2	PVC	427.69
Asthmatic Bronchitis, Unspec.	493.90	Edema	782.3	Rash, Non Specific	782.1
Atrial Fibrillation	427.31	Fever, Unknown Origin	780.6	Seizure Disorder NOS	780.39
Atypical Chest Pain, Unspec.	786.59	Gastritis, Acute w/o Hemorrhage	535.00	Serous Otitis Media, Chronic, Unspec.	381.10
Bronchiolitis, due to RSV	466.11	Gastroenteritis, NOS	558.9	Sinusitis, Acute NOS	461.9
Bronchitis, Acute	466.0	Gastroesophageal Reflux	530.81	Tonsillitis, Acute	463.
Bronchitis, NOS	490	Hepatitis A, Infectious	070.1	Upper Respiratory Infection, Acute NOS	465.9
Cardiac Arrest	427.5	Hypercholesterolemia, Pure	272.0	Urinary Tract Infection, Unspec.	599.0
Cardiopulmonary Disease, Chronic, Unspec.	416.9	Hypertension, Unspec.	401.9	Urticaria, Unspec.	708.9
Cellulitis, NOS	682.9	Hypoglycemia NOS	251.2	Vertigo, NOS	780.4
Congestive Heart Failure, Unspec.	428.0	Hypokalemia	276.8	Viral Infection NOS	079.99
Contact Dermatitis NOS	692.9	Impetigo	684	Weakness, Generalized	780.79
COPD NOS	496	Lymphadenitis, Unspec.	289.3	Weight Loss, Abnormal	783.21
CVA, Acute, NOS	434.91	Mononucleosis	075		
CVA, Old or Healed	438.9	Myocardial Infarction, Acute, NOS	410.9		
Degenerative Arthritis (Specify Site)	715.9	Organic Brain Syndrome	310.9		
		Otitis Externa, Acute NOS	380.10		

ABN: I UNDERSTAND THAT MEDICARE PROBABLY WILL NOT COVER THE SERVICES LISTED BELOW

A. _____   B. _____   C. _____
                          Patient
Date _____   Signature _____

Doctor's Signature   LD Heath

RETURN: _____ Days _____   2   (Weeks) _____ Months

DOUGLASVILLE MEDICINE ASSOCIATES
5076 BRAND BLVD., SUITE 401
DOUGLASVILLE, NY 01234
PHONE No. (123) 456-7890
☒ L.D. HEATH, M.D.   ☐ D.J. SCHWARTZ, M.D.
NPI# 9995010111   NPI# 9995020212
EIN# 00-1234560

REF# 122949 SB (05.07.09)   TO REORDER CALL INHEALTH RECORD SYSTEMS 800-477-7374

(Used with permission. InHealth Record Systems, Inc. 5076 Winters Chapel Road, Atlanta, GA 30360, 800-477-7374. http://www.inhealthrecords.com)

SOURCE DOCUMENT WB6-2

Devon Trimble
774 Marble Way #206
Douglasville, NY 01234

9-5678/1234

1734

DATE ___10/20/2009___

PAY TO THE
ORDER OF ___L.D Heath, MD_____ $ | 10.00

___Exactly Ten Dollars_____ DOLLARS 🔒 Security features Included. Details on back.

Memo **Co-pay**_____ ___*Devon Trimble*___ MP

⑆ 1 2 3 4 5 6 7 8 0 ⑆ 1 2 3 ⑈ 4 5 6 ⑈ 7 ⑈

(Delmar/Cengage Learning)

SOURCE DOCUMENT WB6-3

PLEASE RETURN THIS FORM TO RECEPTIONIST	NAME Harold Engleman

Ref # WB002

| PLACE OF SERVICE: | (X) OFFICE
( ) NEW YORK COUNTY HOSPITAL
( ) COMMUNITY GENERAL HOSPITAL | ( ) RETIREMENT INN NURSING HOME
( ) _____ | DATE OF SERVICE 10/22/2009 |

A. OFFICE VISITS - New Patient

Code	History	Exam	Dec.	Time	
___ 99201	Prob. Foc.	Prob. Foc.	Straight	10 min.	_____
___ 99202	Ex. Prob. Foc.	Ex. Prob. Foc.	Straight	20 min.	_____
___ 99203	Detail	Detail	Low	30 min.	_____
___ 99204	Comp.	Comp.	Mod.	45 min.	_____
X 99205	Comp.	Comp.	High	60 min.	1, 2

B. OFFICE VISIT - Established Patient

Code	History	Exam	Dec.	Time	
___ 99211	Minimal	Minimal	Minimal	5 min.	_____
___ 99212	Prob. Foc.	Prob. Foc.	Straight	10min.	_____
___ 99213	Ex. Prob. Foc.	Ex. Prob. Foc.	Low	15 min.	_____
___ 99214	Detail	Detail	Mod.	25 min.	_____
___ 99215	Comp.	Comp.	High	40 min.	_____

C. HOSPITAL CARE

		Dx	Units	
1.	Initial Hospital Care (30 min)	___ ___ 99221	_____
2.	Subsequent Care	___ ___ 99231	_____
3.	Critical Care (30-74 min)	___ ___ 99291	_____
4.	each additional 30 min.	___ ___ 99292	_____
5.	Discharge Services	___ ___ 99238	_____
6.	Emergency Room	___ ___ 99282	_____

D. NURSING HOME CARE

		Dx	Units	
Initial Care - New Pt.				
1.	Expanded	___ ___ 99322	_____
2.	Detailed	___ ___ 99323	_____
Subsequent Care - Estab. Pt.				
3.	Problem Focused	___ ___ 99307	_____
4.	Expanded	___ ___ 99308	_____
5.	Detailed	___ ___ 99309	_____
5.	Comprehensive	___ ___ 99310	_____

E. PROCEDURES

		Dx		
1.	Arthrocentesis, Small Jt.	___	20600	_____
2.	Colonoscopy		45378	_____
3.	EKG w/interpretation	___	93000	_____
4.	X-Ray Chest, PA/LAT	___	71020	_____

F. LAB

1.	Blood Sugar	___	82947	_____
2.	CBC w/differential	___	85031	_____
3.	Cholesterol	___	82465	_____
4.	Comprehensive Metabolic Panel	___	80053	_____
5.	ESR	___	85651	_____
6.	Hematocrit	___	85014	_____
7.	Mono Screen	___	86308	_____
8.	Pap Smear	___	88150	_____
9.	Potassium	___	84132	_____
10.	Preg. Test, Quantitative	___	84702	_____
11.	Routine Venipuncture	___	36415	_____

F. Cont'd

		Dx	Units	
12.	Strep Screen	___	87081	_____
13.	UA, Routine w/Micro	___	81000	_____
14.	UA, Routine w/o Micro	___	81002	_____
15.	Uric Acid	___	84550	_____
16.	VDRL	___	86592	_____
17.	Wet Prep	___	82710	_____
18.	_____	___	___	_____

G. INJECTIONS

1.	Influenza Virus Vaccine	_____	90658	_____
2.	Pneumoccocal Vaccine	_____	90772	_____
3.	Tetanus Toxoids	_____	90703	_____
4.	Therapeutic Subcut/IM	_____	90732	_____
5.	Vaccine Administration	_____	90471	_____
6.	Vaccine - each additional	_____	90472	_____

H. MISCELLANEOUS

1. _____ ____ _____
2. _____ ____ _____

AMOUNT PAID $ ____ 0

Mark diagnosis with (1=Primary, 2=Secondary, 3=Tertiary)	DIAGNOSIS NOT LISTED _____ BELOW _____

DIAGNOSIS	ICD-9-CM 1, 2, 3	DIAGNOSIS	ICD-9-CM 1, 2, 3	DIAGNOSIS	ICD-9-CM 1, 2, 3
Abdominal Pain	789.0_	Dehydration	276.51 ____	Otitis Media, Acute NOS	382.9 ____
Allergic Rhinitis, Unspec.	477.9	Depression, NOS	311 ____	Peptic Ulcer Disease	536.9 ____
Angina Pectoris, Unspec.	413.9	Diabetes Mellitus, Type II Controlled	250.00 ____	Peripheral Vascular Disease NOS	443.9 ____
Anemia, Iron Deficiency, Unspec.	280.9	Diabetes Mellitus, Type II Controlled	250.02 ____	Pharyngitis, Acute	462 ____
Anemia, NOS	285.9	Drug Reaction, NOS	995.29 ____	Pneumonia, Organism Unspec.	486 ____
Anemia, Pernicious	281.0	Dysuria	788.1 ____	Prostatitis, NOS	601.9 ____
Asthma w/ Exacerbation	493.92	Eczema, NOS	692.2 ____	PVC	427.69 ____
Asthmatic Bronchitis, Unspec.	493.90	Edema	782.3 ____	Rash, Non Specific	782.1 ____
Atrial Fibrillation	427.31	Fever, Unknown Origin	780.6 ____	Seizure Disorder NOS	780.39 ____
Atypical Chest Pain, Unspec.	786.59	Gastritis, Acute w/o Hemorrhage	535.00 ____	Serous Otitis Media, Chronic, Unspec.	381.10 ____
Bronchiolitis, due to RSV	466.11	Gastroenteritis, NOS	558.9 ____	Sinusitis, Acute NOS	461.9 ____
Bronchitis, Acute	466.0	Gastroesophageal Reflux	530.81	1	Tonsillitis, Acute	463. ____
Bronchitis, NOS	490	Hepatitis A, Infectious	070.1 ____	Upper Respiratory Infection, Acute NOS	465.9 ____
Cardiac Arrest	427.5	Hypercholesterolemia, Pure	272.0 ____	Urinary Tract Infection, Unspec.	599.0 ____
Cardiopulmonary Disease, Chronic, Unspec.	416.9	Hypertension, Unspec.	401.9	2	Urticaria, Unspec.	708.9 ____
Cellulitis, NOS	682.9	Hypoglycemia NOS	251.2 ____	Vertigo, NOS	780.4 ____
Congestive Heart Failure, Unspec.	428.0	Hypokalemia	276.8 ____	Viral Infection NOS	079.99 ____
Contact Dermatitis NOS	692.9	Impetigo	684 ____	Weakness, Generalized	780.79 ____
COPD NOS	496	Lymphadenitis, Unspec.	289.3 ____	Weight Loss, Abnormal	783.21 ____
CVA, Acute, NOS	434.91	Mononucleosis	075 ____		
CVA, Old or Healed	438.9	Myocardial Infarction, Acute, NOS	410.9 ____		
Degenerative Arthritis (Specify Site) _____	715.9	Organic Brain Syndrome	310.9 ____		
		Otitis Externa, Acute NOS	380.10 ____		

ABN: I UNDERSTAND THAT MEDICARE PROBABLY WILL NOT COVER THE SERVICES LISTED BELOW	
A. _____ B. _____ C. _____ Patient Date _____ Signature _____ Doctor's Signature *DJ Schwartz MD* RETURN: _____ Days _____ Weeks _1_ (Months)	**DOUGLASVILLE MEDICINE ASSOCIATES** 5076 BRAND BLVD., SUITE 401 DOUGLASVILLE, NY 01234 PHONE No. (123) 456-7890 ☐ L.D. HEATH, M.D. ☒ D.J. SCHWARTZ, M.D. NPI# 9995010111 NPI# 9995020212 EIN# 00-1234560

REF# 122949 SB (05.07.09) TO REORDER CALL INHEALTH RECORD SYSTEMS 800-477-7374

(Used with permission. InHealth Record Systems, Inc. 5076 Winters Chapel Road, Atlanta, GA 30360, 800-477-7374. http://www.inhealthrecords.com)

SOURCE DOCUMENT WB6-4

PLEASE RETURN THIS FORM TO RECEPTIONIST	NAME Derek Wallace

Ref # WB003

PLACE OF SERVICE:
(X) OFFICE
( ) NEW YORK COUNTY HOSPITAL
( ) COMMUNITY GENERAL HOSPITAL
( ) RETIREMENT INN NURSING HOME
( ) _____

DATE OF SERVICE 10/22/2009

A. OFFICE VISITS - New Patient

Code	History	Exam	Dec.	Time	
____ 99201	Prob. Foc.	Prob. Foc.	Straight	10 min.	_____
____ 99202	Ex. Prob. Foc.	Ex. Prob. Foc.	Straight	20 min.	_____
____ 99203	Detail	Detail	Low	30 min.	_____
____ 99204	Comp.	Comp.	Mod.	45 min.	_____
____ 99205	Comp.	Comp.	High	60 min.	_____

B. OFFICE VISIT - Established Patient

Code	History	Exam	Dec.	Time	
____ 99211	Minimal	Minimal	Minimal	5 min.	_____
X 99212	Prob. Foc.	Prob. Foc.	Straight	10 min.	1
____ 99213	Ex. Prob. Foc.	Ex. Prob. Foc.	Low	15 min.	_____
____ 99214	Detail	Detail	Mod.	25 min.	_____
____ 99215	Comp.	Comp.	High	40 min.	_____

C. HOSPITAL CARE

		Dx Units	
1. Initial Hospital Care (30 min)	____ ___	99221	_____
2. Subsequent Care	____ ___	99231	_____
3. Critical Care (30-74 min)	____ ___	99291	_____
4. each additional 30 min.	____ ___	99292	_____
5. Discharge Services	____ ___	99238	_____
6. Emergency Room	____ ___	99282	_____

D. NURSING HOME CARE

		Dx	Units	
Initial Care - New Pt.				
1. Expanded		____	99322	_____
2. Detailed		____ ___	99323	
Subsequent Care - Estab. Pt.				
3. Problem Focused		____ ___	99307	
4. Expanded		____ ___	99308	
5. Detailed		____ ___	99309	
5. Comprehensive		____ ___	99310	

E. PROCEDURES

1. Arthrocentesis, Small Jt.	____	20600	_____
2. Colonoscopy	____	45378	_____
3. EKG w/interpretation	____	93000	_____
4. X-Ray Chest, PA/LAT	____	71020	_____

F. LAB

1. Blood Sugar	____	82947	_____
2. CBC w/differential	____	85031	_____
3. Cholesterol	____	82465	_____
4. Comprehensive Metabolic Panel	____	80053	_____
5. ESR	____	85651	_____
6. Hematocrit	____	85014	_____
7. Mono Screen	____	86308	_____
8. Pap Smear	____	88150	_____
9. Potassium	____	84132	_____
10. Preg. Test, Quantitative	____	84702	_____
11. Routine Venipuncture	____	36415	_____

F. Cont'd

		Dx	Units
12. Strep Screen	____	87081	_____
13. UA, Routine w/Micro	____	81000	_____
14. UA, Routine w/o Micro	____	81002	_____
15. Uric Acid	____	84550	_____
16. VDRL	____	86592	_____
17. Wet Prep	____	82710	_____
18. _____	____	____	_____

G. INJECTIONS

1. Influenza Virus Vaccine	____	90658	_____
2. Pneumoccocal Vaccine	____	90772	_____
3. Tetanus Toxoids	____	90703	_____
4. Therapeutic Subcut/IM	____	90732	_____
5. Vaccine Administration	____	90471	_____
6. Vaccine - each additional	____	90472	_____

H. MISCELLANEOUS

1. _____ ____ ____ _____
2. _____ ____ ____ _____

AMOUNT PAID $ 20.00

Mark diagnosis with
(1=Primary, 2=Secondary, 3=Tertiary)

DIAGNOSIS NOT LISTED _____
BELOW _____

DIAGNOSIS	ICD-9-CM 1, 2, 3	DIAGNOSIS	ICD-9-CM 1, 2, 3	DIAGNOSIS	ICD-9-CM 1, 2, 3
Abdominal Pain	789.0 ___	Dehydration	276.51 ____	Otitis Media, Acute NOS	382.9 ____
Allergic Rhinitis, Unspec.	477.9 ____	Depression, NOS	311 ____	Peptic Ulcer Disease	536.9 ____
Angina Pectoris, Unspec.	413.9 ____	Diabetes Mellitus, Type II Controlled	250.00 ____	Peripheral Vascular Disease NOS	443.9 ____
Anemia, Iron Deficiency, Unspec.	280.9 ____	Diabetes Mellitus, Type II Controlled	250.02 ____	Pharyngitis, Acute	462 ____
Anemia, NOS	285.9 ____	Drug Reaction, NOS	995.29 ____	Pneumonia, Organism Unspec.	486 ____
Anemia, Pernicious	281.0 ____	Dysuria	788.1 ____	Prostatitis, NOS	601.9 ____
Asthma w/ Exacerbation	493.92 ____	Eczema, NOS	692.2 ____	PVC	427.69 ____
Asthmatic Bronchitis, Unspec.	493.90 ____	Edema	782.3 ____	Rash, Non Specific	782.1 ____
Atrial Fibrillation	427.31 ____	Fever, Unknown Origin	780.6 ____	Seizure Disorder NOS	780.39 ____
Atypical Chest Pain, Unspec.	786.59 ____	Gastritis, Acute w/o Hemorrhage	535.00 ____	Serous Otitis Media, Chronic, Unspec.	381.10 ____
Bronchiolitis, due to RSV	466.11 ____	Gastroenteritis, NOS	558.9 ____	Sinusitis, Acute NOS	461.9 ____
Bronchitis, Acute	466.0 ____	Gastroesophageal Reflux	530.81 ____	Tonsillitis, Acute	463. ____
Bronchitis, NOS	490 ____	Hepatitis A, Infectious	070.1 ____	Upper Respiratory Infection, Acute NOS	465.9 ____
Cardiac Arrest	427.5 ____	Hypercholesterolemia, Pure	272.0 ____	Urinary Tract Infection, Unspec.	599.0 ____ 1
Cardiopulmonary Disease, Chronic, Unspec.	416.9 ____	Hypertension, Unspec.	401.9 ____	Urticaria, Unspec.	708.9 ____
Cellulitis, NOS	682.9 ____	Hypoglycemia NOS	251.2 ____	Vertigo, NOS	780.4 ____
Congestive Heart Failure, Unspec.	428.0 ____	Hypokalemia	276.8 ____	Viral Infection NOS	079.99 ____
Contact Dermatitis NOS	692.9 ____	Impetigo	684 ____	Weakness, Generalized	780.79 ____
COPD NOS	496 ____	Lymphadenitis, Unspec.	289.3 ____	Weight Loss, Abnormal	783.21 ____
CVA, Acute, NOS	434.91 ____	Mononucleosis	075 ____		
CVA, Old or Healed	438.9 ____	Myocardial Infarction, Acute, NOS	410.9 ____		
Degenerative Arthritis (Specify Site) ____	715.9 ____	Organic Brain Syndrome	310.9 ____		
		Otitis Externa, Acute NOS	380.10 ____		

ABN: I UNDERSTAND THAT MEDICARE PROBABLY WILL NOT COVER THE SERVICES LISTED BELOW

A. _____ B. _____ C. _____

Patient

Date _____ Signature _____

Doctor's Signature _LD Heath_

RETURN: Prn Days _____ Weeks _____ Months _____

REF# 122949 SB (05.07.09) TO REORDER CALL INHEALTH RECORD SYSTEMS 800-477-7374

DOUGLASVILLE MEDICINE ASSOCIATES
5076 BRAND BLVD., SUITE 401
DOUGLASVILLE, NY 01234
PHONE No. (123) 456-7890
☒ L.D. HEATH, M.D. ☐ D.J. SCHWARTZ, M.D.
NPI# 9995010111   NPI# 9995020212
EIN# 00-1234560

(Used with permission. InHealth Record Systems, Inc. 5076 Winters Chapel Road, Atlanta, GA 30360, 800-477-7374. http://www.inhealthrecords.com)

SOURCE DOCUMENT WB6-5

Derek Wallace
35821 George Place
Douglasville, NY 01234

9-5678/1234

208

DATE **10/22/2009**

PAY TO THE
ORDER OF **L.D. Heath**

$ 20.00

Exactly Twenty Dollars ------------------------ DOLLARS

🔒 Security features included. Details on back.

Memo **Co-pay**

Derek Wallace MP

⑆123456780⑆ 123⑈456⑈7⑈

(Delmar/Cengage Learning)

SOURCE DOCUMENT WB6-6

PLEASE RETURN THIS FORM TO RECEPTIONIST

NAME   Naomi Yamagata

Ref # WB004

PLACE OF SERVICE:
(X) OFFICE
( ) NEW YORK COUNTY HOSPITAL
( ) COMMUNITY GENERAL HOSPITAL
( ) RETIREMENT INN NURSING HOME
( ) _____

DATE OF SERVICE   10/22/2009

A. OFFICE VISITS - New Patient

Code	History	Exam	Dec.	Time	
___ 99201	Prob. Foc.	Prob. Foc.	Straight	10 min.	_____
___ 99202	Ex. Prob. Foc.	Ex. Prob. Foc.	Straight	20 min.	_____
___ 99203	Detail	Detail	Low	30 min.	_____
___ 99204	Comp.	Comp.	Mod.	45 min.	_____
___ 99205	Comp.	Comp.	High	60 min.	_____

B. OFFICE VISIT - Established Patient

Code	History	Exam	Dec.	Time	
___ 99211	Minimal	Minimal	Minimal	5 min.	_____
___ 99212	Prob. Foc.	Prob. Foc.	Straight	10min.	_____
___ 99213	Ex. Prob. Foc.	Ex. Prob. Foc.	Low	15 min.	_____
X 99214	Detail	Detail	Mod.	25 min.	1
___ 99215	Comp.	Comp.	High	40 min.	_____

C. HOSPITAL CARE

		Dx	Units	
1. Initial Hospital Care (30 min)	____ ___ 99221			_____
2. Subsequent Care	____ ___ 99231			_____
3. Critical Care (30-74 min)	____ ___ 99291			_____
4. each additional 30 min.	____ ___ 99292			_____
5. Discharge Services	____ ___ 99238			_____
6. Emergency Room	____ ___ 99282			_____

D. NURSING HOME CARE

		Dx	Units	
Initial Care - New Pt.				
1. Expanded		____ ___	99322	_____
2. Detailed		____ ___	99323	_____
Subsequent Care - Estab. Pt.				
3. Problem Focused		____ ___	99307	_____
4. Expanded		____ ___	99308	_____
5. Detailed		____ ___	99309	_____
5. Comprehensive		____ ___	99310	_____

E. PROCEDURES

1. Arthrocentesis, Small Jt.	____	20600	_____
2. Colonoscopy		45378	_____
3. EKG w/interpretation	____	93000	_____
4. X-Ray Chest, PA/LAT		71020	_____

F. LAB

1. Blood Sugar	____	82947	_____
2. CBC w/differential	____	85031	_____
3. Cholesterol	____	82465	_____
4. Comprehensive Metabolic Panel	____	80053	_____
5. ESR	____	85651	_____
6. Hematocrit	____	85014	_____
7. Mono Screen	____	86308	_____
8. Pap Smear	____	88150	_____
9. Potassium	____	84132	_____
10. Preg. Test, Quantitative	____	84702	_____
11. Routine Venipuncture	____	36415	_____

F. Cont'd

		Dx	Units	
12. Strep Screen	____		87081	_____
13. UA, Routine w/Micro	____		81000	_____
14. UA, Routine w/o Micro	____		81002	_____
15. Uric Acid	____		84550	_____
16. VDRL	____		86592	_____
17. Wet Prep	____		82710	_____
18. _____	____		____	_____

G. INJECTIONS

1. Influenza Virus Vaccine	____	90658	_____
2. Pneumoccocal Vaccine	____	90772	_____
3. Tetanus Toxoids	____	90703	_____
4. Therapeutic Subcut/IM	____	90732	_____
5. Vaccine Administration	____	90471	_____
6. Vaccine - each additional	____	90472	_____

H. MISCELLANEOUS

1. _____   ____   _____
2. _____   ____   _____

AMOUNT PAID $ _10.00_

Mark diagnosis with (1=Primary, 2=Secondary, 3=Tertiary)

DIAGNOSIS NOT LISTED BELOW _____

DIAGNOSIS	ICD-9-CM 1, 2, 3	DIAGNOSIS	ICD-9-CM 1, 2, 3	DIAGNOSIS	ICD-9-CM 1, 2, 3
Abdominal Pain	789.0_	Dehydration	276.51 ____	Otitis Media, Acute NOS	382.9 ____
Allergic Rhinitis, Unspec.	477.9 ____	Depression, NOS	311 ____	Peptic Ulcer Disease	536.9 ____
Angina Pectoris, Unspec.	413.9 ____	Diabetes Mellitus, Type II Controlled	250.00 ____	Peripheral Vascular Disease NOS	443.9 ____
Anemia, Iron Deficiency, Unspec.	280.9 ____	Diabetes Mellitus, Type II Controlled	250.02 ____	Pharyngitis, Acute	462 ____
Anemia, NOS	285.9 ____	Drug Reaction, NOS	995.29 ____	Pneumonia, Organism Unspec.	486 ____
Anemia, Pernicious	281.0 ____	Dysuria	788.1 ____	Prostatitis, NOS	601.9 ____
Asthma w/ Exacerbation	493.92 ____	Eczema, NOS	692.2 ____	PVC	427.69 ____
Asthmatic Bronchitis, Unspec.	493.90 1	Edema	782.3 ____	Rash, Non Specific	782.1 ____
Atrial Fibrillation	427.31 ____	Fever, Unknown Origin	780.6 ____	Seizure Disorder NOS	780.39 ____
Atypical Chest Pain, Unspec.	786.59 ____	Gastritis, Acute w/o Hemorrhage	535.00 ____	Serous Otitis Media, Chronic, Unspec.	381.10 ____
Bronchiolitis, due to RSV	466.11 ____	Gastroenteritis, NOS	558.9 ____	Sinusitis, Acute NOS	461.9 ____
Bronchitis, Acute	466.0 ____	Gastroesophageal Reflux	530.81 ____	Tonsillitis, Acute	463. ____
Bronchitis, NOS	490 ____	Hepatitis A, Infectious	070.1 ____	Upper Respiratory Infection, Acute NOS	465.9 ____
Cardiac Arrest	427.5 ____	Hypercholesterolemia, Pure	272.0 ____	Urinary Tract Infection, Unspec.	599.0 ____
Cardiopulmonary Disease, Chronic, Unspec.	416.9 ____	Hypertension, Unspec.	401.9 ____	Urticaria, Unspec.	708.9 ____
Cellulitis, NOS	682.9 ____	Hypoglycemia NOS	251.2 ____	Vertigo, NOS	780.4 ____
Congestive Heart Failure, Unspec.	428.0 ____	Hypokalemia	276.8 ____	Viral Infection NOS	079.99 ____
Contact Dermatitis NOS	692.9 ____	Impetigo	684 ____	Weakness, Generalized	780.79 ____
COPD NOS	496 ____	Lymphadenitis, Unspec.	289.3 ____	Weight Loss, Abnormal	783.21 ____
CVA, Acute, NOS	434.91 ____	Mononucleosis	075 ____		
CVA, Old or Healed	438.9 ____	Myocardial Infarction, Acute, NOS	410.9 ____		
Degenerative Arthritis		Organic Brain Syndrome	310.9 ____		
(Specify Site) ____	715.9 ____	Otitis Externa, Acute NOS	380.10 ____		

ABN: I UNDERSTAND THAT MEDICARE PROBABLY WILL NOT COVER THE SERVICES LISTED BELOW

A. _____   B. _____   C. _____
Patient

Date _____   Signature _____

Doctor's Signature   _DJ Schwartz, MD_

RETURN: _____ Days _2_   (Weeks) _____ Months

REF# 122949 SB (05.07.09)   TO REORDER CALL INHEALTH RECORD SYSTEMS 800-477-7374

DOUGLASVILLE MEDICINE ASSOCIATES
5076 BRAND BLVD., SUITE 401
DOUGLASVILLE, NY 01234
PHONE No. (123) 456-7890
☐ L.D. HEATH, M.D.   ☒ D.J. SCHWARTZ, M.D.
NPI# 9995010111   NPI# 9995020212
EIN# 00-1234560

(Used with permission. InHealth Record Systems, Inc. 5076 Winters Chapel Road, Atlanta, GA 30360, 800-477-7374. http://www.inhealthrecords.com)

SOURCE DOCUMENT WB6-7

PLEASE RETURN THIS FORM TO RECEPTIONIST	NAME Nancy Herbert

Ref # WB005

PLACE OF SERVICE:
(X) OFFICE
( ) NEW YORK COUNTY HOSPITAL
( ) COMMUNITY GENERAL HOSPITAL
( ) RETIREMENT INN NURSING HOME
( ) _____

DATE OF SERVICE 10/22/2009

A. OFFICE VISITS - New Patient

Code	History	Exam	Dec.	Time	
___ 99201	Prob. Foc.	Prob. Foc.	Straight	10 min.	___
___ 99202	Ex. Prob. Foc.	Ex. Prob. Foc.	Straight	20 min.	___
___ 99203	Detail	Detail	Low	30 min.	___
___ 99204	Comp.	Comp.	Mod.	45 min.	___
___ 99205	Comp.	Comp.	High	60 min.	___

B. OFFICE VISIT - Established Patient

Code	History	Exam	Dec.	Time	
___ 99211	Minimal	Minimal	Minimal	5 min.	___
___ 99212	Prob. Foc.	Prob. Foc.	Straight	10min.	___
___ 99213	Ex. Prob. Foc.	Ex. Prob. Foc.	Low	15 min.	___
___ 99214	Detail	Detail	Mod.	25 min.	___
X 99215	Comp.	Comp.	High	40 min.	1, 2, 3

C. HOSPITAL CARE

		Dx	Units	
1. Initial Hospital Care (30 min)	99221	___	___	___
2. Subsequent Care	99231	___	___	___
3. Critical Care (30-74 min)	99291	___	___	___
4. each additional 30 min.	99292	___	___	___
5. Discharge Services	99238	___	___	___
6. Emergency Room	99282	___	___	___

D. NURSING HOME CARE

	Dx	Units	
Initial Care - New Pt.			
1. Expanded	___ ___	99322	___
2. Detailed	___ ___	99323	___
Subsequent Care - Estab. Pt.			
3. Problem Focused	___ ___	99307	___
4. Expanded	___ ___	99308	___
5. Detailed	___ ___	99309	___
5. Comprehensive	___ ___	99310	___

E. PROCEDURES

1. Arthrocentesis, Small Jt.	___	20600
2. Colonoscopy	___	45378
3. EKG w/interpretation	___	93000
4. X-Ray Chest, PA/LAT	___	71020

F. LAB

1. Blood Sugar	___	82947	___
2. CBC w/differential	___	85031	___
3. Cholesterol	___	82465	___
4. Comprehensive Metabolic Panel	1, 2, 3	80053	X
5. ESR	___	85651	___
6. Hematocrit	3	85014	X
7. Mono Screen	___	86308	___
8. Pap Smear	___	88150	___
9. Potassium	___	84132	___
10. Preg. Test, Quantitative	___	84702	___
11. Routine Venipuncture	___	36415	___

F. Cont'd

	Dx	Units	
12. Strep Screen	___	87081	___
13. UA, Routine w/Micro	___	81000	___
14. UA, Routine w/o Micro	___	81002	___
15. Uric Acid	___	84550	___
16. VDRL	___	86592	___
17. Wet Prep	___	82710	___
18. _____	___	___	___

G. INJECTIONS

1. Influenza Virus Vaccine	___	90658	___
2. Pneumococcal Vaccine	___	90772	___
3. Tetanus Toxoids	___	90703	___
4. Therapeutic Subcut/IM	___	90732	___
5. Vaccine Administration	___	90471	___
6. Vaccine - each additional	___	90472	___

H. MISCELLANEOUS

1. _____ ___ ___
2. _____ ___ ___

AMOUNT PAID $ 0

Mark diagnosis with (1=Primary, 2=Secondary, 3=Tertiary)

DIAGNOSIS NOT LISTED BELOW _____

DIAGNOSIS	ICD-9-CM 1,2,3	DIAGNOSIS	ICD-9-CM 1,2,3	DIAGNOSIS	ICD-9-CM 1,2,3
Abdominal Pain	789.0_ ___	Dehydration	276.51 ___	Otitis Media, Acute NOS	382.9 ___
Allergic Rhinitis, Unspec.	477.9 ___	Depression, NOS	311 ___	Peptic Ulcer Disease	536.9 ___
Angina Pectoris, Unspec.	413.9 ___	Diabetes Mellitus, Type II Controlled	250.00 ___	Peripheral Vascular Disease NOS	443.9 ___
Anemia, Iron Deficiency, Unspec.	280.9 ___	Diabetes Mellitus, Type II Controlled	250.02 ___	Pharyngitis, Acute	462 ___
Anemia, NOS	285.9 3	Drug Reaction, NOS	995.29 ___	Pneumonia, Organism Unspec.	486 ___
Anemia, Pernicious	281.0 ___	Dysuria	788.1 ___	Prostatitis, NOS	601.9 ___
Asthma w/ Exacerbation	493.92 ___	Eczema, NOS	692.2 ___	PVC	427.69 ___
Asthmatic Bronchitis, Unspec.	493.90 ___	Edema	782.3 ___	Rash, Non Specific	782.1 ___
Atrial Fibrillation	427.31 ___	Fever, Unknown Origin	780.6 ___	Seizure Disorder NOS	780.39 ___
Atypical Chest Pain, Unspec.	786.59 ___	Gastritis, Acute w/o Hemorrhage	535.00 ___	Serous Otitis Media, Chronic, Unspec.	381.10 ___
Bronchiolitis, due to RSV	466.11 ___	Gastroenteritis, NOS	558.9 ___	Sinusitis, Acute NOS	461.9 ___
Bronchitis, Acute	466.0 ___	Gastroesophageal Reflux	530.81 ___	Tonsillitis, Acute	463. ___
Bronchitis, NOS	490 ___	Hepatitis A, Infectious	070.1 ___	Upper Respiratory Infection, Acute NOS	465.9 ___
Cardiac Arrest	427.5 ___	Hypercholesterolemia, Pure	272.0 ___	Urinary Tract Infection, Unspec.	599.0 ___
Cardiopulmonary Disease, Chronic, Unspec.	416.9 ___	Hypertension, Unspec.	401.9 2	Urticaria, Unspec.	708.9 ___
Cellulitis, NOS	682.9 ___	Hypoglycemia NOS	251.2 ___	Vertigo, NOS	780.4 ___
Congestive Heart Failure, Unspec.	428.0 ___	Hypokalemia	276.8 ___	Viral Infection NOS	079.99 ___
Contact Dermatitis NOS	692.9 ___	Impetigo	684 ___	Weakness, Generalized	780.79 ___
COPD NOS	496 1	Lymphadenitis, Unspec.	289.3 ___	Weight Loss, Abnormal	783.21 ___
CVA, Acute, NOS	434.91 ___	Mononucleosis	075 ___		
CVA, Old or Healed	438.9 ___	Myocardial Infarction, Acute, NOS	410.9 ___		
Degenerative Arthritis		Organic Brain Syndrome	310.9 ___		
(Specify Site) ___	715.9 ___	Otitis Externa, Acute NOS	380.10 ___		

ABN: I UNDERSTAND THAT MEDICARE PROBABLY WILL NOT COVER THE SERVICES LISTED BELOW

A. _____ B. _____ C. _____
Patient
Date _____ Signature _____

Doctor's Signature *LD Heath*

RETURN: _____ Days _____ Weeks 3 (Months)

DOUGLASVILLE MEDICINE ASSOCIATES
5076 BRAND BLVD., SUITE 401
DOUGLASVILLE, NY 01234
PHONE No. (123) 456-7890
☒ L.D. HEATH, M.D.   ☐ D.J. SCHWARTZ, M.D.
NPI# 9995010111   NPI# 9995020212
EIN# 00-1234560

REF# 122949 SB (05.07.09)   TO REORDER CALL INHEALTH RECORD SYSTEMS 800-477-7374

(Used with permission. InHealth Record Systems, Inc. 5076 Winters Chapel Road, Atlanta, GA 30360, 800-477-7374. http://www.inhealthrecords.com)

SOURCE DOCUMENT WB6-8

PLEASE RETURN THIS FORM TO RECEPTIONIST	NAME Alan Shuman

Ref # WB006

PLACE OF SERVICE:
(X) OFFICE
( ) NEW YORK COUNTY HOSPITAL
( ) COMMUNITY GENERAL HOSPITAL
( ) RETIREMENT INN NURSING HOME
( ) _____

DATE OF SERVICE 10/22/2009

A. OFFICE VISITS - New Patient

Code	History	Exam	Dec.	Time	
___ 99201	Prob. Foc.	Prob. Foc.	Straight	10 min.	___
___ 99202	Ex. Prob. Foc.	Ex. Prob. Foc.	Straight	20 min.	___
___ 99203	Detail	Detail	Low	30 min.	___
___ 99204	Comp.	Comp.	Mod.	45 min.	___
___ 99205	Comp.	Comp.	High	60 min.	___

B. OFFICE VISIT - Established Patient

Code	History	Exam	Dec.	Time	
___ 99211	Minimal	Minimal	Minimal	5 min.	___
___ 99212	Prob. Foc.	Prob. Foc.	Straight	10min.	___
___ 99213	Ex. Prob. Foc.	Ex. Prob. Foc.	Low	15 min.	___
___ 99214	Detail	Detail	Mod.	25 min.	___
X 99215	Comp.	Comp.	High	40 min.	1, 2

C. HOSPITAL CARE

		Dx	Units	
1.	Initial Hospital Care (30 min)	___ ___ 99221	___
2.	Subsequent Care	___ ___ 99231	___
3.	Critical Care (30-74 min)	___ ___ 99291	___
4.	each additional 30 min.	___ ___ 99292	___
5.	Discharge Services	___ ___ 99238	___
6.	Emergency Room	___ ___ 99282	___

D. NURSING HOME CARE

		Dx	Units
	Initial Care - New Pt.		
1.	Expanded	___ ___	99322
2.	Detailed	___ ___	99323
	Subsequent Care - Estab. Pt.		
3.	Problem Focused	___ ___	99307
4.	Expanded	___ ___	99308
5.	Detailed	___ ___	99309
5.	Comprehensive	___ ___	99310

E. PROCEDURES

		Dx	Units
1.	Arthrocentesis, Small Jt.	___	20600
2.	Colonoscopy	___	45378
3.	EKG w/interpretation	___	93000
4.	X-Ray Chest, PA/LAT	___	71020

F. LAB

1.	Blood Sugar	___	82947	___
2.	CBC w/differential	___	85031	___
3.	Cholesterol	___	82465	___
4.	Comprehensive Metabolic Panel	___	80053	___
5.	ESR	___	85651	___
6.	Hematocrit	___	85014	___
7.	Mono Screen	___	86308	___
8.	Pap Smear	___	88150	___
9.	Potassium	___	84132	___
10.	Preg. Test, Quantitative	___	84702	___
11.	Routine Venipuncture	___	36415	___

F. Cont'd

		Dx	Units	
12.	Strep Screen	___	87081	___
13.	UA, Routine w/Micro	___	81000	___
14.	UA, Routine w/o Micro	___	81002	___
15.	Uric Acid	___	84550	___
16.	VDRL	___	86592	___
17.	Wet Prep	___	82710	___
18.	_____	___	___	___

G. INJECTIONS

1.	Influenza Virus Vaccine	1	90658	X
2.	Pneumoccocal Vaccine	1	90772	X
3.	Tetanus Toxoids	___	90703	___
4.	Therapeutic Subcut/IM	___	90732	___
5.	Vaccine Administration	___	90471	___
6.	Vaccine - each additional	___	90472	___

H. MISCELLANEOUS

1. _____ ___ ___
2. _____ ___ ___

AMOUNT PAID $ 20.00

Mark diagnosis with (1=Primary, 2=Secondary, 3=Tertiary)

DIAGNOSIS NOT LISTED BELOW _____

DIAGNOSIS	ICD-9-CM	1,2,3	DIAGNOSIS	ICD-9-CM	1,2,3	DIAGNOSIS	ICD-9-CM	1,2,3
Abdominal Pain	789.0	___	Dehydration	276.51	___	Otitis Media, Acute NOS	382.9	___
Allergic Rhinitis, Unspec.	477.9	___	Depression, NOS	311	___	Peptic Ulcer Disease	536.9	___
Angina Pectoris, Unspec.	413.9	___	Diabetes Mellitus, Type II Controlled	250.00	___	Peripheral Vascular Disease NOS	443.9	___
Anemia, Iron Deficiency, Unspec.	280.9	___	Diabetes Mellitus, Type II Controlled	250.02	___	Pharyngitis, Acute	462	___
Anemia, NOS	285.9	___	Drug Reaction, NOS	995.29	___	Pneumonia, Organism Unspec.	486	___
Anemia, Pernicious	281.0	___	Dysuria	788.1	___	Prostatitis, NOS	601.9	___
Asthma w/ Exacerbation	493.92	___	Eczema, NOS	692.2	___	PVC	427.69	___
Asthmatic Bronchitis, Unspec.	493.90	___	Edema	782.3	___	Rash, Non Specific	782.1	___
Atrial Fibrillation	427.31	___	Fever, Unknown Origin	780.6	___	Seizure Disorder NOS	780.39	___
Atypical Chest Pain, Unspec.	786.59	___	Gastritis, Acute w/o Hemorrhage	535.00	___	Serous Otitis Media, Chronic, Unspec.	381.10	___
Bronchiolitis, due to RSV	466.11	___	Gastroenteritis, NOS	558.9	___	Sinusitis, Acute NOS	461.9	___
Bronchitis, Acute	466.0	___	Gastroesophageal Reflux	530.81	___	Tonsillitis, Acute	463.	___
Bronchitis, NOS	490	___	Hepatitis A, Infectious	070.1	___	Upper Respiratory Infection, Acute NOS	465.9	___
Cardiac Arrest	427.5	___	Hypercholesterolemia, Pure	272.0	___	Urinary Tract Infection, Unspec.	599.0	___
Cardiopulmonary Disease, Chronic, Unspec.	416.9	___	Hypertension, Unspec.	401.9	___	Urticaria, Unspec.	708.9	___
Cellulitis, NOS	682.9	___	Hypoglycemia NOS	251.2	___	Vertigo, NOS	780.4	___
Congestive Heart Failure, Unspec.	428.0	___	Hypokalemia	276.8	___	Viral Infection NOS	079.99	___
Contact Dermatitis NOS	692.9	___	Impetigo	684	___	Weakness, Generalized	780.79	___
COPD NOS	496	1	Lymphadenitis, Unspec.	289.3	___	Weight Loss, Abnormal	783.21	___
CVA, Acute, NOS	434.91	___	Mononucleosis	075	___			
CVA, Old or Healed	438.9	2	Myocardial Infarction, Acute, NOS	410.9	___			
Degenerative Arthritis			Organic Brain Syndrome	310.9	___			
(Specify Site) _____	715.9	___	Otitis Externa, Acute NOS	380.10	___			

ABN: I UNDERSTAND THAT MEDICARE PROBABLY WILL NOT COVER THE SERVICES LISTED BELOW

A. _____ B. _____ C. _____

Patient

Date _____ Signature _____

Doctor's Signature _LD Heath_

RETURN: _____ Days _____ Weeks __2__ Months

DOUGLASVILLE MEDICINE ASSOCIATES
5076 BRAND BLVD., SUITE 401
DOUGLASVILLE, NY 01234
PHONE No. (123) 456-7890
☒ L.D. HEATH, M.D. ☐ D.J. SCHWARTZ, M.D.
NPI# 9995010111 NPI# 9995020212
EIN# 00-1234560

REF# 122949 SB (05.07.09) TO REORDER CALL INHEALTH RECORD SYSTEMS 800-477-7374

(Used with permission. InHealth Record Systems, Inc. 5076 Winters Chapel Road, Atlanta, GA 30360, 800-477-7374. http://www.inhealthrecords.com)

SOURCE DOCUMENT WB6-9

Alan Shuman
5211 Highland Blvd.
Douglasville, NY 01235

9-5678/1234

43991

DATE 10/22/2009

PAY TO THE ORDER OF Dr. L.D. Heath

$ 20.00

Exactly Twenty Dollars------------------------ DOLLARS

Security features included. Details on back.

Memo Co-pay

Alan Shuman MP

⑈123456780⑈ ⑈23ꞮꞮꞮ456ꞮꞮꞮ7ꞮꞮ

(Delmar/Cengage Learning)

SOURCE DOCUMENT WB6-10

PLEASE RETURN THIS FORM TO RECEPTIONIST	NAME Emery Camille

Ref # WB007

PLACE OF SERVICE:
(X) OFFICE   ( ) RETIREMENT INN NURSING HOME
( ) NEW YORK COUNTY HOSPITAL
( ) COMMUNITY GENERAL HOSPITAL   ( ) _____

DATE OF SERVICE 10/22/2009

A. OFFICE VISITS - New Patient

Code	History	Exam	Dec.	Time	
___ 99201	Prob. Foc.	Prob. Foc.	Straight	10 min.	_____
___ 99202	Ex. Prob. Foc.	Ex. Prob. Foc.	Straight	20 min.	_____
___ 99203	Detail	Detail	Low	30 min.	_____
___ 99204	Comp.	Comp.	Mod.	45 min.	_____
___ 99205	Comp.	Comp.	High	60 min.	_____

B. OFFICE VISIT - Established Patient

Code	History	Exam	Dec.	Time	
___ 99211	Minimal	Minimal	Minimal	5 min.	_____
___ 99212	Prob. Foc.	Prob. Foc.	Straight	10min.	_____
X 99213	Ex. Prob. Foc.	Ex. Prob. Foc.	Low	15 min.	1, 2
___ 99214	Detail	Detail	Mod.	25 min.	_____
___ 99215	Comp.	Comp.	High	40 min.	_____

C. HOSPITAL CARE

		Dx	Units	
1. Initial Hospital Care (30 min)	___	___	99221	_____
2. Subsequent Care	___	___	99231	_____
3. Critical Care (30-74 min)	___	___	99291	_____
4. each additional 30 min.	___	___	99292	_____
5. Discharge Services	___	___	99238	_____
6. Emergency Room	___	___	99282	_____

D. NURSING HOME CARE

	Dx	Units	
Initial Care - New Pt.			
1. Expanded	___	___	99322
2. Detailed	___	___	99323
Subsequent Care - Estab. Pt.			
3. Problem Focused	___	___	99307
4. Expanded	___	___	99308
5. Detailed	___	___	99309
5. Comprehensive	___	___	99310

E. PROCEDURES

1. Arthrocentesis, Small Jt.	___	20600
2. Colonoscopy	___	45378
3. EKG w/interpretation	___	93000
4. X-Ray Chest, PA/LAT	___	71020

F. LAB

1. Blood Sugar	___	82947	_____
2. CBC w/differential	1	85031	X
3. Cholesterol	___	82465	_____
4. Comprehensive Metabolic Panel	___	80053	_____
5. ESR	___	85651	_____
6. Hematocrit	___	85014	_____
7. Mono Screen	___	86308	_____
8. Pap Smear	___	88150	_____
9. Potassium	___	84132	_____
10. Preg. Test, Quantitative	___	84702	_____
11. Routine Venipuncture	___	36415	_____

F. Cont'd

	Dx	Units	
12. Strep Screen	___	87081	_____
13. UA, Routine w/Micro	___	81000	_____
14. UA, Routine w/o Micro	___	81002	_____
15. Uric Acid	___	84550	_____
16. VDRL	___	86592	_____
17. Wet Prep	___	82710	_____
18. _____	___	___	_____

G. INJECTIONS

1. Influenza Virus Vaccine	___	90658	_____
2. Pneumoccocal Vaccine	___	90772	_____
3. Tetanus Toxoids	___	90703	_____
4. Therapeutic Subcut/IM	___	90732	_____
5. Vaccine Administration	___	90471	_____
6. Vaccine - each additional	___	90472	_____

H. MISCELLANEOUS

1. _____   ___   _____
2. _____   ___   _____

AMOUNT PAID $ 10.00

Mark diagnosis with (1=Primary, 2=Secondary, 3=Tertiary)

DIAGNOSIS NOT LISTED _____
BELOW _____

DIAGNOSIS	ICD-9-CM 1, 2, 3	DIAGNOSIS	ICD-9-CM 1, 2, 3	DIAGNOSIS	ICD-9-CM 1, 2, 3
Abdominal Pain	789.0 ___	Dehydration	276.51 ___	Otitis Media, Acute NOS	382.9 1
Allergic Rhinitis, Unspec.	477.9 ___	Depression, NOS	311 ___	Peptic Ulcer Disease	536.9 ___
Angina Pectoris, Unspec.	413.9 ___	Diabetes Mellitus, Type II Controlled	250.00 ___	Peripheral Vascular Disease NOS	443.9 ___
Anemia, Iron Deficiency, Unspec.	280.9 ___	Diabetes Mellitus, Type II Controlled	250.02 ___	Pharyngitis, Acute	462 ___
Anemia, NOS	285.9 ___	Drug Reaction, NOS	995.29 ___	Pneumonia, Organism Unspec.	486 ___
Anemia, Pernicious	281.0 ___	Dysuria	788.1 ___	Prostatitis, NOS	601.9 ___
Asthma w/ Exacerbation	493.92 ___	Eczema, NOS	692.2 ___	PVC	427.69 ___
Asthmatic Bronchitis, Unspec.	493.90 ___	Edema	782.3 ___	Rash, Non Specific	782.1 ___
Atrial Fibrillation	427.31 ___	Fever, Unknown Origin	780.6 ___	Seizure Disorder NOS	780.39 ___
Atypical Chest Pain, Unspec.	786.59 ___	Gastritis, Acute w/o Hemorrhage	535.00 ___	Serous Otitis Media, Chronic, Unspec.	381.10 ___
Bronchiolitis, due to RSV	466.11 ___	Gastroenteritis, NOS	558.9 ___	Sinusitis, Acute NOS	461.9 ___
Bronchitis, Acute	466.0 ___	Gastroesophageal Reflux	530.81 ___	Tonsillitis, Acute	463. ___
Bronchitis, NOS	490 ___	Hepatitis A, Infectious	070.1 ___	Upper Respiratory Infection, Acute NOS	465.9 ___
Cardiac Arrest	427.5 ___	Hypercholesterolemia, Pure	272.0 ___	Urinary Tract Infection, Unspec.	599.0 ___
Cardiopulmonary Disease, Chronic, Unspec.	416.9 ___	Hypertension, Unspec.	401.9 ___	Urticaria, Unspec.	708.9 ___
Cellulitis, NOS	682.9 ___	Hypoglycemia NOS	251.2 ___	Vertigo, NOS	780.4 ___
Congestive Heart Failure, Unspec.	428.0 ___	Hypokalemia	276.8 ___	Viral Infection NOS	079.99 2
Contact Dermatitis NOS	692.9 ___	Impetigo	684 ___	Weakness, Generalized	780.79 ___
COPD NOS	496 ___	Lymphadenitis, Unspec.	289.3 ___	Weight Loss, Abnormal	783.21 ___
CVA, Acute, NOS	434.91 ___	Mononucleosis	075 ___		
CVA, Old or Healed	438.9 ___	Myocardial Infarction, Acute, NOS	410.9 ___		
Degenerative Arthritis		Organic Brain Syndrome	310.9 ___		
(Specify Site)	715.9 ___	Otitis Externa, Acute NOS	380.10 ___		

ABN: I UNDERSTAND THAT MEDICARE PROBABLY WILL NOT COVER THE SERVICES LISTED BELOW

A. _____ B. _____ C. _____
Patient
Date _____ Signature _____

Doctor's Signature *DJ Schwartz, MD*

RETURN: _____ Days 1 Weeks _____ Months _____

DOUGLASVILLE MEDICINE ASSOCIATES
5076 BRAND BLVD., SUITE 401
DOUGLASVILLE, NY 01234
PHONE No. (123) 456-7890

❑ L.D. HEATH, M.D.   ☒ D.J. SCHWARTZ, M.D.
NPI# 9995010111   NPI# 9995020212
EIN# 00-1234560

REF# 122949 SB (05.07.09)   TO REORDER CALL INHEALTH RECORD SYSTEMS 800-477-7374

(Used with permission. InHealth Record Systems, Inc. 5076 Winters Chapel Road, Atlanta, GA 30360, 800-477-7374. http://www.inhealthrecords.com)

SOURCE DOCUMENT WB6-11

Gabrielle Camille
1569 Telluride Place
Douglasville, NY 01234

9-5678/1234

1006

DATE ___10/22/2009___

PAY TO THE ORDER OF ___Dr. D.J. Schwartz___ | $ 10.00

___Ten dollars and 00/100___-------------------------- DOLLARS

Security features
included. Details
on back.

Memo ___Co-pay for Emery___   ___Gabrielle Camille___ MP

⑆123456780⑆ 123⑈456⑈71⑉

(Delmar/Cengage Learning)

SOURCE DOCUMENT WB6-12

PLEASE RETURN THIS FORM TO RECEPTIONIST	NAME Deanna Hartsfeld

Ref # WB008

PLACE OF SERVICE:	(X) OFFICE ( ) NEW YORK COUNTY HOSPITAL ( ) COMMUNITY GENERAL HOSPITAL	( ) RETIREMENT INN NURSING HOME ( ) _____ DATE OF SERVICE 10/22/2009

A. OFFICE VISITS - New Patient

Code	History	Exam	Dec.	Time	
99201	Prob. Foc.	Prob. Foc.	Straight	10 min.	
99202	Ex. Prob. Foc.	Ex. Prob. Foc.	Straight	20 min.	
99203	Detail	Detail	Low	30 min.	
99204	Comp.	Comp.	Mod.	45 min.	
99205	Comp.	Comp.	High	60 min.	

B. OFFICE VISIT - Established Patient

Code	History	Exam	Dec.	Time	
99211	Minimal	Minimal	Minimal	5 min.	
99212	Prob. Foc.	Prob. Foc.	Straight	10min.	
99213	Ex. Prob. Foc.	Ex. Prob. Foc.	Low	15 min.	
X 99214	Detail	Detail	Mod.	25 min.	1, 2
99215	Comp.	Comp.	High	40 min.	

C. HOSPITAL CARE

		Dx	Units	
1. Initial Hospital Care (30 min)		____	____	99221
2. Subsequent Care		____	____	99231
3. Critical Care (30-74 min)		____	____	99291
4. each additional 30 min.		____	____	99292
5. Discharge Services		____	____	99238
6. Emergency Room		____	____	99282

D. NURSING HOME CARE

			Dx	Units
Initial Care - New Pt.				
1. Expanded			____ ____	99322
2. Detailed			____ ____	99323
Subsequent Care - Estab. Pt.				
3. Problem Focused			____ ____	99307
4. Expanded			____ ____	99308
5. Detailed			____ ____	99309
5. Comprehensive			____ ____	99310

E. PROCEDURES

		Dx		
1. Arthrocentesis, Small Jt.	____		20600	
2. Colonoscopy			45378	
3. EKG w/interpretation	____		93000	
4. X-Ray Chest, PA/LAT	____		71020	

F. LAB

		Dx		
1. Blood Sugar	____		82947	
2. CBC w/differential	____		85031	
3. Cholesterol	____		82465	
4. Comprehensive Metabolic Panel	____		80053	1
5. ESR	____		85651	
6. Hematocrit	____		85014	
7. Mono Screen	____		86308	
8. Pap Smear	____		88150	
9. Potassium	____		84132	
10. Preg. Test, Quantitative	____		84702	
11. Routine Venipuncture	____		36415	

F. Cont'd

		Dx	Units	
12. Strep Screen	____		87081	
13. UA, Routine w/Micro	____		81000	
14. UA, Routine w/o Micro	____		81002	
15. Uric Acid	____		84550	
16. VDRL	____		86592	
17. Wet Prep	____		82710	
18. _____	____		_____	

G. INJECTIONS

1. Influenza Virus Vaccine	____		90658	
2. Pneumococcal Vaccine	____		90772	
3. Tetanus Toxoids	____		90703	
4. Therapeutic Subcut/IM	____		90732	
5. Vaccine Administration	____		90471	
6. Vaccine - each additional	____		90472	

H. MISCELLANEOUS

1. _____
2. _____

AMOUNT PAID $ 0

Mark diagnosis with (1=Primary, 2=Secondary, 3=Tertiary)

DIAGNOSIS NOT LISTED _____
BELOW _____

DIAGNOSIS	ICD-9-CM 1, 2, 3	DIAGNOSIS	ICD-9-CM 1, 2, 3	DIAGNOSIS	ICD-9-CM 1, 2, 3
Abdominal Pain	789.0	Dehydration	276.51	Otitis Media, Acute NOS	382.9
Allergic Rhinitis, Unspec.	477.9	Depression, NOS	311	Peptic Ulcer Disease	536.9
Angina Pectoris, Unspec.	413.9	Diabetes Mellitus, Type II Controlled	250.00	Peripheral Vascular Disease NOS	443.9
Anemia, Iron Deficiency, Unspec.	280.9	Diabetes Mellitus, Type II Controlled	250.02	Pharyngitis, Acute	462
Anemia, NOS	285.9	Drug Reaction, NOS	995.29	Pneumonia, Organism Unspec.	486
Anemia, Pernicious	281.0	Dysuria	788.1	Prostatitis, NOS	601.9
Asthma w/ Exacerbation	493.92	Eczema, NOS	692.2	PVC	427.69
Asthmatic Bronchitis, Unspec.	493.90	Edema	782.3	Rash, Non Specific	782.1
Atrial Fibrillation	427.31	Fever, Unknown Origin	780.6	Seizure Disorder NOS	780.39
Atypical Chest Pain, Unspec.	786.59	Gastritis, Acute w/o Hemorrhage	535.00	Serous Otitis Media, Chronic, Unspec.	381.10
Bronchiolitis, due to RSV	466.11	Gastroenteritis, NOS	558.9	Sinusitis, Acute NOS	461.9
Bronchitis, Acute	466.0	Gastroesophageal Reflux	530.81	Tonsillitis, Acute	463.
Bronchitis, NOS	490	Hepatitis A, Infectious	070.1	Upper Respiratory Infection, Acute NOS	465.9
Cardiac Arrest	427.5	Hypercholesterolemia, Pure	272.0	1	Urinary Tract Infection, Unspec.	599.0
Cardiopulmonary Disease, Chronic, Unspec.	416.9	Hypertension, Unspec.	401.9	2	Urticaria, Unspec.	708.9
Cellulitis, NOS	682.9	Hypoglycemia NOS	251.2	Vertigo, NOS	780.4
Congestive Heart Failure, Unspec.	428.0	Hypokalemia	276.8	Viral Infection NOS	079.99
Contact Dermatitis NOS	692.9	Impetigo	684	Weakness, Generalized	780.79
COPD NOS	496	Lymphadenitis, Unspec.	289.3	Weight Loss, Abnormal	783.21
CVA, Acute, NOS	434.91	Mononucleosis	075		
CVA, Old or Healed	438.9	Myocardial Infarction, Acute, NOS	410.9		
Degenerative Arthritis		Organic Brain Syndrome	310.9		
(Specify Site)	715.9	Otitis Externa, Acute NOS	380.10		

ABN: I UNDERSTAND THAT MEDICARE PROBABLY WILL NOT COVER THE SERVICES LISTED BELOW

A. _____ B. _____ C. _____

Patient

Date _____ Signature _____

Doctor's Signature *LD Heath*

RETURN: _____ Days _____ Weeks 2 Months _____

REF# 122949 SB (05.07.09) TO REORDER CALL INHEALTH RECORD SYSTEMS 800-477-7374

DOUGLASVILLE MEDICINE ASSOCIATES
5076 BRAND BLVD., SUITE 401
DOUGLASVILLE, NY 01234
PHONE No. (123) 456-7890
☒ L.D. HEATH, M.D.   ☐ D.J. SCHWARTZ, M.D.
NPI# 9995010111   NPI# 9995020212
EIN# 00-1234560

(Used with permission. InHealth Record Systems, Inc. 5076 Winters Chapel Road, Atlanta, GA 30360, 800-477-7374. http://www.inhealthrecords.com)

SOURCE DOCUMENT WB6-13

PLEASE RETURN THIS FORM TO RECEPTIONIST

NAME *Aimee Bradley*

Ref # WB009

PLACE OF SERVICE:
(X) OFFICE
( ) NEW YORK COUNTY HOSPITAL
( ) COMMUNITY GENERAL HOSPITAL
( ) RETIREMENT INN NURSING HOME
( ) _____

DATE OF SERVICE *10/22/2009*

A. OFFICE VISITS - New Patient

Code	History	Exam	Dec.	Time	
___ 99201	Prob. Foc.	Prob. Foc.	Straight	10 min.	_____
___ 99202	Ex. Prob. Foc.	Ex. Prob. Foc.	Straight	20 min.	_____
___ 99203	Detail	Detail	Low	30 min.	_____
___ 99204	Comp.	Comp.	Mod.	45 min.	_____
___ 99205	Comp.	Comp.	High	60 min.	_____

B. OFFICE VISIT - Established Patient

Code	History	Exam	Dec.	Time	
___ 99211	Minimal	Minimal	Minimal	5 min.	_____
___ 99212	Prob. Foc.	Prob. Foc.	Straight	10min.	_____
___ 99213	Ex. Prob. Foc.	Ex. Prob. Foc.	Low	15 min.	_____
X 99214	Detail	Detail	Mod.	25 min.	1, 2
___ 99215	Comp.	Comp.	High	40 min.	_____

C. HOSPITAL CARE   Dx Units

1. Initial Hospital Care (30 min) ___ ___ 99221 _____
2. Subsequent Care ___ ___ 99231 _____
3. Critical Care (30-74 min) ___ ___ 99291 _____
4. each additional 30 min. ___ ___ 99292 _____
5. Discharge Services ___ ___ 99238 _____
6. Emergency Room ___ ___ 99282 _____

D. NURSING HOME CARE   Dx Units

Initial Care - New Pt.
1. Expanded ___ ___ 99322 _____
2. Detailed ___ ___ 99323 _____

Subsequent Care - Estab. Pt.
3. Problem Focused ___ ___ 99307 _____
4. Expanded ___ ___ 99308 _____
5. Detailed ___ ___ 99309 _____
5. Comprehensive ___ ___ 99310 _____

E. PROCEDURES

1. Arthrocentesis, Small Jt. ___ 20600 _____
2. Colonoscopy ___ 45378 _____
3. EKG w/interpretation ___ 93000 _____
4. X-Ray Chest, PA/LAT ___ 71020 _____

F. LAB

1. Blood Sugar ___ 82947 _____
2. CBC w/differential ___ 85031 _____
3. Cholesterol ___ 82465 _____
4. Comprehensive Metabolic Panel ___ 80053 _____
5. ESR ___ 85651 _____
6. Hematocrit ___ 85014 _____
7. Mono Screen ___ 86308 _____
8. Pap Smear ___ 88150 _____
9. Potassium ___ 84132 _____
10. Preg. Test, Quantitative ___ 84702 _____
11. Routine Venipuncture ___ 36415 _____

F. Cont'd   Dx Units

		Dx		
12. Strep Screen		2	87081	X
13. UA, Routine w/Micro			81000	_____
14. UA, Routine w/o Micro			81002	_____
15. Uric Acid			84550	_____
16. VDRL			86592	_____
17. Wet Prep			82710	_____
18. _____			_____	_____

G. INJECTIONS

1. Influenza Virus Vaccine ___ 90658 _____
2. Pneumoccocal Vaccine ___ 90772 _____
3. Tetanus Toxoids ___ 90703 _____
4. Therapeutic Subcut/IM ___ 90732 _____
5. Vaccine Administration ___ 90471 _____
6. Vaccine - each additional ___ 90472 _____

H. MISCELLANEOUS

1. _____ _____ _____
2. _____ _____ _____

AMOUNT PAID $ ____0____

Mark diagnosis with (1=Primary, 2=Secondary, 3=Tertiary)

DIAGNOSIS NOT LISTED BELOW _____

DIAGNOSIS	ICD-9-CM	1, 2, 3	DIAGNOSIS	ICD-9-CM	1, 2, 3	DIAGNOSIS	ICD-9-CM	1, 2, 3
Abdominal Pain	789.0		Dehydration	276.51		Otitis Media, Acute NOS	382.9	
Allergic Rhinitis, Unspec.	477.9		Depression, NOS	311		Peptic Ulcer Disease	536.9	
Angina Pectoris, Unspec.	413.9		Diabetes Mellitus, Type II Controlled	250.00		Peripheral Vascular Disease NOS	443.9	
Anemia, Iron Deficiency, Unspec.	280.9		Diabetes Mellitus, Type II Controlled	250.02		Pharyngitis, Acute	462	2
Anemia, NOS	285.9		Drug Reaction, NOS	995.29		Pneumonia, Organism Unspec.	486	
Anemia, Pernicious	281.0		Dysuria	788.1		Prostatitis, NOS	601.9	
Asthma w/ Exacerbation	493.92		Eczema, NOS	692.2		PVC	427.69	
Asthmatic Bronchitis, Unspec.	493.90		Edema	782.3		Rash, Non Specific	782.1	
Atrial Fibrillation	427.31		Fever, Unknown Origin	780.6		Seizure Disorder NOS	780.39	
Atypical Chest Pain, Unspec.	786.59		Gastritis, Acute w/o Hemorrhage	535.00		Serous Otitis Media, Chronic, Unspec.	381.10	
Bronchiolitis, due to RSV	466.11		Gastroenteritis, NOS	558.9		Sinusitis, Acute NOS	461.9	
Bronchitis, Acute	466.0		Gastroesophageal Reflux	530.81		Tonsillitis, Acute	463	1
Bronchitis, NOS	490		Hepatitis A, Infectious	070.1		Upper Respiratory Infection, Acute NOS	465.9	
Cardiac Arrest	427.5		Hypercholesterolemia, Pure	272.0		Urinary Tract Infection, Unspec.	599.0	
Cardiopulmonary Disease, Chronic, Unspec.	416.9		Hypertension, Unspec.	401.9		Urticaria, Unspec.	708.9	
Cellulitis, NOS	682.9		Hypoglycemia NOS	251.2		Vertigo, NOS	780.4	
Congestive Heart Failure, Unspec.	428.0		Hypokalemia	276.8		Viral Infection NOS	079.99	
Contact Dermatitis NOS	692.9		Impetigo	684		Weakness, Generalized	780.79	
COPD NOS	496		Lymphadenitis, Unspec.	289.3		Weight Loss, Abnormal	783.21	
CVA, Acute, NOS	434.91		Mononucleosis	075				
CVA, Old or Healed	438.9		Myocardial Infarction, Acute, NOS	410.9				
Degenerative Arthritis (Specify Site) ___	715.9		Organic Brain Syndrome	310.9				
			Otitis Externa, Acute NOS	380.10				

ABN: I UNDERSTAND THAT MEDICARE PROBABLY WILL NOT COVER THE SERVICES LISTED BELOW

A. _____ B. _____ C. _____

Date _____ Patient Signature _____

Doctor's Signature *DJ Schwartz, MD*

RETURN: _____ Days ___3___ Weeks _____ Months _____

DOUGLASVILLE MEDICINE ASSOCIATES
5076 BRAND BLVD., SUITE 401
DOUGLASVILLE, NY 01234
PHONE No. (123) 456-7890
❑ L.D. HEATH, M.D.   ☒ D.J. SCHWARTZ, M.D.
NPI# 9995010111   NPI# 9995020212
EIN# 00-1234560

REF# 122949 SB (05.07.09)   TO REORDER CALL INHEALTH RECORD SYSTEMS 800-477-7374

(Used with permission. InHealth Record Systems, Inc. 5076 Winters Chapel Road, Atlanta, GA 30360, 800-477-7374. http://www.inhealthrecords.com)

SOURCE DOCUMENT WB6-14

PLEASE RETURN THIS FORM TO RECEPTIONIST

NAME   Tina Rizzo

Ref # WB010

PLACE OF SERVICE:
(X) OFFICE
( ) NEW YORK COUNTY HOSPITAL
( ) COMMUNITY GENERAL HOSPITAL
( ) RETIREMENT INN NURSING HOME
( ) _____

DATE OF SERVICE   10/22/2009

A. OFFICE VISITS - New Patient

Code	History	Exam	Dec.	Time	
___ 99201	Prob. Foc.	Prob. Foc.	Straight	10 min.	___
___ 99202	Ex. Prob. Foc.	Ex. Prob. Foc.	Straight	20 min.	___
___ 99203	Detail	Detail	Low	30 min.	___
___ 99204	Comp.	Comp.	Mod.	45 min.	___
___ 99205	Comp.	Comp.	High	60 min.	___

B. OFFICE VISIT - Established Patient

Code	History	Exam	Dec.	Time	
___ 99211	Minimal	Minimal	Minimal	5 min.	___
___ 99212	Prob. Foc.	Prob. Foc.	Straight	10min.	___
___ 99213	Ex. Prob. Foc.	Ex. Prob. Foc.	Low	15 min.	___
X 99214	Detail	Detail	Mod.	25 min.	1, 2
___ 99215	Comp.	Comp.	High	40 min.	___

C. HOSPITAL CARE

		Dx	Units	
1.	Initial Hospital Care (30 min)	___	___ 99221	___
2.	Subsequent Care	___	___ 99231	___
3.	Critical Care (30-74 min)	___	___ 99291	___
4.	each additional 30 min.	___	___ 99292	___
5.	Discharge Services	___	___ 99238	___
6.	Emergency Room	___	___ 99282	___

D. NURSING HOME CARE

		Dx	Units	
Initial Care - New Pt.				
1.	Expanded	___	___ 99322	
2.	Detailed	___	___ 99323	
Subsequent Care - Estab. Pt.				
3.	Problem Focused	___	___ 99307	
4.	Expanded	___	___ 99308	
5.	Detailed	___	___ 99309	
5.	Comprehensive	___	___ 99310	

E. PROCEDURES

		Dx		
1.	Arthrocentesis, Small Jt.	___	20600	___
2.	Colonoscopy		45378	___
3.	EKG w/interpretation	___	93000	___
4.	X-Ray Chest, PA/LAT	___	71020	___

F. LAB

		Dx		
1.	Blood Sugar	___	82947	___
2.	CBC w/differential	1, 2	85031	X
3.	Cholesterol	___	82465	___
4.	Comprehensive Metabolic Panel	___	80053	___
5.	ESR	___	85651	___
6.	Hematocrit	___	85014	___
7.	Mono Screen	___	86308	___
8.	Pap Smear	___	88150	___
9.	Potassium	___	84132	___
10.	Preg. Test, Quantitative	___	84702	___
11.	Routine Venipuncture	2	36415	X

F. Cont'd

		Dx		Units
12.	Strep Screen	___	87081	___
13.	UA, Routine w/Micro	___	81000	___
14.	UA, Routine w/o Micro	___	81002	___
15.	Uric Acid	___	84550	___
16.	VDRL	___	86592	___
17.	Wet Prep	___	82710	___
18.	_____	___	_____	___

G. INJECTIONS

1.	Influenza Virus Vaccine	___	90658	___
2.	Pneumoccocal Vaccine	___	90772	___
3.	Tetanus Toxoids	___	90703	___
4.	Therapeutic Subcut/IM	___	90732	___
5.	Vaccine Administration	___	90471	___
6.	Vaccine - each additional	___	90472	___

H. MISCELLANEOUS

1. _____
2. _____

AMOUNT PAID $ 0

Mark diagnosis with
(1=Primary, 2=Secondary, 3=Tertiary)

DIAGNOSIS NOT LISTED _____
BELOW _____

DIAGNOSIS	ICD-9-CM 1, 2, 3	DIAGNOSIS	ICD-9-CM 1, 2, 3	DIAGNOSIS	ICD-9-CM 1, 2, 3
Abdominal Pain	789.0 ___	Dehydration	276.51 ___	Otitis Media, Acute NOS	382.9 ___
Allergic Rhinitis, Unspec.	477.9 __1__	Depression, NOS	311 ___	Peptic Ulcer Disease	536.9 ___
Angina Pectoris, Unspec.	413.9 ___	Diabetes Mellitus, Type II Controlled	250.00 ___	Peripheral Vascular Disease NOS	443.9 ___
Anemia, Iron Deficiency, Unspec.	280.9 ___	Diabetes Mellitus, Type II Controlled	250.02 ___	Pharyngitis, Acute	462 ___
Anemia, NOS	285.9 ___	Drug Reaction, NOS	995.29 ___	Pneumonia, Organism Unspec.	486 ___
Anemia, Pernicious	281.0 ___	Dysuria	788.1 ___	Prostatitis, NOS	601.9 ___
Asthma w/ Exacerbation	493.92 ___	Eczema, NOS	692.2 ___	PVC	427.69 ___
Asthmatic Bronchitis, Unspec.	493.90 ___	Edema	782.3 ___	Rash, Non Specific	782.1 __2__
Atrial Fibrillation	427.31 ___	Fever, Unknown Origin	780.6 ___	Seizure Disorder NOS	780.39 ___
Atypical Chest Pain, Unspec.	786.59 ___	Gastritis, Acute w/o Hemorrhage	535.00 ___	Serous Otitis Media, Chronic, Unspec.	381.10 ___
Bronchiolitis, due to RSV	466.11 ___	Gastroenteritis, NOS	558.9 ___	Sinusitis, Acute NOS	461.9 ___
Bronchitis, Acute	466.0 ___	Gastroesophageal Reflux	530.81 ___	Tonsillitis, Acute	463. ___
Bronchitis, NOS	490 ___	Hepatitis A, Infectious	070.1 ___	Upper Respiratory Infection, Acute NOS	465.9 ___
Cardiac Arrest	427.5 ___	Hypercholesterolemia, Pure	272.0 ___	Urinary Tract Infection, Unspec.	599.0 ___
Cardiopulmonary Disease, Chronic, Unspec.	416.9 ___	Hypertension, Unspec.	401.9 ___	Urticaria, Unspec.	708.9 ___
Cellulitis, NOS	682.9 ___	Hypoglycemia NOS	251.2 ___	Vertigo, NOS	780.4 ___
Congestive Heart Failure, Unspec.	428.0 ___	Hypokalemia	276.8 ___	Viral Infection NOS	079.99 ___
Contact Dermatitis NOS	692.9 ___	Impetigo	684 ___	Weakness, Generalized	780.79 ___
COPD NOS	496 ___	Lymphadenitis, Unspec.	289.3 ___	Weight Loss, Abnormal	783.21 ___
CVA, Acute, NOS	434.91 ___	Mononucleosis	075 ___		
CVA, Old or Healed	438.9 ___	Myocardial Infarction, Acute, NOS	410.9 ___		
Degenerative Arthritis		Organic Brain Syndrome	310.9 ___		
(Specify Site) ___	715.9 ___	Otitis Externa, Acute NOS	380.10 ___		

ABN: I UNDERSTAND THAT MEDICARE PROBABLY WILL NOT COVER THE SERVICES LISTED BELOW

A. _____ B. _____ C. _____

Patient

Date _____ Signature _____

Doctor's Signature   *LD Heath*

RETURN: _____ Days   2   Weeks _____ Months _____

REF# 122949 SB (05.07.09)   TO REORDER CALL INHEALTH RECORD SYSTEMS 800-477-7374

DOUGLASVILLE MEDICINE ASSOCIATES
5076 BRAND BLVD., SUITE 401
DOUGLASVILLE, NY 01234
PHONE No. (123) 456-7890
☒ L.D. HEATH, M.D.   ❑ D.J. SCHWARTZ, M.D.
NPI# 9995010111   NPI# 9995020212
EIN# 00-1234560

(Used with permission. InHealth Record Systems, Inc. 5076 Winters Chapel Road, Atlanta, GA 30360, 800-477-7374. http://www.inhealthrecords.com)

SOURCE DOCUMENT WB6-15

PLEASE RETURN THIS FORM TO RECEPTIONIST	NAME *Caitlin Barryroe*

Ref # WB011

PLACE OF SERVICE:
(X) OFFICE
( ) NEW YORK COUNTY HOSPITAL
( ) COMMUNITY GENERAL HOSPITAL
( ) RETIREMENT INN NURSING HOME
( ) _____

DATE OF SERVICE _10/23/2009_

A. OFFICE VISITS - New Patient

Code	History	Exam	Dec.	Time	
99201	Prob. Foc.	Prob. Foc.	Straight	10 min.	
99202	Ex. Prob. Foc.	Ex. Prob. Foc.	Straight	20 min.	
99203	Detail	Detail	Low	30 min.	
99204	Comp.	Comp.	Mod.	45 min.	
99205	Comp.	Comp.	High	60 min.	

B. OFFICE VISIT - Established Patient

Code	History	Exam	Dec.	Time	
99211	Minimal	Minimal	Minimal	5 min.	
99212	Prob. Foc.	Prob. Foc.	Straight	10min.	
99213	Ex. Prob. Foc.	Ex. Prob. Foc.	Low	15 min.	
X 99214	Detail	Detail	Mod.	25 min.	1, 2
99215	Comp.	Comp.	High	40 min.	

C. HOSPITAL CARE — Dx Units

1. Initial Hospital Care (30 min)	____ ___	99221	_____
2. Subsequent Care	____ ___	99231	_____
3. Critical Care (30-74 min)	____ ___	99291	_____
4. each additional 30 min.	____ ___	99292	_____
5. Discharge Services	____ ___	99238	_____
6. Emergency Room	____ ___	99282	_____

D. NURSING HOME CARE — Dx Units

Initial Care - New Pt.

1. Expanded	____ ___	99322	_____
2. Detailed	____ ___	99323	_____

Subsequent Care - Estab. Pt.

3. Problem Focused	____ ___	99307	_____
4. Expanded	____ ___	99308	_____
5. Detailed	____ ___	99309	_____
5. Comprehensive	____ ___	99310	_____

E. PROCEDURES

1. Arthrocentesis, Small Jt.	____	20600	_____
2. Colonoscopy		45378	_____
3. EKG w/interpretation		93000	_____
4. X-Ray Chest, PA/LAT		71020	_____

F. LAB

1. Blood Sugar	____	82947	_____
2. CBC w/differential	____	85031	_____
3. Cholesterol		82465	_____
4. Comprehensive Metabolic Panel	1, 2	80053	X
5. ESR		85651	_____
6. Hematocrit	____	85014	_____
7. Mono Screen	____	86308	_____
8. Pap Smear		88150	_____
9. Potassium		84132	_____
10. Preg. Test, Quantitative	____	84702	_____
11. Routine Venipuncture	____	36415	_____

F. Cont'd — Dx Units

12. Strep Screen		87081	_____
13. UA, Routine w/Micro	_1_	81000	X
14. UA, Routine w/o Micro	____	81002	_____
15. Uric Acid		84550	_____
16. VDRL	____	86592	_____
17. Wet Prep	____	82710	_____
18. _____	____	_____	_____

G. INJECTIONS

1. Influenza Virus Vaccine	____	90658	_____
2. Pneumoccocal Vaccine	____	90772	_____
3. Tetanus Toxoids	____	90703	_____
4. Therapeutic Subcut/IM	____	90732	_____
5. Vaccine Administration	____	90471	_____
6. Vaccine - each additional	____	90472	_____

H. MISCELLANEOUS

1. _____	____	_____	_____
2. _____	____	_____	_____

AMOUNT PAID $ _20.00_

Mark diagnosis with (1=Primary, 2=Secondary, 3=Tertiary)

DIAGNOSIS NOT LISTED BELOW _____

DIAGNOSIS	ICD-9-CM	1, 2, 3	DIAGNOSIS	ICD-9-CM	1, 2, 3	DIAGNOSIS	ICD-9-CM	1, 2, 3
Abdominal Pain	789.0_		Dehydration	276.51		Otitis Media, Acute NOS	382.9	
Allergic Rhinitis, Unspec.	477.9		Depression, NOS	311		Peptic Ulcer Disease	536.9	
Angina Pectoris, Unspec.	413.9		Diabetes Mellitus, Type II Controlled	250.00		Peripheral Vascular Disease NOS	443.9	
Anemia, Iron Deficiency, Unspec.	280.9		Diabetes Mellitus, Type II Controlled	250.02		Pharyngitis, Acute	462	
Anemia, NOS	285.9		Drug Reaction, NOS	995.29		Pneumonia, Organism Unspec.	486	
Anemia, Pernicious	281.0		Dysuria	788.1		Prostatitis, NOS	601.9	
Asthma w/ Exacerbation	493.92		Eczema, NOS	692.2		PVC	427.69	
Asthmatic Bronchitis, Unspec.	493.90		Edema	782.3		Rash, Non Specific	782.1	
Atrial Fibrillation	427.31		Fever, Unknown Origin	780.6	2	Seizure Disorder NOS	780.39	
Atypical Chest Pain, Unspec.	786.59		Gastritis, Acute w/o Hemorrhage	535.00		Serous Otitis Media, Chronic, Unspec.	381.10	
Bronchiolitis, due to RSV	466.11		Gastroenteritis, NOS	558.9		Sinusitis, Acute NOS	461.9	
Bronchitis, Acute	466.0		Gastroesophageal Reflux	530.81		Tonsillitis, Acute	463.	
Bronchitis, NOS	490		Hepatitis A, Infectious	070.1		Upper Respiratory Infection, Acute NOS	465.9	
Cardiac Arrest	427.5		Hypercholesterolemia, Pure	272.0		Urinary Tract Infection, Unspec.	599.0	1
Cardiopulmonary Disease, Chronic, Unspec.	416.9		Hypertension, Unspec.	401.9		Urticaria, Unspec.	708.9	
Cellulitis, NOS	682.9		Hypoglycemia NOS	251.2		Vertigo, NOS	780.4	
Congestive Heart Failure, Unspec.	428.0		Hypokalemia	276.8		Viral Infection NOS	079.99	
Contact Dermatitis NOS	692.9		Impetigo	684		Weakness, Generalized	780.79	
COPD NOS	496		Lymphadenitis, Unspec.	289.3		Weight Loss, Abnormal	783.21	
CVA, Acute, NOS	434.91		Mononucleosis	075				
CVA, Old or Healed	438.9		Myocardial Infarction, Acute, NOS	410.9				
Degenerative Arthritis			Organic Brain Syndrome	310.9				
(Specify Site) _____	715.9		Otitis Externa, Acute NOS	380.10				

ABN: I UNDERSTAND THAT MEDICARE PROBABLY WILL NOT COVER THE SERVICES LISTED BELOW

A._____ B._____ C._____

Patient

Date_____ Signature_____

Doctor's Signature _LD Heath_

RETURN: __5__ (Days) _____ Weeks _____ Months

DOUGLASVILLE MEDICINE ASSOCIATES
5076 BRAND BLVD., SUITE 401
DOUGLASVILLE, NY 01234
PHONE No. (123) 456-7890
☒ L.D. HEATH, M.D. ☐ D.J. SCHWARTZ, M.D.
NPI# 9995010111 NPI# 9995020212
EIN# 00-1234560

REF# 122949 SB (05.07.09) TO REORDER CALL INHEALTH RECORD SYSTEMS 800-477-7374

(Used with permission. InHealth Record Systems, Inc. 5076 Winters Chapel Road, Atlanta, GA 30360, 800-477-7374. http://www.inhealthrecords.com)

SOURCE DOCUMENT WB6-16

Caitlin Barryroe
386 Glenwood Court Apt 202
Douglasville, NY 01235

9-5678/1234

361

DATE __10/22/2009__

PAY TO THE
ORDER OF __Dr. Heath__ $ __20.00__

__Twenty dollars exactly__ ----------------------- DOLLARS

🔒 Security features
Included. Details
on back.

Memo __Co-payment__   *Caitlin Barryroe*   MP

⑆123456780⑆ 123⑈456⑈7⑈

(Delmar/Cengage Learning)

SOURCE DOCUMENT WB6-17

PLEASE RETURN THIS FORM TO RECEPTIONIST	NAME Wynona Sheridan

Ref # WB012

	(X) OFFICE	( ) RETIREMENT INN NURSING HOME
PLACE OF	( ) NEW YORK COUNTY HOSPITAL	
SERVICE:	( ) COMMUNITY GENERAL HOSPITAL ( ) _____	DATE OF SERVICE 10/27/2009

A. OFFICE VISITS - New Patient

Code	History	Exam	Dec.	Time	
___ 99201	Prob. Foc.	Prob. Foc.	Straight	10 min.	_____
___ 99202	Ex. Prob. Foc.	Ex. Prob. Foc.	Straight	20 min.	___ 1
X 99203	Detail	Detail	Low	30 min.	___ 1
___ 99204	Comp.	Comp.	Mod.	45 min.	_____
___ 99205	Comp.	Comp.	High	60 min.	_____

B. OFFICE VISIT - Established Patient

Code	History	Exam	Dec.	Time	
___ 99211	Minimal	Minimal	Minimal	5 min.	_____
___ 99212	Prob. Foc.	Prob. Foc.	Straight	10min.	_____
___ 99213	Ex. Prob. Foc.	Ex. Prob. Foc.	Low	15 min.	_____
___ 99214	Detail	Detail	Mod.	25 min.	_____
___ 99215	Comp.	Comp.	High	40 min.	_____

C. HOSPITAL CARE   Dx Units

1. Initial Hospital Care (30 min)	___ ___ 99221	_____
2. Subsequent Care	___ ___ 99231	_____
3. Critical Care (30-74 min)	___ ___ 99291	_____
4. each additional 30 min.	___ ___ 99292	_____
5. Discharge Services	___ ___ 99238	_____
6. Emergency Room	___ ___ 99282	_____

D. NURSING HOME CARE

Dx Units

Initial Care - New Pt.

1. Expanded	___ ___ 99322	_____
2. Detailed	___ ___ 99323	_____

Subsequent Care - Estab. Pt.

3. Problem Focused	___ ___ 99307	_____
4. Expanded	___ ___ 99308	_____
5. Detailed	___ ___ 99309	_____
5. Comprehensive	___ ___ 99310	_____

E. PROCEDURES

1. Arthrocentesis, Small Jt.	___ 20600	_____
2. Colonoscopy	45378	_____
3. EKG w/interpretation	___ 93000	_____
4. X-Ray Chest, PA/LAT	___ 71020	_____

F. LAB

1. Blood Sugar	___ 82947	_____
2. CBC w/differential	85031	_____
3. Cholesterol	82465	_____
4. Comprehensive Metabolic Panel	___ 80053	_____
5. ESR	85651	_____
6. Hematocrit	___ 85014	_____
7. Mono Screen	86308	_____
8. Pap Smear	88150	_____
9. Potassium	84132	_____
10. Preg. Test, Quantitative	___ 84702	_____
11. Routine Venipuncture	___ 36415	_____

F. Cont'd   Dx Units

12. Strep Screen	___	87081	_____
13. UA, Routine w/Micro	___	81000	_____
14. UA, Routine w/o Micro	___	81002	_____
15. Uric Acid	___	84550	_____
16. VDRL	___	86592	_____
17. Wet Prep	___	82710	_____
18. _____	___	___	_____

G. INJECTIONS

1. Influenza Virus Vaccine	___	90658	_____
2. Pneumoccocal Vaccine	___	90772	_____
3. Tetanus Toxoids	___	90703	_____
4. Therapeutic Subcut/IM	___	90732	_____
5. Vaccine Administration	___	90471	_____
6. Vaccine - each additional	___	90472	_____

H. MISCELLANEOUS

1. _____
2. _____

AMOUNT PAID $ ___ 0

Mark diagnosis with
(1=Primary, 2=Secondary, 3=Tertiary)

DIAGNOSIS
NOT LISTED _____
BELOW _____

DIAGNOSIS	ICD-9-CM 1, 2, 3	DIAGNOSIS	ICD-9-CM 1, 2, 3	DIAGNOSIS	ICD-9-CM 1, 2, 3
Abdominal Pain	789.0_ _____	Dehydration	276.51 _____	Otitis Media, Acute NOS	382.9 _____
Allergic Rhinitis, Unspec.	477.9 _____	Depression, NOS	311 _____	Peptic Ulcer Disease	536.9 _____
Angina Pectoris, Unspec.	413.9 _____	Diabetes Mellitus, Type II Controlled	250.00 _____	Peripheral Vascular Disease NOS	443.9 _____
Anemia, Iron Deficiency, Unspec.	280.9 _____	Diabetes Mellitus, Type II Controlled	250.02 _____	Pharyngitis, Acute	462 _____
Anemia, NOS	285.9 _____	Drug Reaction, NOS	995.29 _____	Pneumonia, Organism Unspec.	486 _____
Anemia, Pernicious	281.0 _____	Dysuria	788.1 _____	Prostatitis, NOS	601.9 _____
Asthma w/ Exacerbation	493.92 _____	Eczema, NOS	692.2 _____	PVC	427.69 _____
Asthmatic Bronchitis, Unspec.	493.90 _____	Edema	782.3 _____	Rash, Non Specific	782.1 _____
Atrial Fibrillation	427.31 _____	Fever, Unknown Origin	780.6 _____	Seizure Disorder NOS	780.39 _____
Atypical Chest Pain, Unspec.	786.59 _____	Gastritis, Acute w/o Hemorrhage	535.00 _____	Serous Otitis Media, Chronic, Unspec.	381.10 _____
Bronchiolitis, due to RSV	466.11 _____	Gastroenteritis, NOS	558.9 ___ 1	Sinusitis, Acute NOS	461.9 _____
Bronchitis, Acute	466.0 _____	Gastroesophageal Reflux	530.81 _____	Tonsillitis, Acute	463. _____
Bronchitis, NOS	490 _____	Hepatitis A, Infectious	070.1 _____	Upper Respiratory Infection, Acute NOS	465.9 _____
Cardiac Arrest	427.5 _____	Hypercholesterolemia, Pure	272.0 _____	Urinary Tract Infection, Unspec.	599.0 _____
Cardiopulmonary Disease, Chronic, Unspec.	416.9 _____	Hypertension, Unspec.	401.9 _____	Urticaria, Unspec.	708.9 _____
Cellulitis, NOS	682.9 _____	Hypoglycemia NOS	251.2 _____	Vertigo, NOS	780.4 _____
Congestive Heart Failure, Unspec.	428.0 _____	Hypokalemia	276.8 _____	Viral Infection NOS	079.99 _____
Contact Dermatitis NOS	692.9 _____	Impetigo	684 _____	Weakness, Generalized	780.79 _____
COPD NOS	496 _____	Lymphadenitis, Unspec.	289.3 _____	Weight Loss, Abnormal	783.21 _____
CVA, Acute, NOS	434.91 _____	Mononucleosis	075 _____		
CVA, Old or Healed	438.9 _____	Myocardial Infarction, Acute, NOS	410.9 _____		
Degenerative Arthritis		Organic Brain Syndrome	310.9 _____		
(Specify Site) _____	715.9 _____	Otitis Externa, Acute NOS	380.10 _____		

ABN: I UNDERSTAND THAT MEDICARE PROBABLY WILL NOT COVER THE SERVICES LISTED BELOW

A. _____ B. _____ C. _____

Patient

Date _____ Signature _____

Doctor's
Signature   *LD Heath*

RETURN: _____ Days ___ 1 ___ Weeks _____ Months _____

DOUGLASVILLE
MEDICINE ASSOCIATES
5076 BRAND BLVD., SUITE 401
DOUGLASVILLE, NY 01234
PHONE No. (123) 456-7890
☒ L.D. HEATH, M.D.   ❑ D.J. SCHWARTZ, M.D.
NPI# 9995010111   NPI# 9995020212
EIN# 00-1234560

REF# 122949 SB (05.07.09)   TO REORDER CALL INHEALTH RECORD SYSTEMS 800-477-7374

(Used with permission. InHealth Record Systems, Inc. 5076 Winters Chapel Road, Atlanta, GA 30360, 800-477-7374. http://www.inhealthrecords.com)

SOURCE DOCUMENT WB8-1

	Date(s) of Service	Amount Charged	Amount Allowed	Amount Disallowed	Level One	Level Two	Level Three	Preventative Care	Patient Responsibility	Benefit Paid by HRA	*Remark Codes
Patient: Aimee Bradley		Claim#: 32155460				**Provider: SCHWARTZ**			**Douglasville Medicine Associates**		
	102209	$180.00	$168.70	$11.30	$168.70	0.00	0.00	0.00	$0.00	$168.70	001
	102209	$16.00	$11.00	$5.00	$11.00	0.00	0.00	0.00	$0.00	$11.00	001
Patient: Tina Rizzo		Claim#: 32155461				**Provider: HEATH**			**Douglasville Medicine Associates**		
	102209	$180.00	$168.70	$11.30	$0.00	$168.70	0.00	0.00	$168.70	$0.00	002
	102209	$11.00	$9.00	$2.00	$0.00	$9.00	0.00	0.00	$9.00	$0.00	002
	102509	$18.00	$5.00	$13.00	$0.00	$5.00	0.00	0.00	$5.00	$0.00	002
Patient: Wynona Sheridan		Claim#: 32155462				**Provider: HEATH**			**Douglasville Medicine Associates**		
	102709	$200.00	$196.00	$4.00	$0.00	$196.00	0.00	0.00	$196.00	$0.00	001, 002
Patient: Mark Hedensten		Claim#: 32155463				**Provider: SCHWARTZ**			**Douglasville Medicine Associates**		
	112309	$145.00	$145.00	$0.00	$0.00	$0.00	$116.00	0.00	$29.00	$116.00	003
	TOTALS	$750.00	$703.40	$46.60	$181.70	$386.70	$116.00	0.00	$407.70	$295.70	*

Service Detail – ConsumerONE HRA

*Remark Codes:
001 Level One EPA — Disallowed amount is an in-network provider write-off.
002 Level Two — Patient out-of-pocket responsibility up to $500.00; EPA exhausted
003 Level Three — In-Network 80/20 HRA reimbursement agreement.

(Delmar/Cengage Learning)

SOURCE DOCUMENT WB8-2

Explanation of Medical Benefits   Flexi Health PPO Plan

Service Date	Type of Service	Charge(s) Submitted	Not Covered or Discount	Amount Covered	Patient Co-payment Co-insurance Deductible	Covered Balance	Plan Liability	See Note
Insured Name **BARRYROE, CAITLIN**		Insured/PatientID 999579754				Patient Name **BARRYROE, CAITLIN**		
Provider Name: L.D.Heath, MD – In-Network Provider								
Reference Number: 987680								
10/23/2009	99214 Office Service	$180.00	$20.00	$160.00	$20.00 co-pay	$140.00	$140.00	A
10/23/2009	80053 Laboratory	$ 47.00	$15.00	$ 32.00	$ 0.00	$ 32.00	$ 32.00	A
10/23/2009	81000 Laboratory	$ 12.00	$ 3.00	$ 9.00	$ 0.00	$ 9.00	$ 9.00	A
						Total Paid:	$181.00	
Insured Name **SHUMAN, ROSE**		Insured/PatientID 999213562-02				Patient Name **SHUMAN, ALAN**		
Provider Name: L.D.Heath, MD – In-Network Provider								
Reference Number: 987681								
10/22/2009	99215 Office Service	$249.00	$38.60	$210.40	$20.00 co-pay	$190.40	$190.40	A
10/22/2009	90658 Influenza	$ 22.00	$ 0.00	$ 22.00	$ 0.00	$ 22.00	$ 22.00	A
10/22/2009	90772 Pneumovax	$ 81.00	$10.00	$ 71.00	$ 0.00	$ 71.00	$ 71.00	A
						TotalPaid:	$283.40	
Insured Name **WALLACE, DEREK**		Insured/PatientID 999611257				Patient Name **WALLACE, DEREK**		
Provider Name: L.D.Heath, MD – In-Network Provider								
Reference Number: 987682								
10/20/2009	99212 Office Service	$ 80.00	$12.00	$ 68.00	$20.00 co-pay	$ 48.00	$ 48.00	A
						TotalPaid:	$ 48.00	

Notes on Benefit Determination:

A — Preferred provider discount.Patient is not required to pay this amount.

B — Patient is responsible for non-covered amounts for Out-of-Network providers

(Delmar/Cengage Learning)

SOURCE DOCUMENT WB8-3

Explanation of Medical Benefits   FlexiHealth PPO Plan

Service Date	Type of Service	Charge(s) Submitted	Not Covered or Discount	Amount Covered	Patient Co-payment Co-insurance Deductible	Covered Balance	Plan Liability	See Note
Insured Name **JOHNSEN, DENNIS**			Insured/Patient ID **999529842-01**		Patient Name **JOHNSEN, DENNIS**			
Provider Name: L.D. Heath, MD – In-Network Provider Reference Number: 988754								
11/09/2009	99282 ER Service	$147.00	$12.00	$135.00	$135.00 Deductible	$0.00	$0.00	A
					Total Paid:		**$0.00**	
Insured Name **JOUHARIAN, SIRAN**			Insured/Patient ID **999571164-02**		Patient Name **JOUHARIAN, SIRAN**			
Provider Name: L.D. Heath, MD – In-Network Provider Reference Number: 988755								
11/12/2009	99282 ER Service	$147.00	$12.00	$135.00	$ 27.00 Co-insurance	$108.00	$108.00	A
					Total Paid:		**$108.00**	
Insured Name **ROSS, THOMAS**			Insured/Patient ID **999321611-02**		Patient Name **ROSS, KAREN**			
Provider Name: L.D. Heath, MD – In-Network Provider Reference Number: 988756								
11/17/2009	99221 Inpt. Hospital Svc	$145.00	$11.40	$133.60	$133.60 Deductible	$ 0.00	$ 0.00	A
					Total Paid:		**$ 0.00**	

Notes on Benefit Determination:
A — Preferred provider discount. Patient is not required to pay this amount.
B — Patient is responsible for non-covered amounts for Out-of-Network providers.

(Delmar/Cengage Learning)

SOURCE DOCUMENT WB8-4

Explanation of Medical Benefits

FlexiHealth PPO Plan

Insured Name
ENGLEMAN, HAROLD

Insured/Patient ID
999811169-01

Patient Name
ENGLEMAN, HAROLD

Provider Name: D.J. Schwartz MD – Out-of-Network Provider

Reference Number: 987801

Service Date	Type of Service	Charge(s) Submitted	Not Covered or Discount	Amount Covered	Patient Co-payment Co-insurance Deductible	Covered Balance	Plan Liability	See Note
10/22/2009	99205 Office Service	$358.00	$32.00	$260.80	$65.20 co-ins	$326.00	$260.80	B
						Total Paid:	**$260.80**	

Notes on Benefit Determination:

A — Preferred provider discount. Patient is not required to pay this amount.

B — Patient is responsible for non-covered amounts for Out-of-Network providers.

(Delmar/Cengage Learning)

SOURCE DOCUMENT WB8-5

<table>
<tr><td colspan="9" align="center">**PROVIDER PAYMENT ADVICE**
Signal HMO
Student 1</td></tr>
<tr><td colspan="9">**Patient Name: Devon Trimble (TRI001)**</td></tr>
<tr><td>*Claim ID*</td><td>*DOS*</td><td>*Procedure*</td><td>*Charges*</td><td>*Allowed Amount*</td><td>*Patient Responsibility*</td><td>*Rejected Amount*</td><td>*Paid to Provider*</td><td>*Remarks*</td></tr>
<tr><td>1000396</td><td>10/20/2009</td><td>81002</td><td>$9.00</td><td>$7.97</td><td>$0.00</td><td>$0.00</td><td>$7.97</td><td>A</td></tr>
<tr><td>1000395</td><td>10/20/2009</td><td>80053</td><td>$47.00</td><td>$41.60</td><td>$0.00</td><td>$0.00</td><td>$41.60</td><td>A</td></tr>
<tr><td>1000394</td><td>10/20/2009</td><td>99204</td><td>$283.00</td><td>$250.46</td><td>$10.00</td><td>$0.00</td><td>$240.46</td><td>A</td></tr>
<tr><td>**Patient Totals**</td><td></td><td></td><td>$339.00</td><td>$300.02</td><td>$10.00</td><td>$0.00</td><td>$290.02</td><td></td></tr>
<tr><td colspan="9">**Patient Name: Emery Camille (CAM001)**</td></tr>
<tr><td>*Claim ID*</td><td>*DOS*</td><td>*Procedure*</td><td>*Charges*</td><td>*Allowed Amount*</td><td>*Patient Responsibility*</td><td>*Rejected Amount*</td><td>*Paid to Provider*</td><td>*Remarks*</td></tr>
<tr><td>1000407</td><td>10/22/2009</td><td>85031</td><td>$11.00</td><td>$9.74</td><td>$0.00</td><td>$0.00</td><td>$9.74</td><td>A</td></tr>
<tr><td>1000406</td><td>10/22/2009</td><td>99213</td><td>$111.00</td><td>$98.24</td><td>$10.00</td><td>$0.00</td><td>$88.24</td><td>A</td></tr>
<tr><td>**Patient Totals**</td><td></td><td></td><td>$122.00</td><td>$107.98</td><td>$10.00</td><td>$0.00</td><td>$97.98</td><td></td></tr>
<tr><td colspan="9">**Patient Name: Naomi Yamagata (YAM001)**</td></tr>
<tr><td>*Claim ID*</td><td>*DOS*</td><td>*Procedure*</td><td>*Charges*</td><td>*Allowed Amount*</td><td>*Patient Responsibility*</td><td>*Rejected Amount*</td><td>*Paid to Provider*</td><td>*Remarks*</td></tr>
<tr><td>1000399</td><td>10/22/2009</td><td>99214</td><td>$180.00</td><td>$159.30</td><td>$10.00</td><td>$0.00</td><td>$149.30</td><td>A</td></tr>
<tr><td>**Patient Totals**</td><td></td><td></td><td>$180.00</td><td>$159.30</td><td>$10.00</td><td>$0.00</td><td>$149.30</td><td></td></tr>
<tr><td colspan="9">**Patient Name: Janet Souza (SOU001)**</td></tr>
<tr><td>*Claim ID*</td><td>*DOS*</td><td>*Procedure*</td><td>*Charges*</td><td>*Allowed Amount*</td><td>*Patient Responsibility*</td><td>*Rejected Amount*</td><td>*Paid to Provider*</td><td>*Remarks*</td></tr>
<tr><td>1000424</td><td>11/10/2009</td><td>99282</td><td>$147.00</td><td>$130.10</td><td>$0.00</td><td>$0.00</td><td>$130.10</td><td>A</td></tr>
<tr><td>**Patient Totals**</td><td></td><td></td><td>$147.00</td><td>$130.10</td><td>$0.00</td><td>$0.00</td><td>$130.10</td><td></td></tr>
</table>

(Delmar/Cengage Learning)

SOURCE DOCUMENT WB8-6

```
Medicare Remittance Advice (MOSS Sample)
------------------------------------------------------------------------
12-01-2009 MEDICARE CLAIMS SUBMITTED FOR L.D. Heath, MD 999501
------------------------------------------------------------------------
HARTSFELD, DEANNA           BILLED ALLOWED DEDUCT   COINS PROV-PD MC-ADJUSTMENT
HIC        999613122B       ASG Y  ICN    97333672
ACNT       BER001

1022       102209 11 99214  180.00 104.46  75.00    5.89  23.57   75.54
1022       102209 11 80053   47.00  14.77   0.00    0.00  14.77   32.23
           CLAIM TOTALS:227.00 119.23      0.00     5.89  38.34  107.77
HERBERT,   NANCY            BILLED ALLOWED DEDUCT   COINS PROV-PD MC-ADJUSTMENT
HIC        999316512B       ASG Y  ICN    97333671
ACNT       HER001

1022       102209 11 99215  249.00 140.31   0.00   28.06 112.25  108.69
1022       102209 11 80053   47.00  14.77   0.00    0.00  14.77   32.23
1022       102209 11 85014    7.00   3.31   0.00    0.00   3.31    3.69
           CLAIM TOTALS:303.00 158.39      0.00     0.00 130.33  144.61

TOTAL PAID TO PROVIDER: $168.67
```

(Delmar/Cengage Learning)

SOURCE DOCUMENT WB8-7

```
Medicare Remittance Advice (MOSS Sample)
---------------------------------------------------------------------
12-01-2009 MEDICARE CLAIMS SUBMITTED FOR L.D. Heath, MD 999501
---------------------------------------------------------------------
---------------------------------------------------------------------
BERNARDO, WILLIAM          BILLED ALLOWED DEDUCT   COINS PROV-PD MC-ADJUSTMENT
HIC      999328652A        ASG Y  ICN     97333055
ACNT     BER001

1109       110909  23 99282 147.00 65.80   0.00    13.16 52.64      81.20

             CLAIM TOTALS: 147.00 65.80   0.00    13.16 52.64      81.20


DURAND,    ISABEL          BILLED ALLOWED DEDUCT   COINS PROV-PD MC-ADJUSTMENT
HIC      999621132D        ASG Y  ICN     97333056
ACNT     DUR001

1113       111309  31 99307  68.00 35.62   0.00     7.12 28.50      32.38

             CLAIM TOTALS:  68.00 35.62   0.00     7.12 28.50      32.38


ROYZIN,    JOEL            BILLED ALLOWED DEDUCT   COINS PROV-PD MC-ADJUSTMENT
HIC      999139877A        ASG Y  ICN     97333057
ACNT     ROY001

1113       111309  31 99308 113.00 59.06   0.00    11.81 47.25      53.94

             CLAIM TOTALS: 113.00 59.06   0.00    11.81 47.25      53.94


MCKAY,     SEAN            BILLED ALLOWED DEDUCT   COINS PROV-PD MC-ADJUSTMENT
HIC      999325576A        ASG Y  ICN     97333058
ACNT     ROY001

1120       112009  21 99221 145.00 92.33   0.00    18.47 73.86      52.67

             CLAIM TOTALS: 145.00 92.33   0.00    18.47 73.86      52.67

TOTAL PAID TO PROVIDER: $202.25
```

(Delmar/Cengage Learning)

SOURCE DOCUMENT WB9-1

Sean Mckay
521 E. Marble Way
Douglasville, NY 01235

9-5678/1234

8799

DATE 12/21/2009

PAY TO THE ORDER OF Douglasville Medicine Associates $ 18.47

Eighteen and 47/100   DOLLARS   Security features included. Details on back.

Memo MCK001   *Sean Mckay*   MP

⑆123456780⑆ 123⑈456⑉7⑈

(Delmar/Cengage Learning)

SOURCE DOCUMENT WB9-2

Joel Royzin
14321 Wilson Dr.
Douglasville, NY 01234

9-5678/1234

3567880

DATE 12/21/2009

PAY TO THE ORDER OF Douglasville Medicine Assoc. $ 11.81

Eleven and eighty one cents   DOLLARS   Security features included. Details on back.

Memo ROY001   *Joel Royzin*   MP

⑆123456780⑆ 123⑈456⑉7⑈

(Delmar/Cengage Learning)

SOURCE DOCUMENT WB9-3

Siran Jouharian
11234 Long Point.
Douglasville, NY 01234

9-5678/1234

204

DATE 12/21/2009

PAY TO THE ORDER OF Douglasville Medicine Associates $ 27.00

Exactly twenty-seven   DOLLARS   Security features included. Details on back.

Memo JOU001   *Siran Jouharian*   MP

⑆123456780⑆ 123⑈456⑉7⑈

(Delmar/Cengage Learning)

SOURCE DOCUMENT WB9-4

Mark Hedensten
12341 State Court
Douglasville, NY 01235

9-5678/1234

9943

DATE __12/21/2009__

PAY TO THE
ORDER OF __Douglasville Med Associates__ | $ __29.00__

__Twenty-nine and 00/100__ ------------------ DOLLARS

Security features included. Details on back.

Memo __HED001__   *Mark Hedensten* MP

⑆123456780⑆ 123⑈456⑉7⑈

(Delmar/Cengage Learning)

SOURCE DOCUMENT WB9-5

Karen Ross
5831 Pebble Way
Douglasville, NY 01235

9-5678/1234

44326

DATE __12/21/2009__

PAY TO THE
ORDER OF __Dr. Heath__ | $ __133.60__

__One hundred thirty-three and 60/100__ DOLLARS

Security features included. Details on back.

Memo __ROS001__   *Karen Ross* MP

⑆123456780⑆ 123⑈456⑉7⑈

(Delmar/Cengage Learning)

SOURCE DOCUMENT WB9-6

Anthony Rizzo
5831 Pebble Way
Douglasville, NY 01235

9-5678/1234

44326

DATE __12/21/2009__

PAY TO THE
ORDER OF __Dr. DJ Schwartz__ | $ __182.70__

__One hundred eighty two and 70/100__ DOLLARS

Security features included. Details on back.

Memo __RIZ001 - Tina Rizzo__   *Anthony Rizzo* MP

⑆123456780⑆ 123⑈456⑉7⑈

(Delmar/Cengage Learning)

SOURCE DOCUMENT WB9-7

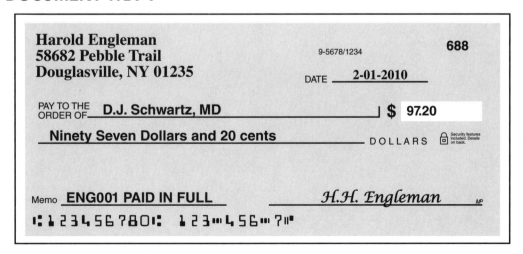

Wynona Sheridan
12390 Marble Way
Douglasville, NY 01234

9-5678/1234

2456

DATE **February 1, 2010**

PAY TO THE ORDER OF **Douglasville Medicine Associates** | $ **25.00**

Twenty-five dollars 00/100 --------------- DOLLARS

Security features included. Details on back.

Memo **SHE002 Payment #1**   *Wynona Sheridan*   MP

⑆123456780⑆ 123⑈456⑈7⑊

(Delmar/Cengage Learning)

SOURCE DOCUMENT WB9-8

Dennis Johnsen
9865 Pebble Way
Douglasville, NY 01235

9-5678/1234

2456

DATE **1-28-10**

PAY TO THE ORDER OF **Douglasville Medicine Associates** | $ **67.50**

Sixty-seven and 50/100 --- DOLLARS

Security features included. Details on back.

Memo **JOH002 #1 of 2**   *Dennis Johnsen*   MP

⑆123456780⑆ 123⑈456⑈7⑊

(Delmar/Cengage Learning)

SOURCE DOCUMENT WB9-9

Harold Engleman
58682 Pebble Trail
Douglasville, NY 01235

9-5678/1234

688

DATE **2-01-2010**

PAY TO THE ORDER OF **D.J. Schwartz, MD** | $ **97.20**

Ninety Seven Dollars and 20 cents DOLLARS

Security features included. Details on back.

Memo **ENG001 PAID IN FULL**   *H.H. Engleman*   MP

⑆123456780⑆ 123⑈456⑈7⑊

(Delmar/Cengage Learning)

SOURCE DOCUMENT WB10-1

Century SeniorGap
4500 Old Town Way
Lowville, NY 01453

Medigap Explanation of Benefits

January 4, 2010
Check Number: 10554549921

Patient Name	Provider	Services Dates From	To	Provider Charged Amt	Medicare Allowed Amt	Medicare Paid Amt	Deductible	SeniorGap Paid
Hartsfeld, Dea	Heath	1022	102209	180.00	104.46	23.57	75.00	80.89
999613122B	Heath	1022	102209	47.00	14.77	14.77	0.00	0.00

SeniorGap Claim
Number: 06988

Check Total: $80.89

(Delmar/Cengage Learning)

SOURCE DOCUMENT WB10-2

Century SeniorGap
4500 Old Town Way
Lowville, NY 01453

Medigap Explanation of Benefits

January 4, 2010
Check Number: 10554587845532

Patient Name	Provider	Services Dates From	To	Provider Charged Amt	Medicare Allowed Amt	Medicare Paid Amt	Deductible	SeniorGap Paid
Herbert, Nancy	Heath	1022	102209	147.00	140.31	112.25	0.00	28.06
999316512B		1022	102209	47.00	14.77	14.77	0.00	0.00
		1022	102209	7.00	3.31	3.31	0.00	0.00

SeniorGap Claim
Number: 06919

Check Total: $28.06

(Delmar/Cengage Learning)

SOURCE DOCUMENT WB10-3

Century SeniorGap
4500 Old Town Way
Lowville, NY 01453

Medigap Explanation of Benefits

January 4, 2010
Check Number: 10554587845532

Patient Name	Provider	Services Dates From	Services Dates To	Provider Charged Amt	Medicare Allowed Amt	Medicare Paid Amt	Deductible	SeniorGap Paid
Bernardo, Wm 999328652A	Heath	1109	110909	147.00	65.80	52.64	0.00	13.16
SeniorGap Claim Number: 06955								

Check Total: $13.16

(Delmar/Cengage Learning)

SOURCE DOCUMENT WB10-4

Medicare Beneficiary Services (MOSS Sample)

As of 01052010

RA Number 10333

Claim Type: MBS

**STATE DEPARTMENT OF MEDICAID SERVICES
MEDICAID MANAGEMENT INFORMATION SYSTEM
REMITTANCE ADVICE**

* PAID CLAIMS *

Provider Name: LD Heath
Provider ID: 890012

Recipient Identification Name	Number	Qty	Claim Services Dates From	Thru	Billed Charges	Deductable Amount	Coinsurance Amount	Pmt Amt
DURAND, I PROC: 99307	999621132D	1	11/13/2009	11/13/2009	68.00	0.00	7.12	7.12

Medicare Paid Date: 12/01/2009

Medicare Approved Amt: 35.62
Medicare Paid Amt: 28.50

Claim Paid on this RA: 1   Total Billed: 7.12   Total Paid: 7.12

(Delmar/Cengage Learning)

SOURCE DOCUMENT WB11-1

```
Medicare Remittance Advice (MOSS Sample)
01-07-2010 MEDICARE CLAIMS SUBMITTED FOR L.D. Heath, MD 999501
```

Mandeville, Joan			BILLED	ALLOWED	DEDUCT	COINS	PROV-PD	MC-ADJUSTMENT
HIC	999613122B		ASG Y	ICN	97333671			
ACNT	MAN009							
1217	121709 11	99214	180.00	72.50	0	14.50	58.00	107.50
1217	121709 11	80053	47.00	14.77	0	0.00	14.77	32.23
	CLAIM TOTALS:		227.00	87.27	0	14.50	72.77	139.73

```
TOTAL PAID TO PROVIDER: $72.77
```

(Delmar/Cengage Learning)

SOURCE DOCUMENT WB11-2

DEPARTMENT OF HEALTH AND HUMAN SERVICES
CENTERS FOR MEDICARE & MEDICAID SERVICES

MEDICARE REDETERMINATION REQUEST FORM

1. Beneficiary's Name: _____

2. Medicare Number: _____

3. Description of Item or Service in Question: _____

4. Date the Service or Item was Received: _____

5. I do not agree with the determination of my claim. MY REASONS ARE:

_____

_____

_____

6. Date of the initial determination notice _____
   (If you received your initial determination notice more than 120 days ago, include your reason for not making this request earlier.)

_____

_____

_____

7. Additional Information Medicare Should Consider: _____

_____

_____

_____

8. Requester's Name: _____

9. Requester's Relationship to the Beneficiary: _____

10. Requester's Address: _____

_____

11. Requester's Telephone Number: _____

12. Requester's Signature: _____

13. Date Signed: _____

14. ❑ I have evidence to submit. (Attach such evidence to this form.)
   ❑ I do not have evidence to submit.

NOTICE: Anyone who misrepresents or falsifies essential information requested by this form may upon conviction be subject to fine or imprisonment under Federal Law.

Form CMS-20027 (05/05) EF 05/2005

(Courtesy of the Centers for Medicare & Medicaid Services)

SOURCE DOCUMENT WB11-3

```
Medicare Remittance Advice (MOSS Sample)
-------------------------------------------------------------------------
01-07-2010 MEDICARE CLAIMS SUBMITTED FOR L.D. Heath, MD 999501
-------------------------------------------------------------------------

Ritter, Franklin        BILLED  ALLOWED DEDUCT   COINS  PROV-PD  MC-ADJUSTMENT
HIC    999231125A       ASG Y    ICN     97333671
ACNT   RIT009

1221    122109 11 99215 249.00   98.20   0         19.64  78.56    150.80

1221    122109 11 80053  47.00   14.77   0          0.00  14.77     32.23

          CLAIM TOTALS: 296.00  112.97   0         19.64  93.33    183.03

TOTAL PAID TO PROVIDER: $93.33
```

(Delmar/Cengage Learning)

SOURCE DOCUMENT WB11-4

DEPARTMENT OF HEALTH AND HUMAN SERVICES
CENTERS FOR MEDICARE & MEDICAID SERVICES

MEDICARE REDETERMINATION REQUEST FORM

1. Beneficiary's Name: _____

2. Medicare Number: _____

3. Description of Item or Service in Question: _____

4. Date the Service or Item was Received: _____

5. I do not agree with the determination of my claim. MY REASONS ARE:

_____

_____

_____

6. Date of the initial determination notice _____

(If you received your initial determination notice more than 120 days ago, include your reason for not making this request earlier.)

_____

_____

_____

7. Additional Information Medicare Should Consider: _____

_____

_____

_____

8. Requester's Name: _____

9. Requester's Relationship to the Beneficiary: _____

10. Requester's Address: _____

_____

11. Requester's Telephone Number: _____

12. Requester's Signature: _____

13. Date Signed: _____

14. ❑ I have evidence to submit. (Attach such evidence to this form.)
      ❑ I do not have evidence to submit.

NOTICE: Anyone who misrepresents or falsifies essential information requested by this form may upon conviction be subject to fine or imprisonment under Federal Law.

Form CMS-20027 (05/05) EF 05/2005

(Courtesy of the Centers for Medicare & Medicaid Services)